FOOD AS MEDICINE

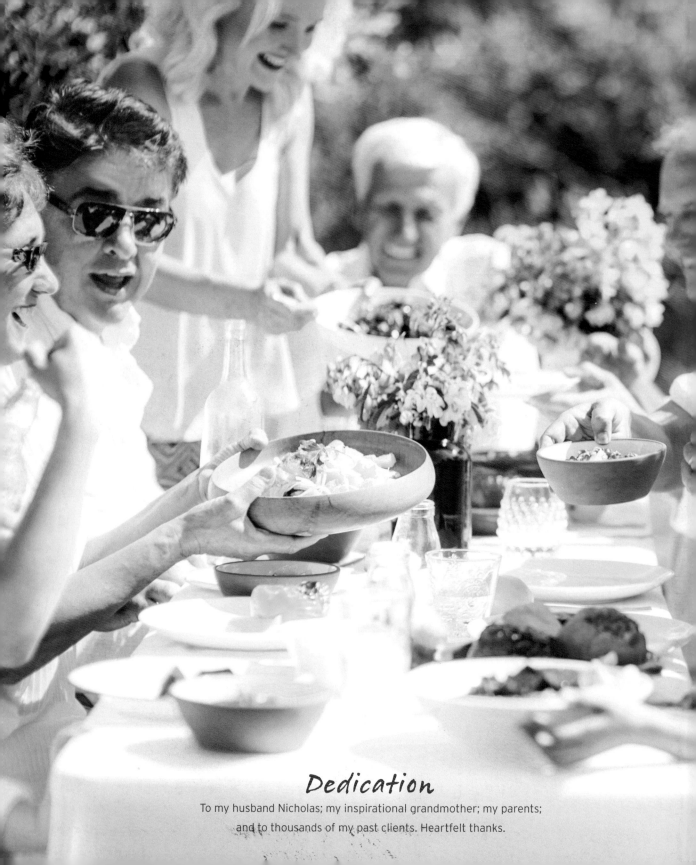

Dedication

To my husband Nicholas; my inspirational grandmother; my parents;
and to thousands of my past clients. Heartfelt thanks.

FOOD AS MEDICINE

150 Plant-Based Recipes for:
- Optimal Health
- Disease Prevention
- Management of Chronic Illness

Sue Radd, PhD

Skyhorse Publishing

CONTENTS

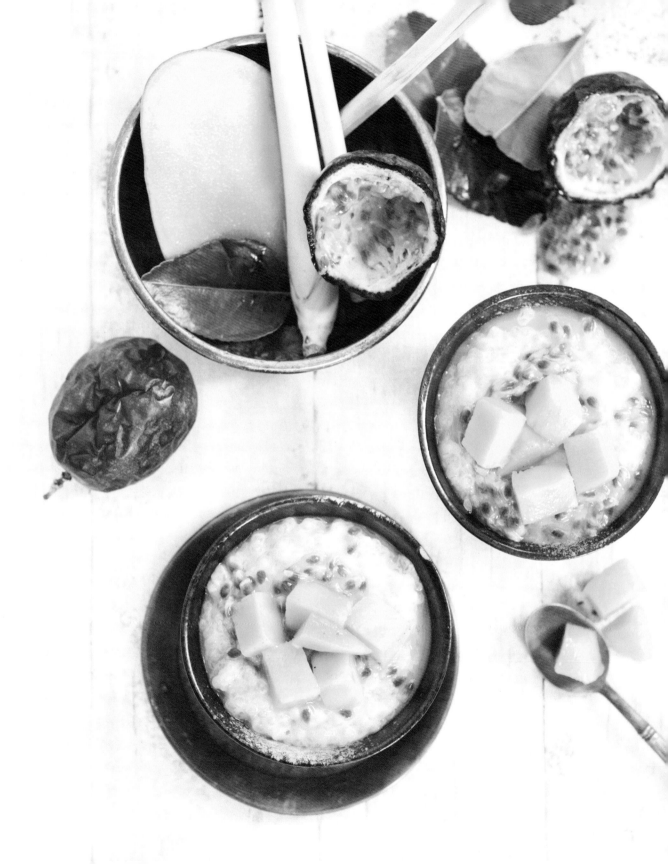

WELCOME TO THE FOOD AS MEDICINE COOKBOOK

Good nutrition—and your best health—starts in your kitchen!

In my earliest memories of cooking, I picture my grandmother at her wood stove and kitchen garden in Croatia—and me climbing her sour cherry trees! She was always teaching me the value of homemade food and "unsprayed" produce.

For years after graduating as a dietitian, I prescribed medical nutrition therapy to my patients. But when scientists began reporting more and more clinical trials showing the amazing health benefits of whole plant foods, I became more passionate about teaching people how to use food as medicine in a practical way.

In 2009, I started running Culinary Medicine Cookshops from the demo kitchen at my Sydney clinic. This was not to replace important clinical nutrition interventions, but as an extra service to help patients connect their nutrition prescriptions with delicious healing meals they could make easily at home. Since then we have had the pleasure of hosting more than 120 events with 2400 attendees!

What have I discovered?

Learning about how to enjoy the foods you should eat can be your motivator for change. And understanding what they can do for you can make all the difference.

Often at my Cookshops, doctors excitedly say they have learned more in one night about how to eat to fight chronic disease than in their entire medical training, and leave inspired to improve their lifestyle.

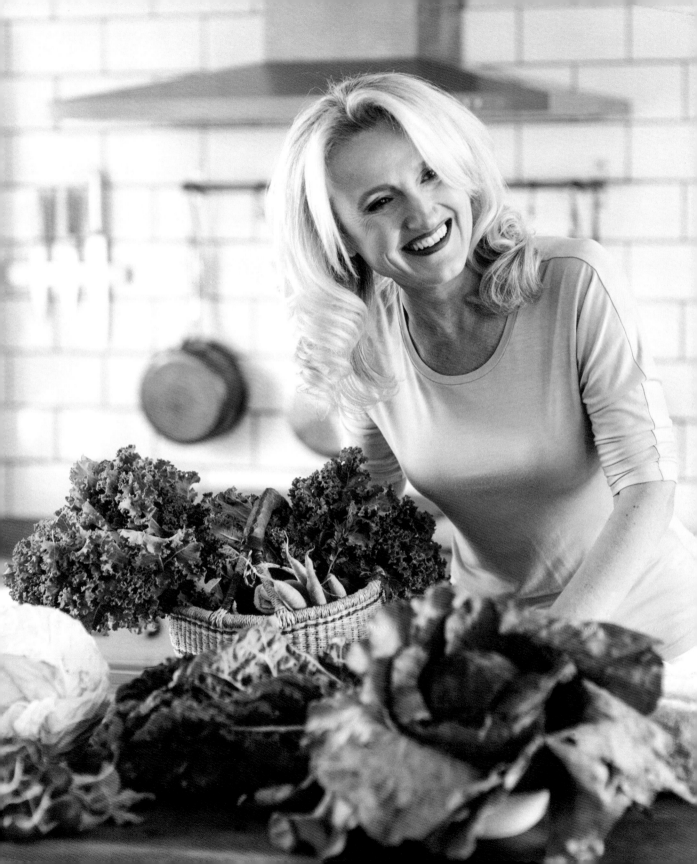

That's what this book is for. This book will help you have a better quantity and quality of life by eating real, tasty foods that attack the silent, deadly disease processes driven by poor diet. Applying the findings from nutrition science can vastly reduce the need for drugs and surgery, and help prevent or even reverse the chronic diseases that kill too many of us.

Unfortunately, despite significant advances in medicine in recent years, the value of food as a form of medicine is still under-recognised. Few universities or hospitals offer culinary medicine classes to help their graduates and patients learn how to stay well. But imagine if hospitals showed each patient with a chronic disease how to cook tasty, healthy food as part of their treatment and rehabilitation program.

As an experienced nutritionist and dietitian with a doctorate in the area of diet and how it can influence memory and thinking problems to lower the risk of dementia, I have spent countless hours reading thousands of scientific research studies to present you with the latest thinking about how food can be your medicine. Research consistently shows that adopting a natural, minimally processed, plant-based diet (page 334) is best because it can simultaneously impact multiple pathways to disease (page 322), rather than just tinkering with symptoms.

What we put in our mouths becomes even more important as we get older. What you eat will either speed up or slow down disease in your body. There is no neutral ground. Scientific evidence shows that you can add 10 good years to your life by regular physical activity, a plant-based diet, a handful of nuts most days, maintaining a healthy weight and not smoking.

The best part is, whether you are looking to stay well and prevent disease or influence the progression of an advanced medical condition, it's never too late to start reaping benefits. Your diet is the cornerstone of health improvement.

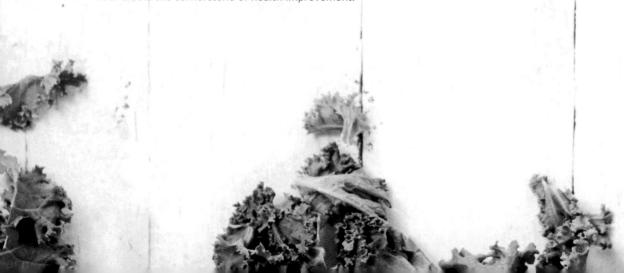

So here is my gift to you: 150 of my best recipes showing you how to use food as medicine in your own home and, at the back of the book, a summary of the scientific evidence. You can read it from cover to cover or dip in and out, trying recipes and reading sections that appeal to you.

I hope you will often thumb through these pages as you plan your family meals. My recipes are also useful if you cook regularly for larger groups. Or if you are a health professional or educator, wanting to place something practical into the hands of your patients or food and nutrition students to empower them.

Whether you use this cookbook by yourself or in conjunction with your health practitioner, I hope it will be your roadmap to wellness with less detours to hospitals, a reduced need for medication and improved energy. Enjoy these recipes and enjoy your best health.

For life,

Sue

Sue Radd, PhD
Advanced Accredited Practising Dietitian & Advanced Nutritionist
Director, Nutrition and Wellbeing Clinic

www.sueradd.com

What you will learn

Enjoy plant-based recipes (page 27) adapted from traditional societies, and the advantages they offer, as shown by modern science.

Re-stock your pantry (page 16) and master easy meal ideas (page 312).

Discover why every meal matters (page 322) and how your food choices control the expression of your genes (page 327). This is even more important if you have a strong family history of disease.

Learn how healthy diets can deliver a list of positive effects like those of medications (page 328).

See why your wellbeing is affected by when you eat (page 325) and why mindless eating is dangerous.

From organics (page 370), raw-food trends (page 372) and alcohol (page 370) to red meat (page 364), sugary drinks (page 369) and supplements (page 368), get the low-down on the major issues people are talking about today so you can decide for yourself how much and what to eat.

Learn the healthiest methods of cooking (page 378), and what cookware and containers to use (page 20) to help you minimize your exposure to toxic chemicals that can leach into your food (page 381). You'll never look at a non-stick pan the same way again!

My key message is that the quality of your calories (or kilojoules) is most important, not just the quantity. If you maintain the healthy way of eating described in these pages, you might never need to diet again. My patients tell me they feel satisfied even while losing weight. This is because unrefined plant-based meals are bulky and make you feel full. Going on a popular diet plan might help you lose a little weight in the short term by dictating what you will eat for each meal (page 332), but my approach is to teach you how and why to adopt your own plant-based eating pattern so the health rewards will remain for life.

Conditions that may be helped by recipes in this cookbook

As you enjoy the delicious foods and flavours in this cookbook, you can feel great about the growing scientific evidence that shows plant-based diets may help reduce the risks of developing–or better manage–a host of chronic conditions linked to the modern diet, including:

- **anxiety**
- **asthma**
- **cataracts**
- **constipation**
- **declining kidney function**
- **dementia (including Alzheimer's disease)**
- **depression**
- **diabetes**
- **diverticulosis**
- **emphysema**
- **fatty liver**
- **gallstones**
- **gout**
- **heart disease (including elevated cholesterol and blood pressure)**
- **inflammatory bowel disease (Crohn's disease and ulcerative colitis)**
- **insulin resistance**
- **kidney stones**
- **macular degeneration**
- **metabolic syndrome**
- **multiple sclerosis (MS)**
- **obesity**
- **Parkinson's disease**
- **PCOS (polycystic ovarian syndrome)**
- **rheumatoid arthritis**

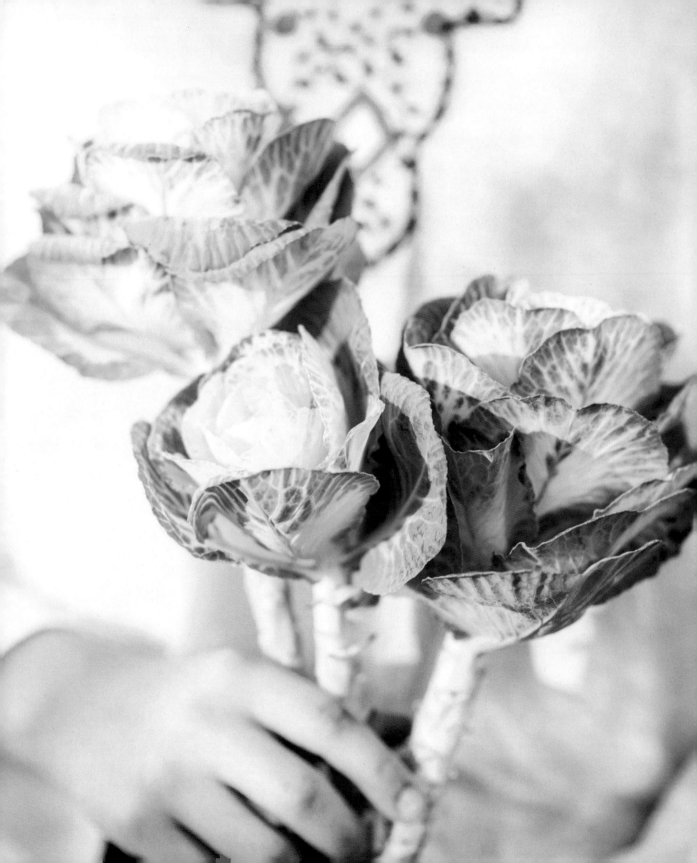

FOODS
THAT HARM
FOODS
THAT HEAL

*your food choices can make
a world of difference*

What you eat matters and every mouthful counts!

The good news: your body has an innate tendency to mend itself and maintain good health. But both the damaging effects and the processes required to fix them kick in more quickly than previously imagined. The sooner you start reversing existing damage with your fork the better! Healthy people also live happier lives. The Mediterranean diet, an example of plant-based eating, has been linked with lower risks of depression, stroke and dementia—conditions plaguing the modern world.

10 FOOD RULES TO LIVE BY

Some foods heal; some foods harm. Here's what you can do to eat well:

1. *Enjoy colourful meals based on natural or minimally processed plant foods with no or minimal additives. They're better for your health, kinder to animals and place less pressure on planetary resources.*
2. *Plan your meals at least one day ahead. This will help you achieve dietary variety.*
3. *Eat three satisfying meals each day, at similar times and not too late. Avoid grazing on processed snacks, even if labelled "organic."*
4. *Emphasise seasonal produce in your cooking: it will taste better, usually contains more nutrients and is cheaper.*
5. *If you're too busy to cook every night, prepare three recipes in bulk over the weekend— examples: dal, curry or thick soup. Portion out and refrigerate/freeze for the week ahead. When serving your meals, round off with a fresh salad.*
6. *Pack your lunch—even breakfast—if you work away from home. Homemade leftovers are ideal.*
7. *Sit around the table and enjoy your dinner with someone you love or can have a good conversation with. Don't eat in front of the TV or with electronic gadgets. Be a good role model to your children.*
8. *Eat slowly and mindfully, consulting your tummy before you take more. Wait for 20 minutes before going for seconds.*
9. *Eat more ethnically. Pick the best of Indian, Japanese, Lebanese, Greek, Italian and other cuisines. Learn to cook traditional plant-based dishes from your family and friends.*
10. *Don't look for magic bullets. It's the total dietary pattern (based on wholefoods) that matters most. Food quality is more important than quantity, at any weight.*

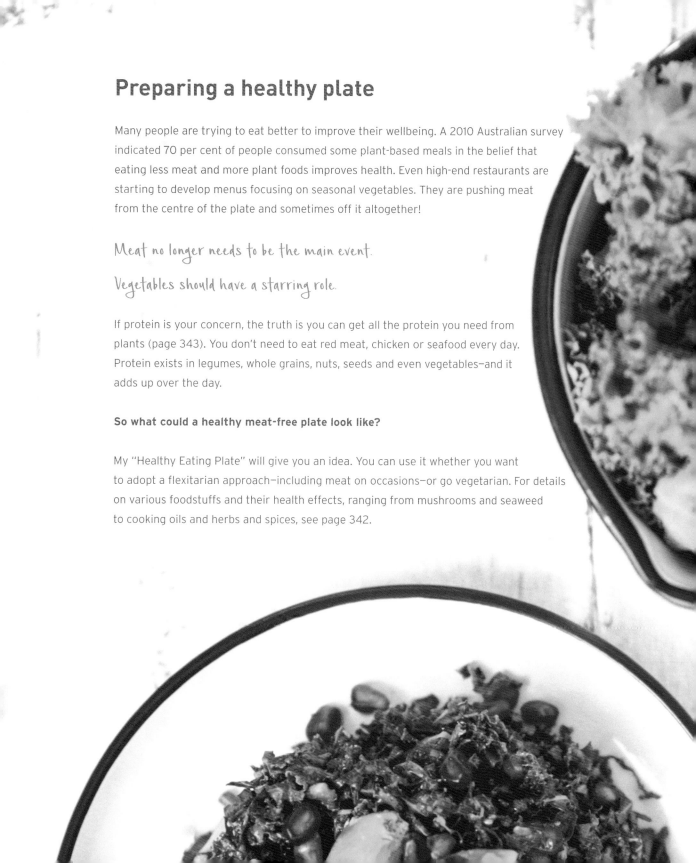

Preparing a healthy plate

Many people are trying to eat better to improve their wellbeing. A 2010 Australian survey indicated 70 per cent of people consumed some plant-based meals in the belief that eating less meat and more plant foods improves health. Even high-end restaurants are starting to develop menus focusing on seasonal vegetables. They are pushing meat from the centre of the plate and sometimes off it altogether!

Meat no longer needs to be the main event.

Vegetables should have a starring role.

If protein is your concern, the truth is you can get all the protein you need from plants (page 343). You don't need to eat red meat, chicken or seafood every day. Protein exists in legumes, whole grains, nuts, seeds and even vegetables—and it adds up over the day.

So what could a healthy meat-free plate look like?

My "Healthy Eating Plate" will give you an idea. You can use it whether you want to adopt a flexitarian approach—including meat on occasions—or go vegetarian. For details on various foodstuffs and their health effects, ranging from mushrooms and seaweed to cooking oils and herbs and spices, see page 342.

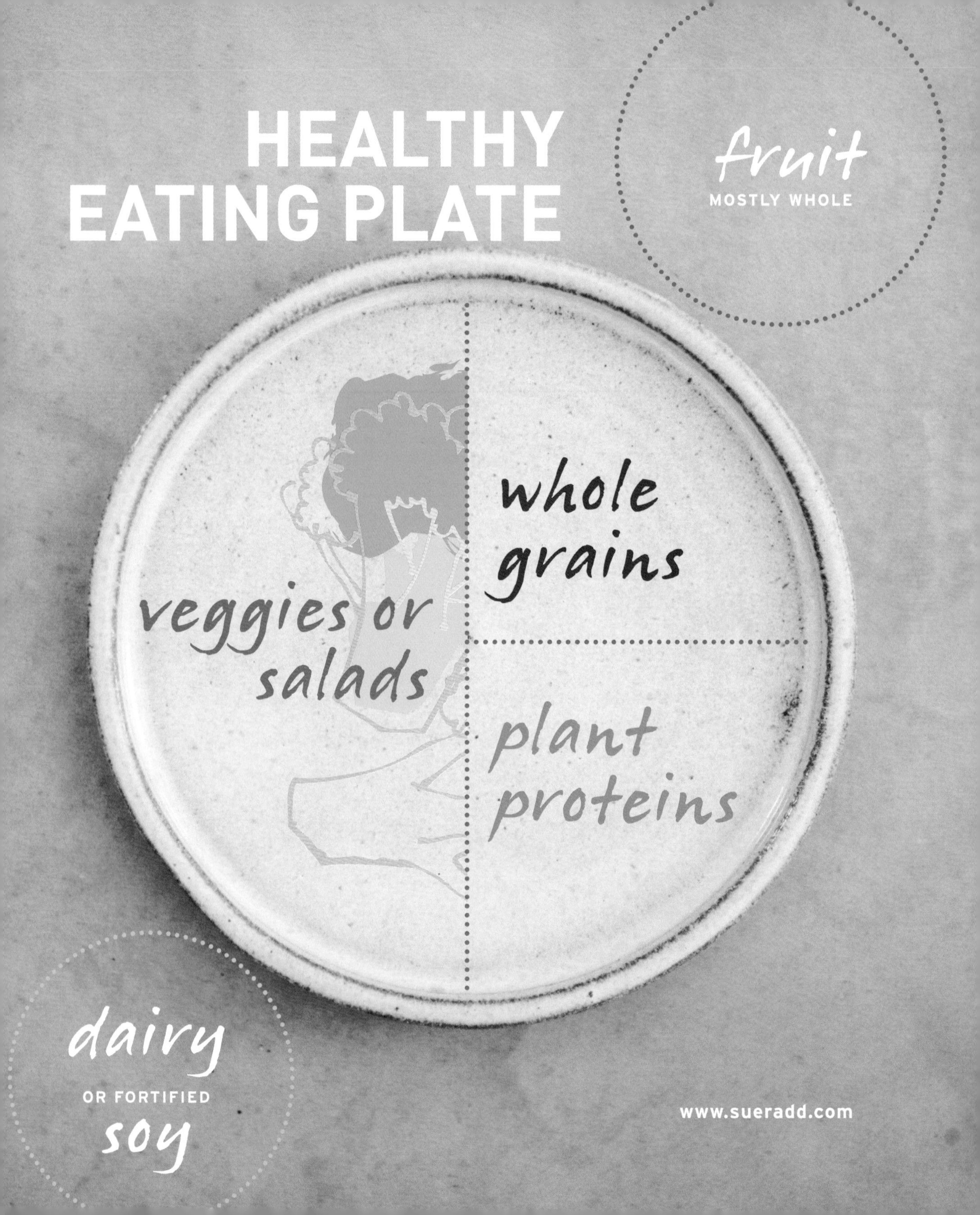

HEALTHY EATING PLATE

fruit
MOSTLY WHOLE

whole grains

veggies or salads

plant proteins

dairy
OR FORTIFIED
soy

www.sueradd.com

Should I go vegetarian?

Your body can usually get enough of most nutrients even on a total plant-based (vegan) diet, according to a 2013 scientific supplement to the *Medical Journal of Australia* titled "Is a Vegetarian Diet Adequate?" If you wish to adopt a vegan diet however, some nutrients might need more attention, including calcium, zinc, vitamin B12 and omega 3. Fortified foods and/or supplements (page 368) taken at dietary levels can provide a top up. It's always best to seek professional advice as poorly planned diets can lead to nutritional deficiencies. A dietitian (page 386) or nutritionist experienced in plant-based nutrition can ensure you have a good grasp of meal planning for your needs.

The importance of starting early

Chronic diseases like cancer take decades to develop. So it's best to get in early and make every plateful count. While you can't change your past, you can make things right for yourself—and your family—going forward. Why not give yourself a fighting chance at slowing or even reversing disease?

You don't have to be overweight and 40 to be paving the way for a heart attack. Hardening of the arteries begins in toddlers! Yet it can be difficult to kick-start motivation, since most of the immediate damage from unhealthy food choices occurs silently. If it were obvious, more people would pay attention to how they eat.

One of the downsides of getting older is that our repair processes slow down and we can begin to accumulate more damage than the body can deal with. If you're no longer a spring chicken, or your waistline has thickened with middle age, it's important to begin eating healing meals right away. Improving your diet is not as difficult as you might think and it can also be delicious.

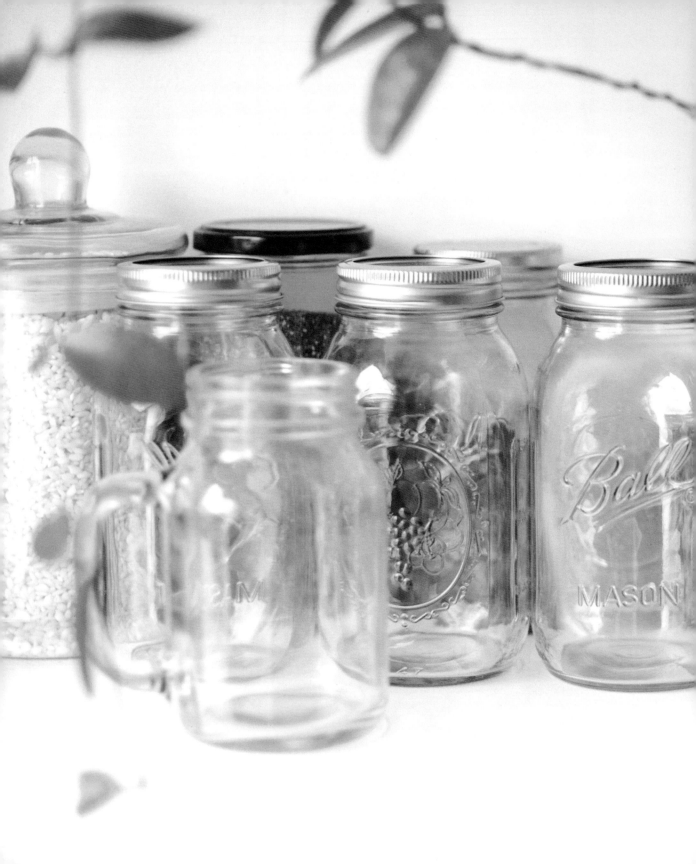

FOOD AS MEDICINE IN YOUR KITCHEN

Does your kitchen need an audit?

Is your pantry, fridge or freezer sabotaging your health goals?

If you've been diagnosed with a chronic disease, have existing risk factors or simply want to feed your family right to stay well, it's time for a pantry audit:

1. **Remove items from the shelves that do not support your health goals.**
2. **Take a closer look inside your pantry and identify any missing wholefoods from the checklist below. Create a list and take yourself shopping.**

Despite our good intentions, we can't rely on willpower. According to research from Cornell University, people make about 250 food-related decisions each day. Most of these are made on autopilot, so it's impossible for all of them to be perfect! Creating a supportive environment, at home, at your workplace and in your car, will prevent sabotage of your health goals.

Foods to keep in your pantry, fridge and freezer

To help me stay focused on using wholefoods, I like to keep the following staples in my kitchen. You can adjust the ingredients for any food allergies or intolerances in your family or how plant-based you want to go. Even if you want to include some animal products, my handy list will help you include important wholefoods to fight chronic disease.

Planning and preparation is the key to success with lifestyle change.

I give preference and prominence to foods I should eat regularly. I shelve legumes and whole grains in separate glass containers at eye level, so I will be prompted to use and rotate these.

As for fresh produce, I try to visit farmers' markets regularly to remind me of what's in season. You can also download seasonal lists from the websites of major city markets.

While some of the foods on these lists might be unfamiliar to you, the first step is to get them into your kitchen. You can then learn to use them, starting with my satisfying recipes.

pantry

> Whole grains—including intact, cracked or rolled whole grains—of all types, such as oats, spelt, wheat, rice, buckwheat, barley, quinoa, millet and other grains. Think steel-cut oats, freekeh and bulgur, to name a few. Also include whole-grain pasta varieties in various shapes and wholemeal flours/meals (preferably coarsely milled), such as polenta (mielimeel).

> Soba noodles (100% buckwheat), bean thread (mung bean vermicelli), kelp noodles.

> Konjac (konnyaku) products such as noodles, spaghetti, rice, blocks or balls.

> Pumpernickel bread, whole-grain/heavily-seeded crispbreads/pappadums.

> Potatoes of all types (Carisma, Nicola and baby/chat potatoes have a low GI).

> Legumes and dry beans of all types, including chickpeas, black beans, borlotti, cannellini, black-eyed, kidney, lentils (red, brown, puy), Lima, mung, split peas and more. Also include their flours, such as besan (chickpea) and lupin flour.

> Textured vegetable protein (dehydrated soy mince), falafel mix.

> Whole unroasted seeds and nuts, including chia seeds, linseeds (flaxseeds), walnuts, almonds and peanuts. Also psyllium husks.

> Dried fruit, such as dates, figs, prunes, pears, apricots, cranberries, goji berries and Inca berries.

> Honey (darker varieties contain a higher antioxidant content), natural maple syrup, raw agave syrup.

> Herbal/non-caffeinated teas, including rooibos, lemon and ginger, chamomile, rosehip and hibiscus, and spearmint.

> Raw cacao powder, raw carob powder.

> Herbs and spices of all types, including blends like Arabic seven spices and zataar. Vegetable-based stocks and seasoning agents, including miso paste, light and dark soy sauce/tamari/shoyu, nutritional yeast seasoning, dried mushrooms, dried fungus, dulse granules and seaweed flakes from shakers.

> Tomato—pasta sauce, passata, paste, semi-dried and sun-dried.

> Oil—extra virgin, cold extracted, including olive, macadamia, avocado, mustard seed and pumpkin seed.

> Souring agents, including lemon and lime juices, vinegar (examples: apple cider, balsamic), sumac, pomegranate molasses and verjuice (store last two in fridge after opening).

fridge

> Seasonal fruit, vegetables, shoots, roots, sprouts and herbs of all types.

> Spreads, including hummus, baba ganoush, nut/seed pastes, ajvar and fresh avocado.

> Sprouted-grain breads (examples: multigrain, khorasan, Ezekiel 4:9).

> Soy milk and yogurt/almond milk/rice milk—fortified with calcium and vitamin B12, where possible.

> Tofu (firm, regular, silken or pre-marinated), tempeh.

> Commercially prepared lentil burgers, soy luncheon meats and veggie sausages, for "emergencies."

> Seeds, including sesame, pumpkin (pepitas), sunflower, linseed (flaxseed) meal and chia bran.

> Tahini.

> Oil—extra virgin, cold extracted flaxseed or chia seed (perishable due to high omega-3 content).

KNOW YOUR SOY SAUCES

Soy sauce supplies less sodium per teaspoon than salt and adds an "umami" flavour to food, with a unique savoury profile.

Chinese soy sauce is labelled dark or light. The darker one is thicker, usually contains more sodium and is used mostly for its colour. The lighter one is thinner, with less sodium and used mostly for flavouring. Dishes often call for a combination of light and dark Chinese soy sauces.

Japanese soy sauces are broadly categorised into two types: shoyu and tamari. Shoyu is the all-purpose natural soy sauce, whereas tamari is usually wheat-free (but check labels). Tamari has a thicker texture, deeper colour and stronger taste than shoyu, which is why it is often used for dipping, rather than just cooking.

All soy sauces contain large amounts of sodium—even salt-reduced varieties—so use sparingly. If you want to avoid added chemicals, choose those naturally fermented/brewed—over six months to two years—rather than the mass-produced commercial varieties of soy sauce, which are induced to ferment in as little as six weeks and contain many additives like colouring, sugars and preservatives. Bragg's Liquid Aminos, sold in health-food stores, is often promoted as a healthier alternative to soy sauce, but it's still high in sodium and not a naturally brewed product.

freezer

> Sliced breads or wraps, including whole grain, stoneground wholemeal and sourdough with plenty of seeds/cracked grains, such as soy and linseed, dark rye, spelt sourdough with sunflower seeds.

> Select fruit—fresh berries, dried barberries, overripe bananas and mango flesh.

> Select vegetables—corn cobs, peas, edamame, mixed family packs and chopped herbs.

> Fresh ginger, fresh turmeric, fresh chillies, curry leaves, kaffir lime leaves.

> Shelled nuts/seeds, including walnuts, cashews, macadamias, almonds and Brazil nuts. (Storing in the freezer reduces oxidation, preserving both their nutrition and flavour.)

> Frozen Quorn (meat substitute made from mycoprotein, a member of the funghi family) and other vegetable protein products.

HOW TO STORE LINSEEDS

Grind small quantities of linseed (flaxseed) in a coffee grinder and store in a glass jar in your fridge or freezer, using it as required. This will protect the delicate omega-3 fats from oxidation. Avoid buying pre-ground linseed meal as it is often bitter, suggesting it has been sitting on the shelf, exposed to heat and light, for extended periods.

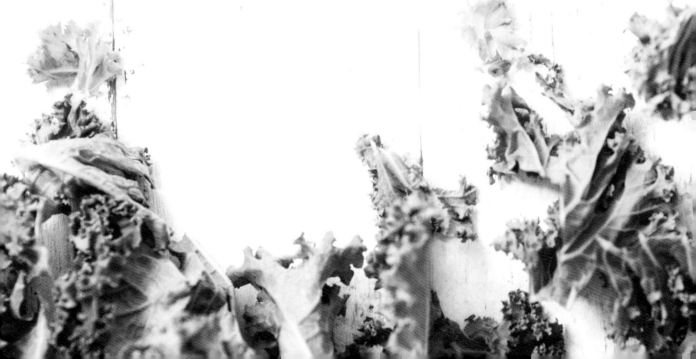

Makeover your storage containers and cookware

It's not only what you cook, but how you store food that may influence your health. While it's impossible to eliminate all sources of potentially toxic chemicals from our environment, it's a good idea to reduce exposure to those under your control. Some cookware and containers are easier to replace than others.

Safer food storage tips
- Go plastic-free as much as possible.
- Buy acidic ingredients, such as tomato paste, in glass jars. You can re-use or recycle these containers.
- Limit exposure to drinks in aluminium cans and canned foods. Seek out BPA-free cans where available.
- Store pantry ingredients in glass or ceramic jars and bottles.
- Store cooked meals in glass or ceramic bowls.
- Use a glass or stainless steel water bottle.
- If you need to use plastic, choose BPA-free bottles and storage containers.

Safer cookware tips
The best choices are those with the most non-reactive surfaces.
- Use stainless steel pots and pans with some oil, juice, stock or water.
- Use enamelled cast-iron pots and ovenware as these are virtually non-stick.
- Use cast-iron pots and pans, seasoned to prevent rusting. With time, these will develop a natural non-stick surface (patina).
- Use glass or ceramic pots, pans and bakeware.
- Use carbon steel woks and frypans for a lightweight solution.
- Use PFOA-free non-stick cookware and bakeware.

Handy kitchen equipment and gadgets

Make it easier for your kitchen to be a healthy zone. Invest in time-saving equipment to motivate you to cook more wholefoods. Here are some of my favourite helpers:

• Pressure cooker

A pressure cooker is a must if you plan to cook legumes and whole grains regularly as it can cut up to 75 per cent from the cooking time. Modern versions are easy to use and have safety valves, so there is no risk of accidents. Buy a good quality stainless steel pressure cooker and it will last a lifetime. For most families, I recommend a 6- or 8-litre (6- or 8-quart) capacity, as this is more versatile to also make soups.

• Rice cooker

Not only for rice, this is the easiest way to cook most whole grains, including barley, quinoa and buckwheat. Create your own whole-grain blends (page 76) using a similar proportion of water in most cases as you would cooking rice. I love this gadget as it effortlessly produces a side dish of *al dente* whole grains without the need for any supervision.

• Steamer

Steamed food is underrated but absolutely delicious! Use a stainless steel basket (cleans easily, lasts longer) or a bamboo steamer (cheaper, looks impressive) that fits on top of your saucepan or wok.

• Slow cooker

Another healthy way to cook foods like stews and curries, but you need to plan ahead. Most recipes take between 4 and 12 hours on low heat.

• Salad spinner

Taking a minute to freshen and dry off leaves and herbs in this neat device enables them to absorb salad dressing better. Salad leaves will also be crisper after washing, helping your family eat more green leaves.

• High-powered blender

Unlike ordinary blenders, these blenders grind and chop without effort and raw foodists swear by them. Compared to ordinary blenders, the sharp blades operate at very high speeds so your final product is velvety smooth.

- **Food processor**

A bowl food processor is ideal for recipes where you need to chop or puree foods into a more solid texture. It has a larger blade and wider brim than a blender, making it easier to scoop out thicker consistencies.

- **Mandoline**

While food processors can shred or slice almost anything, there is a lot more cleaning up compared to a mandoline. I use mandolines to rapidly slice small quantities of everything from radishes and onions to cucumbers and lemons—or chip, crinkle cut, dice and julienne, depending on the attachments. Adjustable knobs allow you to select the desired thickness.

- **Microplane**

This is a super-sharp, rasp-like grater with options for fine zesting through to coarse grating. After you've used one, you might never want to go back to a box grater.

Smart shopping tips

With more than 30,000 food and drink items to choose from, navigating the average supermarket can be a challenge. Understanding the typical layout of a store and how food labels are designed to grab your attention, however, can help you stay healthier.

6 tips for navigating the supermarket:

1. *Always make a shopping list. Plan for at least three main meals that you will cook that week. Be realistic in your plans.*
2. *Shop the perimeter of the store for fresh, refrigerated and frozen wholefoods, and stay out of the middle where more-processed foods lurk. Buy seasonal and local produce. It tastes better and it's usually cheaper.*
3. *Keep away from impulse stands. Stores use psychological tactics to get you to spend more, usually on the most profitable and least healthy foods.*
4. *Don't rely on convenience meals. It's smarter to cook your own and store in meal-sized portions in the fridge or freezer for the week ahead.*
5. *Don't instantly trust packaging claims, stars, ticks and logos. Check the ingredients list first and the nutrition information panel for a breakdown of the figures.*
6. *Avoid buying highly processed items with long lists of additives. It's safer to pick a range of colours in the produce aisle.*

Healthy food does not need to cost more

Some people believe eating healthy food is more expensive. Research from Harvard University suggests it costs only US$1.50 more per person per day. But if you learn to cook foods like legumes from scratch, it can be cheaper than relying on convenience products or fast-food options. Home-cooked food also came out cheaper every time compared to takeaway, according to Australian research. And it usually tastes better. By planning and preparing a few meals ahead–perhaps over the weekend–you can keep yourself on track during a busy week.

Where to shop

While supermarkets might be convenient, they don't always supply the freshest produce and can be a trap for ultra-processed foods. I love farmers' markets as they remind me of what's in season and tastes best at the time. They can also help your family connect with how real food is grown. Eth-nic grocery stores and greengrocers can provide good-value, fresh ingredients. Health-food stores are good for sourcing those difficult-to-find whole-foods. But beware, not everything sold in a health-food store or aisle is necessarily healthy! Always read the fine print.

Take the kids along for an excursion

Food preferences start to form while we're very young, so it's important to take your children grocery shopping to model healthy choices. A study published in *Archives of Internal Medicine* looked into the food preferences of 2-6 year olds whose parents usually took them grocery shopping. When allowed to "buy" food from a play shop–with a choice of 133 items–the researchers discovered that even the youngest children mirrored their parents' usual choices! The conclusion: Children who selected the healthiest food items imitated their parents who preferred these foods.

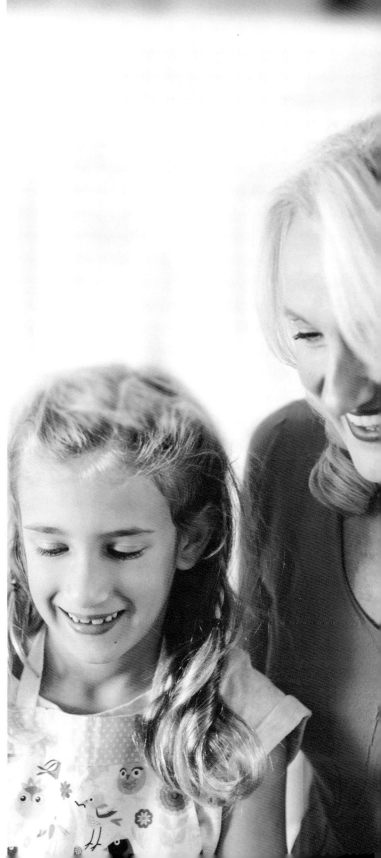

Cooking for your best health

Time spent in food preparation is time well spent. But many people today seem less willing to prioritise food preparation. A century ago and in some cultures, six hours were dedicated to preparing family dinner. The decline and devaluing of cooking—except as a spectator sport on popular TV programs—with the simultaneous increase in convenience foods, has become a recipe for poor health.

According to research published in the *American Journal of Preventive Medicine*, the time spent on home food preparation is an indicator of healthy eating. Spending more time cooking at home is linked with a higher-quality diet—and more frequent intake of fruits and vegetables. But investing less than one hour daily in home food preparation results in more frequent use of fast-food restaurants and greater costs for food purchased away from home.

When college students and young adults cook for themselves, they are less likely to eat fast food on a regular basis, and more likely to meet their food and nutrient goals for whole grains, fruits, vegetables and calcium, according to a study published in the *Journal of the American Dietetics Association*.

In another study, improving the cooking skills of older Australian men resulted in an improvement of their diet. It's never too late to learn to cook and start reaping the benefits.

So how much time are you investing in your kitchen to help your family stay well?

ENGAGE THE WHOLE FAMILY

If you're serious about eating smarter for life, engage the whole family and take them on the journey with you. Cooking for a family can be onerous for one person. Ask family members to share in the responsibility of buying, preparing, cooking and serving food.

Teach your kids to cook

Cooking and other culinary skills are being shared less often between generations and in schools. Yet showing children how to make simple wholesome meals to share with the family can help them eat better for life and positively influence their skill development, attitudes and knowledge.

Showing kids how to grow and cook meals from scratch will increase their willingness to try new foods and eat a greater variety of vegetables, according to findings from the Stephanie Alexander Kitchen Garden National Program rolled out to 177 government primary schools across Australia for more than two years. This program was considered particularly successful at engaging the "non-academic" learners and those with challenging behaviours. The kids' confidence to cook improved. They also learned to safely use a knife, wash up, set the table, adopt table manners and to work as a team.

Here is my suggestion: As soon as your children are old enough, allocate one cooking night per week for each child and give them a budget and some guidance to plan a menu. They will learn lots, appreciate the food more and eat a healthier diet. Plus you might get a night off!

WHAT TO DO WITH FUSSY EATERS

If you struggle to get small children to eat good food, don't give up! Research shows it can take 10 repeated exposures to a new food for it to become acceptable. So keep persevering. A "Veggies Reward" chart might help. Each time your child tries a new vegetable—or eats one they find challenging—present them with a sticker. When they reach their sticker goal, give them a small non-food reward.

Benefits of family meals

Enjoying good food around the table, away from the overstimulation of screens, will prevent hurried or mindless eating that promotes weight gain. It helps you to eat more slowly with full attention. (Start your own "slow-food movement" in the dining room!)

Having set meal times will assist with digestion and regularity, as well as keeping your biological clocks in sync, which is important for disease prevention (page 325). Children exposed to three household routines—eating regular evening meals with the family, getting enough sleep at night, having limited screen time on week days—have about a 40 per cent lower risk of obesity.

But it's not only the kids who benefit. Research shows that more frequent family dinners increase fruit and vegetable intake among parents too. Plus, fathers end up eating less fast food, and mothers diet and binge less. It's a win for the whole family.

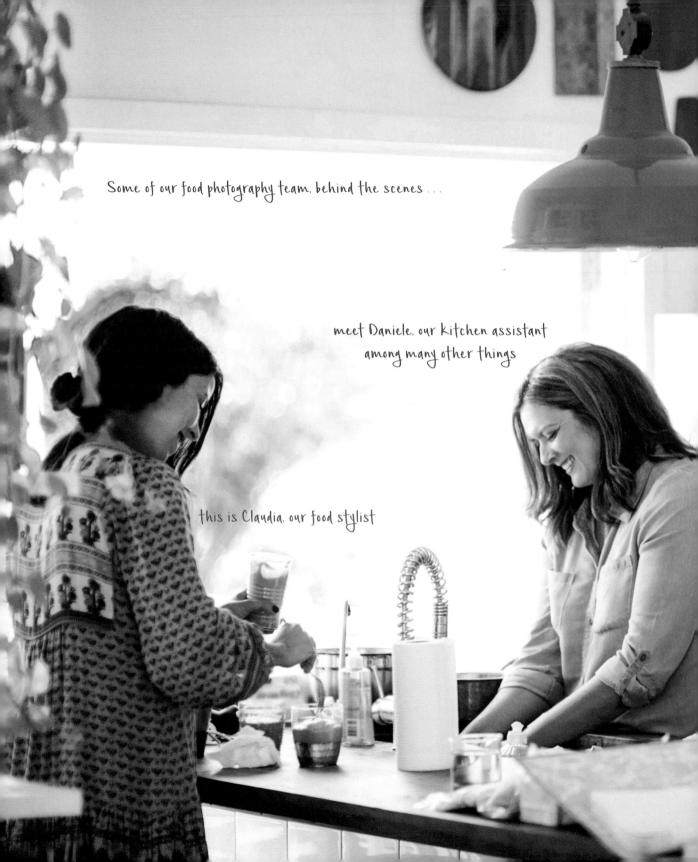

Some of our food photography team, behind the scenes . . .

meet Daniele, our kitchen assistant
among many other things

this is Claudia, our food stylist

meet Bryelle,
ready to help with anything

chef Michael sharing his talent
in the kitchen

RECIPES

"The cook is the forerunner of the doctor."

−Professor Maurizio Bifulco, University of Salerno, Italy

My delicious recipes focus on natural, minimally refined plant foods. There are already plenty of cookbooks that show healthier ways with meat and dairy, but few devote their pages to inspiring you to cook more meals based on legumes, whole grains, nuts, fruits and vegetables. Yet this is where most people need help as more and more people seek to reduce their meat consumption.

Many of my recipes are based on simple peasant fare from countries I have visited and "aunties" who have invited me into their kitchens. In traditional cultures, everybody thrived if they had enough food from their garden. Animal products played a much smaller role and refined plant foods, like white bread, were non-existent. These days, even some vegetarian cookbooks disappoint when their recipes call for liberal amounts of cheese, eggs, butter and white flour. Just because a recipe is meat- or dairy-free doesn't mean it's automatically healthy.

While my recipes are designed to reduce the risks of disease and to better manage existing chronic disease, for certain conditions like irritable bowel disease (IBS), you might need to temporarily lay off certain high-fibre, prebiotic (page 324) foods. Your dietitian or nutritionist can advise when this is required. But it's important to have these foods back on your plate as soon as possible. They are a key to feeding your hungry microbiome (page 324) and keeping your immune system in top shape. If you need to avoid or cut down on certain constituents, such as gluten or salt, choose recipes that suit or adapt them to your needs.

My recipes are designed for the home cook. They use a limited number of common ingredients (with some valuable new ones to discover), simple preparation steps, and fewer pots and pans than most chef-authored cookbooks. Most are quick enough to make on a weeknight with the help of some handy equipment (page 21). For recipes that take a little longer, you will produce more serves, so you can cook once and eat twice!

The stated time requirement is often an overestimate as you can complete some steps while cooking a stage of the recipe. The preparation time is what you will need after all the ingredients, measuring devices and pots are out on the bench ready for you to start. I have tested the cooking time using a gas burner but please note that cooking times will vary with different stoves and ovens. Many of the recipes include water added as needed in the method steps, but I assume that this will be easily accessible in your kitchen.

Standard Australian measuring cups and spoons have been used. The tablespoon is slightly larger than its US equivalent.

1 Australian tablespoon is 20 ml or 4 teaspoons
1 Australian teaspoon is 5 ml
1 Australian cup is 250 ml

Thankfully, my recipes are not low in total fat. Fat carries flavour. But they are low in saturated fats from animal products, which are linked with chronic disease. I also avoid refined vegetable oils as they are deficient in antioxidants. Rather than using butter and cream, I emphasise healthy unrefined plant fats such as nuts, avocado and extra virgin oils, proven to fight underlying disease processes. I use only a little dairy and eggs, and provide alternatives so nobody need miss out.

Added sugar is generally low in my recipes—or much lower than commonly used. I prefer fresh dates and honey for sweetness but at times also use some natural maple syrup or raw agave syrup. I prefer their flavours, but these sweeteners also supply some antioxidant phytonutrients, with a lower GI (page 346) than sugar.

An analysis for each recipe is provided so you can see just how beneficial it is to provide you with key nutrients, such as dietary fibre or calcium.

Finally, you can choose to cook from this book entirely or mix-and-match with other favourites. Feel free to experiment and adjust my recipes to your taste. Whether your preference is to adopt more of a Mediterranean diet or go meat-free on Mondays, I hope my ideas will open your eyes a little wider. A greater variety is possible by incorporating unrefined plant-based meals and you will feel good immediately after eating them!

What you eat matters and every mouthful counts! My goal for you is to maximise your nutritional benefits per bite. Knowing these recipes and recommendations are informed by reputable scientific studies, you can relax and enjoy each scrumptious dish.

SALADS &VEGGIE SIDES

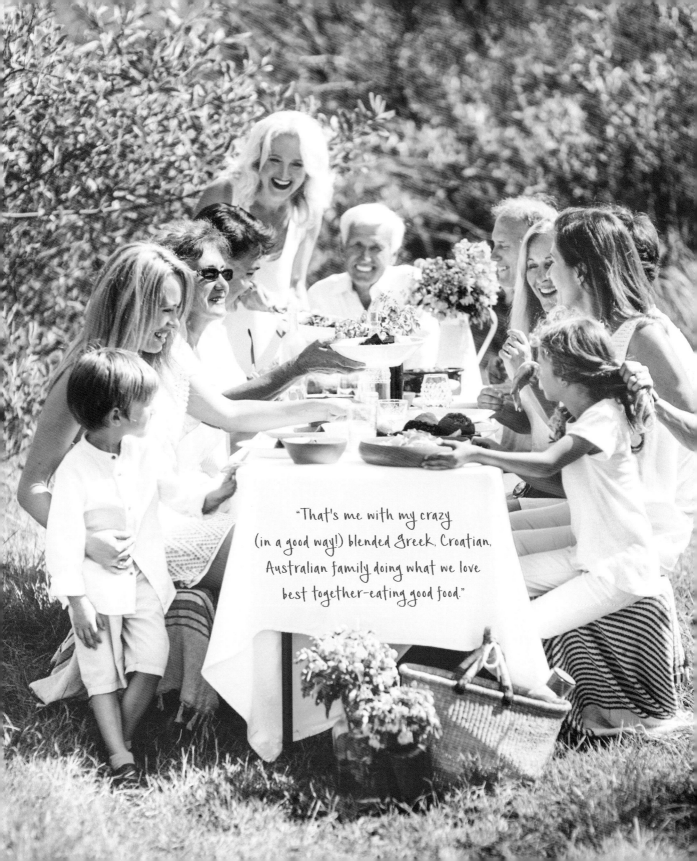

"That's me with my crazy (in a good way!) blended Greek, Croatian, Australian family doing what we love best together-eating good food."

This lively salad is an ideal cancer-fighting food! It was designed to be served as a "raw food" lunch or a side to cooked dishes. The sprouts add a hint of bitterness that is contrasted by the sweet and succulent red papaya. Compared with their mature seeds, sprouts are more nutrient-dense with higher vitamin, mineral and antioxidant levels. Sprouting is also known to boost iron and zinc absorption into the body and make the protein more digestible. Compared with cooked legumes, sprouted legumes are better tolerated by people with irritable bowel syndrome.

SPROUTED BEAN, AVOCADO AND RED PAPAYA SALAD

PREPARATION: 20 MINUTES, COOKING: 0 MINUTES, SERVES 4

Dressing
3 tablespoons lemon juice
3 tablespoons extra virgin olive oil
1 tablespoon natural maple syrup
1 small clove garlic, crushed
1 red birdseye chilli, finely chopped
¼ teaspoon salt

Salad
2 cups sprouted mixed legumes, such as mung beans, lentils or peas
1 medium red papaya, cubed
1 ripe avocado, cubed
1 small bunch chives, finely chopped
½ bunch fresh coriander (cilantro), chopped
80 g (3 oz) rocket (arugula) or small dark green leaves
60 g (2 oz) raw macadamia nuts

1. Place dressing ingredients in a glass jar and shake until well combined. Set aside.
2. Rinse sprouts using a fine-mesh strainer and dab dry, then place in a large salad bowl.
3. Add papaya, avocado, chives and coriander, and pour over dressing. Toss gently using a large spoon.
4. Fold in green leaves just prior to serving, and garnish with nuts and an extra drizzle of olive oil, if desired. Store leftovers in the fridge for up to 24 hours.

Per serve: energy 1828 kJ (437 Cal); protein 6 g; fat 38 g; saturated fat 7 g; cholesterol 0 mg; carbohydrate 14 g; sugars 14 g; fibre 8 g; calcium 75 mg; iron 2.5 mg; sodium 181 mg

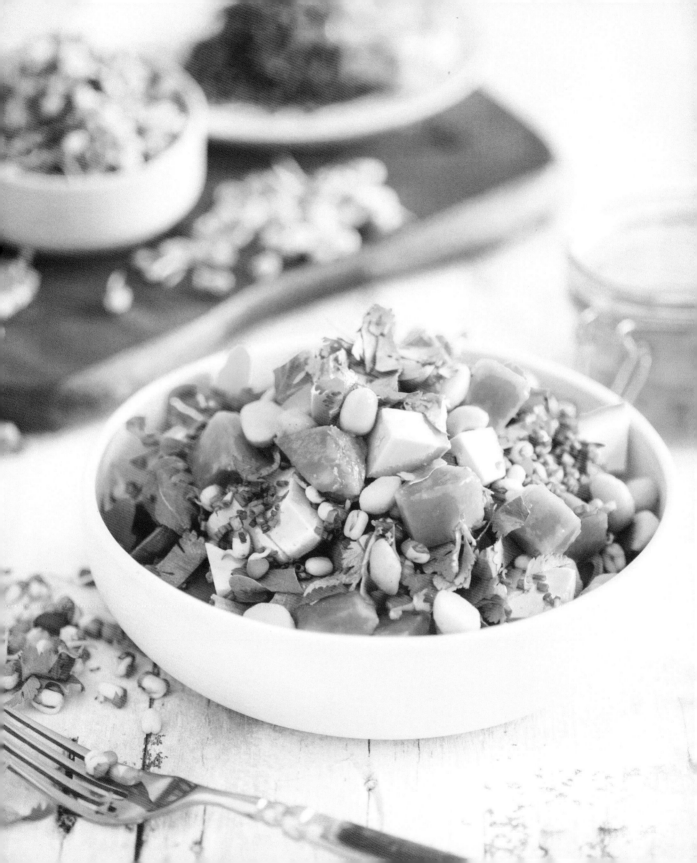

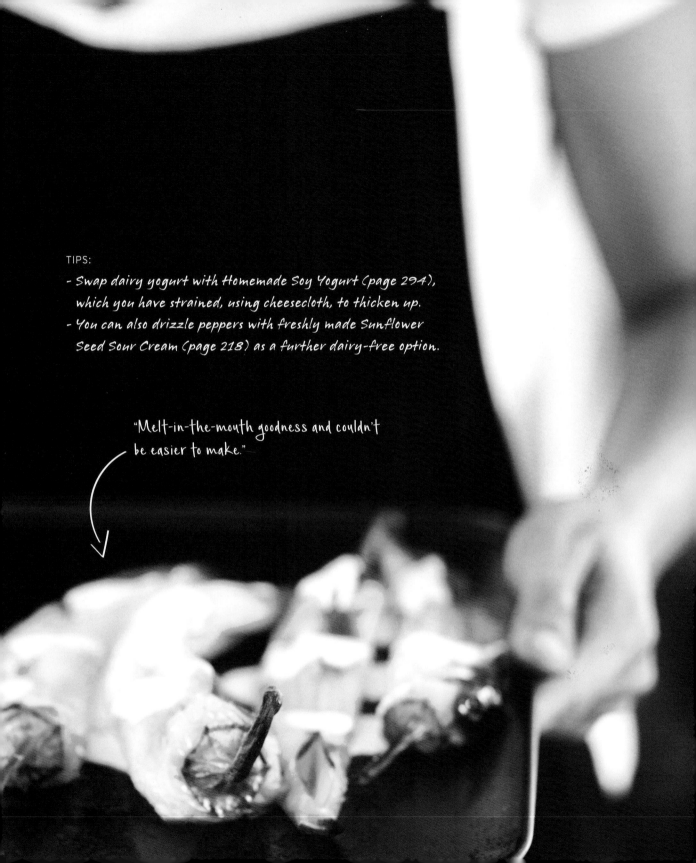

TIPS:
- Swap dairy yogurt with Homemade Soy Yogurt (page 294), which you have strained, using cheesecloth, to thicken up.
- You can also drizzle peppers with freshly made Sunflower Seed Sour Cream (page 218) as a further dairy-free option.

"Melt-in-the-mouth goodness and couldn't be easier to make."

This is a simple way to enjoy banana peppers when they are in season and boost your vegetable intake at the same time. Banana peppers are shaped and coloured like a banana and taste sweet, rather than hot. When baked, they become soft and succulent.

BAKED YELLOW BANANA PEPPERS WITH YOGURT SAUCE

PREPARATION: 4 MINUTES, COOKING: 20 MINUTES, SERVES 5

10 yellow banana peppers
1 tablespoon extra virgin olive oil
pinch salt
200 g (7 oz) natural European-style yogurt
1 clove garlic, crushed

1. Pre-heat oven to 220°C (420°F).

2. Wash peppers and lay a row in a large baking dish. Drizzle with olive oil and rub peppers so all sides are coated. Sprinkle with salt.

3. Bake for about 20 minutes until peppers start to turn golden brown. Remove from oven and allow to rest for 10 minutes.

4. Meanwhile, mix crushed garlic into yogurt to make a creamy sauce.

5. Drizzle yogurt sauce over the baked peppers and serve.

Peppers store well in the fridge for several days but are unsuitable for freezing.

Per serve: energy 416 kJ (99 Cal); protein 5 g; fat 5 g; saturated fat 1 g; cholesterol 6 mg; carbohydrate 8 g; sugars 8 g; fibre 3 g; calcium 91 mg; iron 0.5 mg; sodium 192 mg

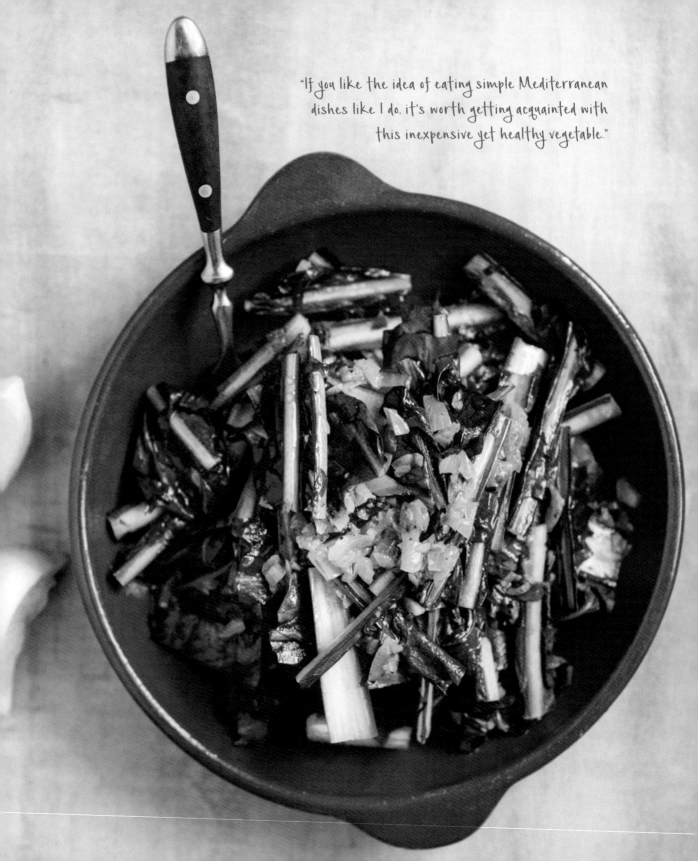

"If you like the idea of eating simple Mediterranean dishes like I do, it's worth getting acquainted with this inexpensive yet healthy vegetable."

Arab and Italian cooks are fond of chicory and its bitterness, which they counterbalance with a fruity olive oil. This home-style Lebanese recipe is a delicious way to prepare this highly nutritious dark-green leafy vegetable. Traditionally, people ate this dish as a simple meal with flatbread, but you can serve it as a side of greens with other foods. Chicory is naturally rich in inulin, an important prebiotic that stimulates the growth of good bacteria in your bowel.

GREEN CHICORY LEAVES WITH GARLIC IN OLIVE OIL

PREPARATION: 15 MINUTES, COOKING: 30 MINUTES, SERVES 6

1 teaspoon salt for cooking water +
   ½ teaspoon for seasoning
1 bunch (about 660 g/23 oz) green
   chicory
2 tablespoons extra virgin olive oil
1 medium onion, chopped
2 cloves garlic, crushed
½ teaspoon ground cumin
½ teaspoon Arabic seven spices
pinch salt
1 lemon, cut into wedges for serving

1. Add salt for cooking to a large pot containing at least 4 litres (1 gallon) of water and bring to boil.

2. Trim chicory base to separate stalks and chop them into 5-centimetre (2-inch) pieces using a cleaver. Wash well, changing the water 3 times or until there is no sand/dirt residue.

3. Add chicory pieces to boiling water, making sure they are at least half submerged. Cover and bring back to boil, then cook for 5 minutes until the chicory softens. (Cooking in salted water reduces bitterness.) Drain chicory in a colander.

4. Heat oil in a large frypan and sauté onion until translucent. Add garlic and cook for another 30 seconds. Stir in cumin, spices and remaining salt, followed by chicory pieces. Continue sautéeing on medium heat for a few minutes, until flavours combine and chicory has softened further.

5. Remove from heat and rest the dish, covered, for at least 5 minutes before serving. Serve on a platter with lemon wedges for drizzling. Chicory stores well in the fridge for several days but is unsuitable for freezing.

TIP:

- Purchase Arabic seven spices from greengrocers, a good delicatessen or Middle Eastern grocery store.

Per serve: energy 338 kJ (81 Cal); protein 2 g; fat 6 g; saturated fat 1 g; cholesterol 0 mg; carbohydrate 2 g; sugars 2 g; fibre 3 g; calcium 41 mg; iron 2.1 mg; sodium 233 mg

A dazzling salad with minimal calories that will bring you accolades at the table! Because of its intense colours, you can be sure this salad is loaded with disease-fighting phytonutrients, such as betacyanins. Beetroot is also an excellent source of nitrates–blood vessel relaxants–that lower high blood pressure and extend endurance during exercise.

FRESH BEETROOT, CARROT AND MINT SALAD

PREPARATION: 20 MINUTES, COOKING: 0 MINUTES, SERVES 6

500 g (17½ oz) raw beetroot bulbs
2 carrots
1 small onion, very finely chopped
½ bunch fresh mint, chopped
1½ tablespoons balsamic vinegar
1 tablespoon apple cider vinegar
2 teaspoons whole-grain mustard
2 tablespoons extra virgin olive oil
1 teaspoon honey

1. Peel beetroots and carrots, and grate finely. Tip: As raw beets are very hard, use your food processor if it has a grating disc.
2. Transfer grated vegetables to a mixing bowl, together with onion and mint.
3. To make the dressing, place vinegar, mustard, olive oil and honey in a jar with a screw-top lid and shake vigorously until well blended.
4. Pour dressing over salad and mix well using clean hands so there are no clumps of beetroot or carrot. Serve immediately as a side dish or refrigerate and use over several days. Recipe is unsuitable for freezing.

TIPS:

- Use leftovers in sandwiches–kids will love the bright colour and slightly sweet flavour.
- To avoid purple hands, wear disposable kitchen gloves!

Per serve: energy 454 kJ (108 Cal); protein 2 g; fat 6 g; saturated fat 1 g; cholesterol 0 mg; carbohydrate 10 g; sugars 9 g; fibre 4 g; calcium 27 mg; iron 0.9 mg; sodium 77 mg

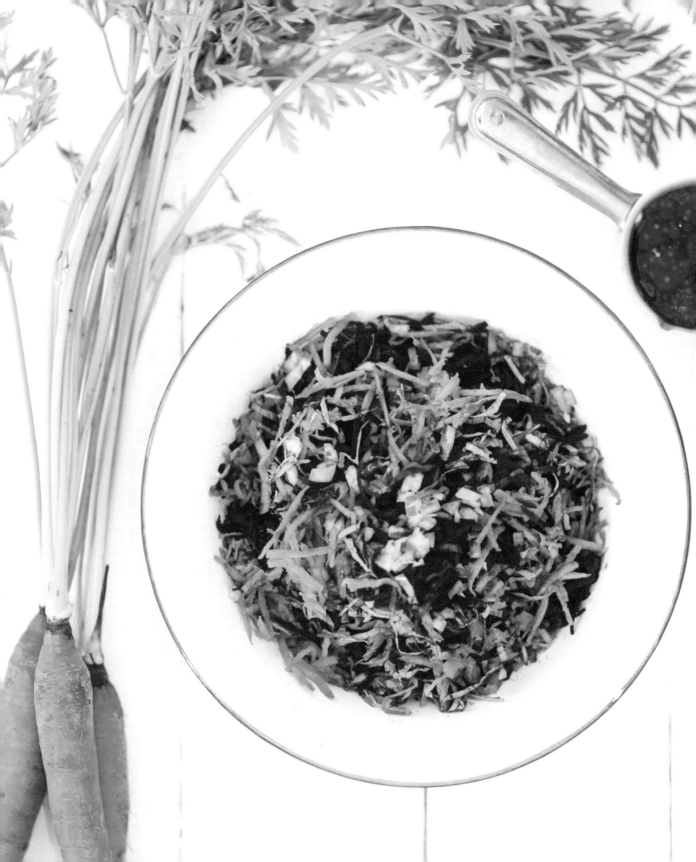

Now served in Middle Eastern restaurants almost everywhere, this refreshing salad originated from Syria and Lebanon. It's full of phytonutrient goodness—and one of my favourites! Radishes belong to the cruciferous family of vegetables and provide potent anti-cancer effects when eaten raw.

FATTOUSH SALAD WITH TOASTED BREAD AND SUMAC

PREPARATION: 20 MINUTES, COOKING: 3 MINUTES, SERVES 6

Dressing
2 cloves garlic, crushed
¼ teaspoon salt
1 tablespoon ground sumac
3 tablespoons extra virgin olive oil
1 lemon, juiced (approximately ¼ cup)

Salad
1½ wholemeal Lebanese breads
1 baby Cos lettuce, sliced into
  2.5-centimetre (1-inch) ribbons
3 medium tomatoes, cut into small
  chunks
3 small Lebanese cucumbers, cut in
  half lengthwise then sliced
5 radishes, finely sliced
½ red capsicum (bell pepper), chopped
4 shallots (scallions), sliced
½ bunch flat leaf parsley, chopped
large handful of mint leaves, chopped

1. Open up Lebanese bread at the seam making thin rounds. Toast in a hot oven for 3 minutes until crisp and dried. Break up the toasted bread into bite-size pieces. Set aside.

2. Place dressing ingredients in a small jar and shake vigorously until combined. Set aside.

3. Prepare salad vegetables and place in a large mixing bowl. Pour over dressing and toss gently with tongs until ingredients are well coated, then transfer to a serving bowl.

4. Just prior to serving, fold through the toasted bread pieces.

Note: If you add the bread earlier, it will go soggy.

Per serve: energy 732 kJ (175 Cal); protein 4 g; fat 10 g; saturated fat 2 g; cholesterol 0 mg; carbohydrate 15 g; sugars 6 g; fibre 4 g; calcium 76 mg; iron 1.4 mg; sodium 219 mg

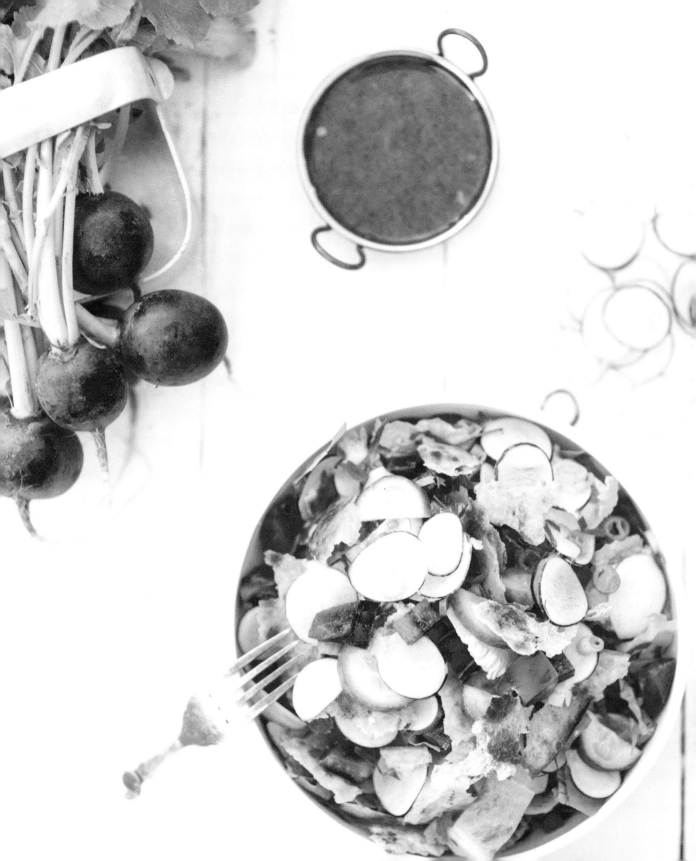

Make this fabulous salt-free salad when eggplants are in season. It's beautiful on bread or as a complement to other dishes. Eggplant is rich in viscous fibres, which lower elevated cholesterol. Garlic has anti-inflammatory properties and may help lower high blood pressure.

EGGPLANT SALAD WITH MINT AND RED CAPSICUM

PREPARATION: 15 MINUTES, COOKING: 40 MINUTES, SERVES 6

3 large purple eggplants (aubergines)
½ red capsicum (bell pepper), finely
   chopped
1 clove garlic, crushed
juice of ½ lemon
2 tablespoons extra virgin olive oil
½ bunch fresh mint, chopped

1. Pre-heat oven to 200ºC (390ºF). Place washed whole eggplants on a baking tray and prick with a fork. Bake for 30-40 minutes until eggplant is cooked and softens but doesn't blacken. Remove from oven and allow to cool slightly, then peel and dice or cut into strips. Place in a mixing bowl.

2. Add capsicum, garlic, lemon juice, olive oil and mint, and mix gently to combine.

3. Serve on a flat platter or shallow salad bowl. Salad can be enjoyed at room temperature or chilled. Store in the fridge for several days but recipe is unsuitable for freezing.

TIPS:

- To get the most medicinal benefits from garlic, crush and allow to sit for 10 minutes before adding to food or cooking.
- Don't like garlic breath? Try chewing on fresh parsley or fennel seeds or bite into a wedge of lemon to help neutralise the odour.

Per serve: energy 537 kJ (128 Cal); protein 4 g; fat 7 g; saturated fat 1 g; cholesterol 0 mg; carbohydrate 9 g; sugars 9 g; fibre 8 g; calcium 82 mg; iron 0.8 mg; sodium 17 mg

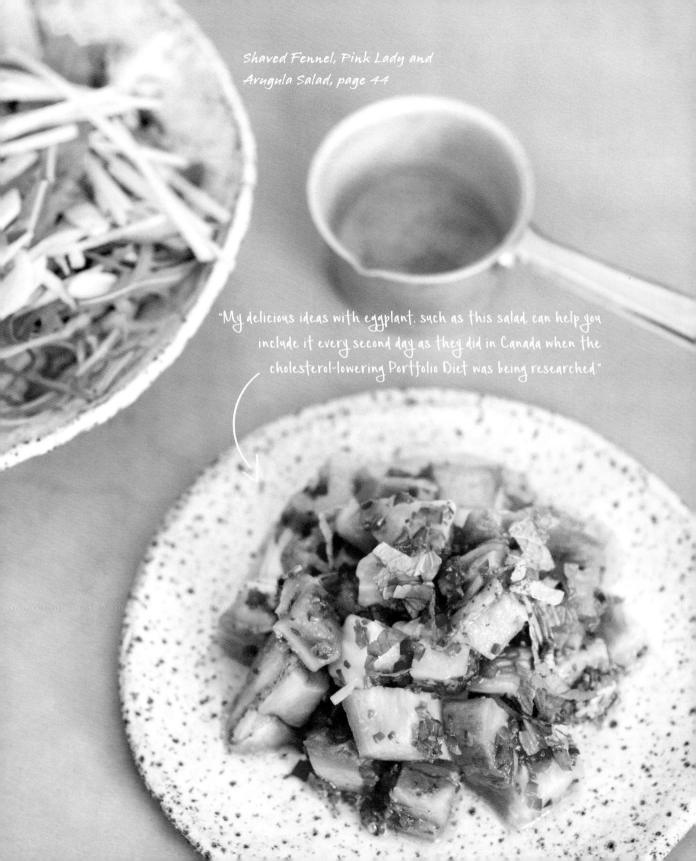

Shaved Fennel, Pink Lady and
Arugula Salad, page 44

"My delicious ideas with eggplant, such as this salad, can help you
include it every second day as they did in Canada when the
cholesterol-lowering Portfolio Diet was being researched."

This refreshing salad, with a hint of aniseed, will cleanse your palate and lighten a heavier meal. Salads are also perfect for dropping high blood pressure! (Recipe image, page 43.)

SHAVED FENNEL, PINK LADY AND ARUGULA SALAD

PREPARATION: 15 MINUTES, COOKING: 0 MINUTES, SERVES 6

Dressing
⅓ cup extra virgin olive oil
3 tablespoons lemon juice
freshly crushed pepper, optional

Salad
1 small bulb fresh fennel, sliced very
    thinly
½ medium Spanish onion, sliced thinly
2 small Pink Lady apples, cored, halved
    and julienned
80 g (6 oz) arugula (rocket)
2 tablespoons freshly chopped mint

1. Place dressing ingredients in a glass jar, screw on lid and shake vigorously until well combined.
2. Combine sliced fennel, onions and julienned apples in a mixing bowl and pour over dressing. Toss until well combined. Just prior to serving, mix through rocket and mint. Pile salad onto a large serving platter. Salad is best served immediately but can be stored, almost completed, for up to 24 hours as the lemon acts as a preservative.

TIPS:

- To prepare fennel for slicing, remove stalks, cut in half vertically and remove the core from both halves using a sharp knife.
- To slice the fennel paper thin, use a mandoline. Many mandolines also have a julienne setting.

Per serve: energy 623 kJ (149 Cal); protein 1 g; fat 13 g; saturated fat 2 g; cholesterol 0 mg; carbohydrate 7 g; sugars 7 g; fibre 2 g; calcium 23 mg; iron 0.4 mg; sodium 25 mg

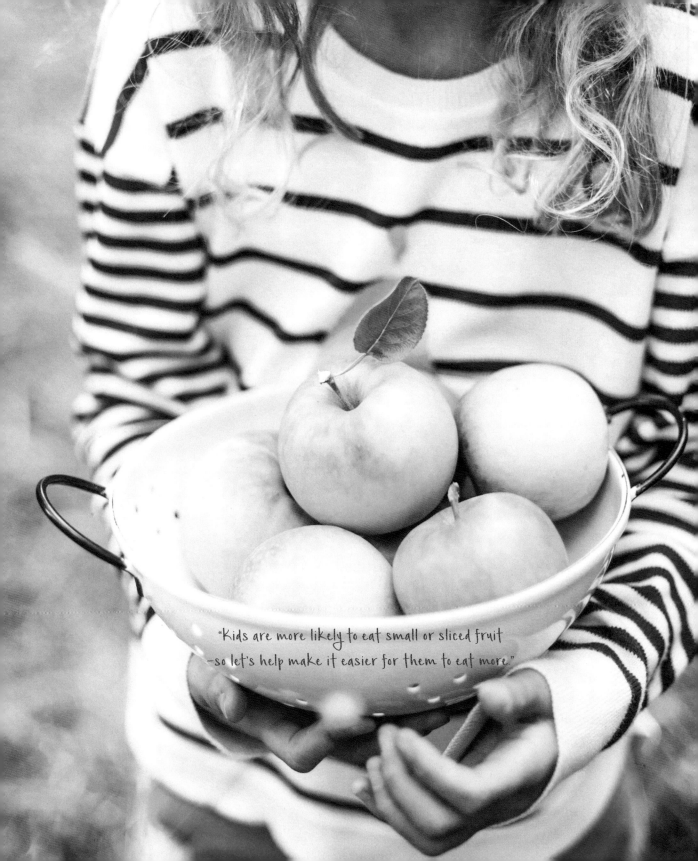

"Kids are more likely to eat small or sliced fruit —so let's help make it easier for them to eat more."

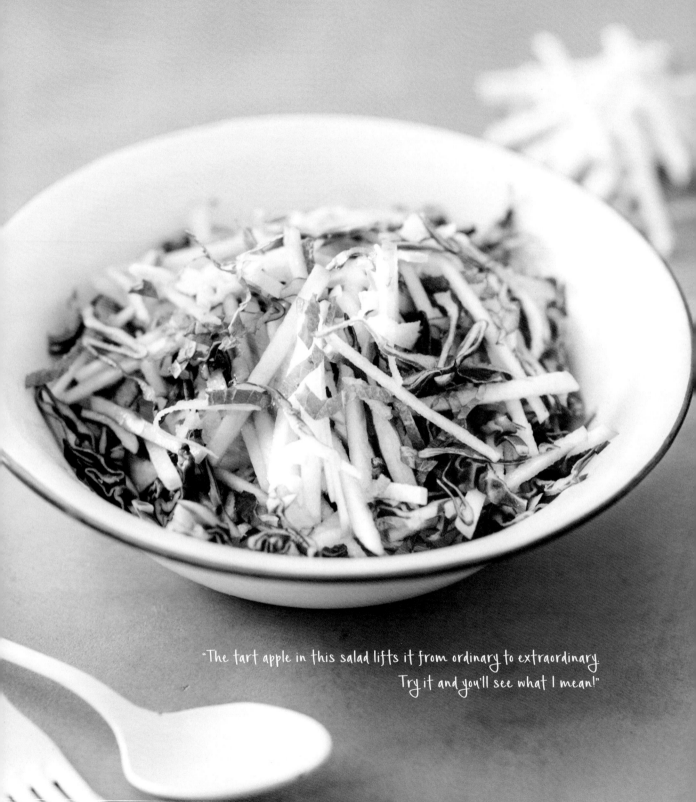

"The tart apple in this salad lifts it from ordinary to extraordinary. Try it and you'll see what I mean!"

The perfect winter salad to complement a hot meal. Kohlrabi—also known as German turnip or turnip cabbage, as it grows above ground—is from the cruciferous family. Like broccoli, cauliflower and watercress, it provides a rich source of anti-cancer phytonutrients when consumed raw!

KOHLRABI, GREEN APPLE AND MINT SALAD

PREPARATION: 15 MINUTES, COOKING: 0 MINUTES, SERVES 6

Salad
300 g (10 oz) purple cabbage
2 medium kohlrabi, peeled and grated
1 large granny smith apple, finely
  julienned
¼ red onion, thinly sliced
3 tablespoons coarsely chopped mint

Dressing
2 tablespoons lemon juice
2 tablespoons extra virgin olive oil
2 teaspoons apple cider vinegar

1. Finely shred cabbage using a mandoline.
2. Add grated kohlrabi, apple and onion.
3. Whisk together dressing ingredients and pour over salad. Using clean hands, mix to combine and evenly distribute salad ingredients.
4. Transfer to a serving bowl and sprinkle with mint. Drizzle with more olive oil, if desired, just prior to serving. Serve immediately or store in the fridge and use within 24 hours as apple may discolour.

TIPS:
- Kohlrabi can also be steamed, baked or sautéed.
- Variation: Instead of kohlrabi, use white radish (daikon) or swede (rutabaga).

Per serve: energy 452 kJ (108 Cal); protein 3 g; fat 6 g; saturated fat 1 g; cholesterol 0 mg; carbohydrate 8 g; sugars 8 g; fibre 4 g; calcium 38 mg; iron 0.8 mg; sodium 18 mg

I adore this easy way to prepare succulent beetroot. This dish is usually served cold but Greeks also eat it warm, when freshly cooked, with a main course. The simple dressing complements the sweet beet flavour and acts as a preservative.

GREEK-STYLE BEETROOT WITH LEMON AND OLIVE OIL

PREPARATION: 30 MINUTES, COOKING: 20 MINUTES INCLUDING PRESSURE COOKER, SERVES 8

2 bunches of fresh beetroot
2 tablespoons fruity extra virgin olive oil
juice of 1 lemon

1. Cut off beetroot stalks, leaving about 2.5 centimetres (about 1 inch) on each beet to minimize "bleeding" during cooking.
2. Wash any dirt from beetroot bulbs and place them in a pressure cooker, half submerged in water. Cover and turn up heat to bring to pressure, then turn down to very low and cook under pressure for 5 minutes. (Alternatively, cook the beetroot conventionally for approximately 1 hour or until soft.) Allow for natural pressure release before opening the pressure cooker, then drain and allow beets to cool slightly.
3. Meanwhile, wash stalks with their leaves, changing the water 3 times to ensure all dirt and sand is removed. Place in a large saucepan containing about 2.5 centimetres (1 inch) of boiling water and simmer for 15 minutes until wilted. Pick up cooked leaves with tongs to drain excess water, then arrange them on a serving platter.
4. Wearing disposable kitchen gloves, peel each cooked beet, then cut into chunks. Place on top of leaves and drizzle with olive oil followed by lemon juice.
5. Serve immediately or cover, refrigerate and enjoy over several days.

TIP:

- *After eating beetroot, as many as 15 per cent of people notice a temporary discolouration when using the bathroom. This is normal and no cause for concern.*

Per serve: energy 573 kJ (137 Cal); protein 4 g; fat 5 g; saturated fat 1 g; cholesterol 0 mg; carbohydrate 17 g; sugars 17 g; fibre 7 g; calcium 16 mg; iron 1.8 mg; sodium 104 mg

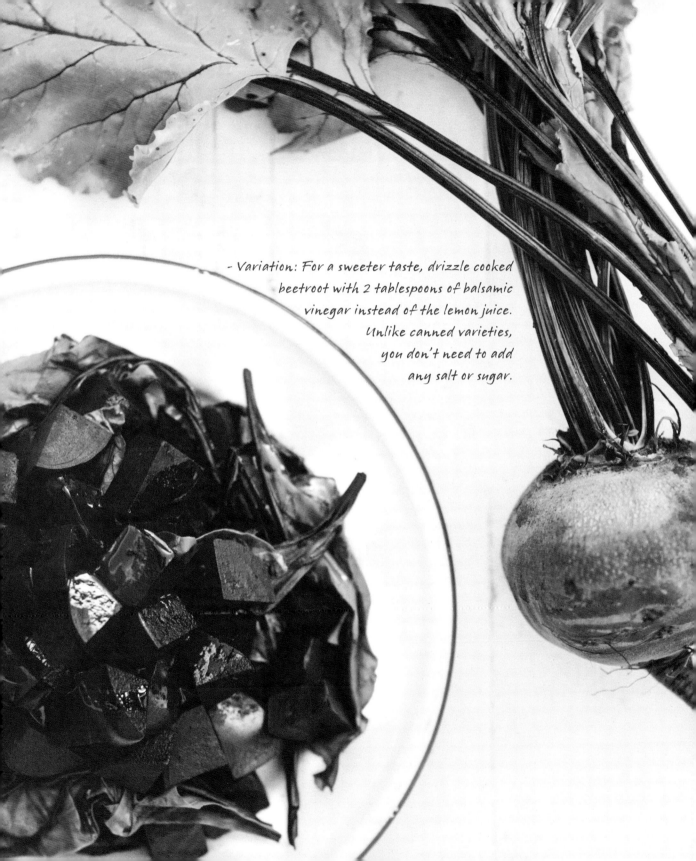

- Variation: For a sweeter taste, drizzle cooked beetroot with 2 tablespoons of balsamic vinegar instead of the lemon juice. Unlike canned varieties, you don't need to add any salt or sugar.

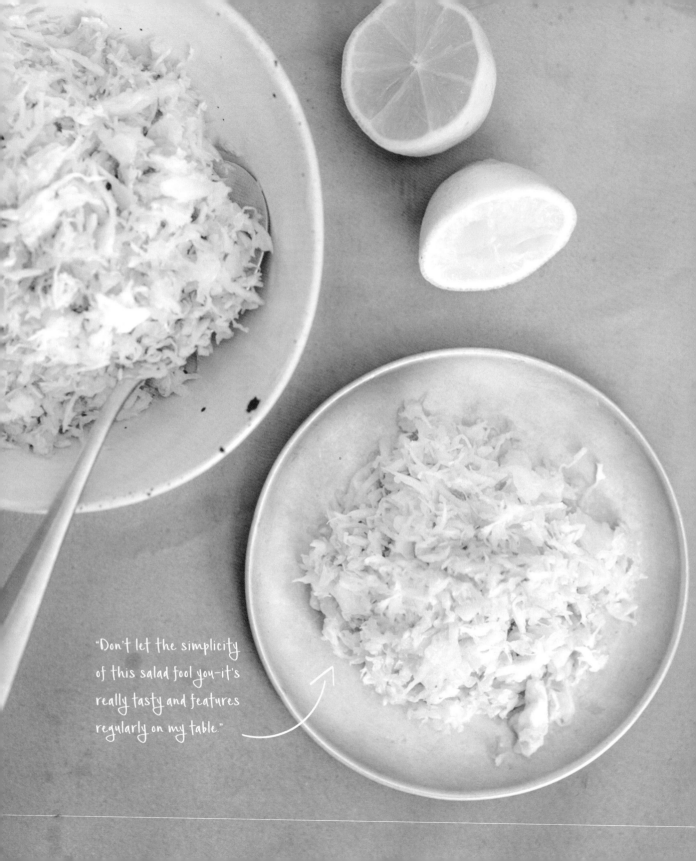

"Don't let the simplicity of this salad fool you–it's really tasty and features regularly on my table."

Raw cabbage is extremely good for you—and this is the simplest and most delicious way to enjoy it! Cabbage has strong anti-cancer properties and has been eaten traditionally with main meals across Eastern Europe and throughout the Mediterranean. The red variety of cabbage also contains anthocyanins, the purple pigment with strong antioxidant activity commonly found in blueberries.

SHAVED SAVOY CABBAGE WITH LEMON DRESSING

PREPARATION: 12 MINUTES, COOKING: 0 MINUTES, SERVES 6

1 kg (2 lb 3 oz) savoy cabbage
⅓ cup lemon juice (about 2 juiced lemons)
⅓ cup extra virgin olive oil
1 teaspoon salt

1. Discard the outer leaf of cabbage if dirty, then cut cabbage in half through its core. Using light pressure on a mandoline, finely shred both cabbage halves into a large bowl.
2. Add remaining ingredients and massage cabbage for 1 minute using a clean hand, until it just softens and the dressing is well dispersed. Transfer to a salad bowl and enjoy immediately or within several hours. Cabbage salad can also be refrigerated and consumed within the next 24 hours, although it will soften further.

TIPS:

- Variation: Rather than Savoy, which has a wrinkly appearance and is softer, you can also use ordinary white or purple cabbage.
- You can shred the cabbage a day in advance and store in the fridge, undressed, until required.
- Cabbage can also be juiced. Fresh cabbage juice contains high myrosinase activity (page 375).

Per serve: energy 658 kJ (157 Cal); protein 3 g; fat 13 g; saturated fat 2 g; cholesterol 0 mg; carbohydrate 6 g; sugars 6 g; fibre 5 g; calcium 60 mg; iron 1 mg; sodium 407 mg

This is a beautiful salad I fell in love with in Sicily. Fennel has the texture of celery but the taste of liquorice or aniseed. While high in fibre, vitamin C, folate and potassium, fennel is low in calories and also contains properties that help lower blood pressure and improve heart health. One of the most fascinating phytonutrients in fennel is anethole, which accounts for the sweet liquorice taste and has been repeatedly shown in animal studies to lower inflammation and help prevent cancer.

SICILIAN ORANGE AND FENNEL SALAD

PREPARATION: 7 MINUTES, COOKING: 0 MINUTES, SERVES 4

2 very large oranges, peeled with the pith removed
250 g (9 oz) fresh fennel, trimmed of stalks
2 tablespoons extra virgin olive oil
flat parsley leaves pulled from stalks, for garnish

1. Segment oranges and cut each segment into 3 chunks. Place into a salad bowl together with any juice.
2. Slice fennel as desired and add to bowl.
3. Drizzle with olive oil and toss. Sprinkle with parsley leaves and serve. Salad stores well in the fridge for up to a day.

TIPS:
- There is no right or wrong way to cut fennel. Slice thinly if you prefer a lighter flavour or into small chunks for a more robust aniseed hit.
- Add a few black olives for extra colour and flavour, before serving.

Per serve: energy 572 kJ (137 Cal); protein 2 g; fat 9 g; saturated fat 1 g; cholesterol 0 mg; carbohydrate 10 g; sugars 10 g; fibre 4 g; calcium 40 mg; iron 0.6 mg; sodium 28 mg

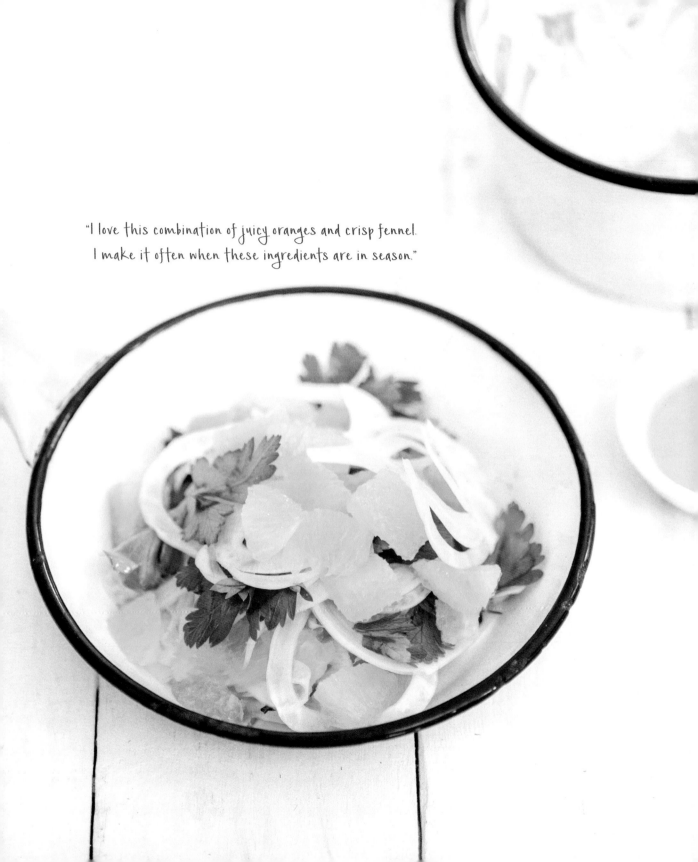

"I love this combination of juicy oranges and crisp fennel.
I make it often when these ingredients are in season."

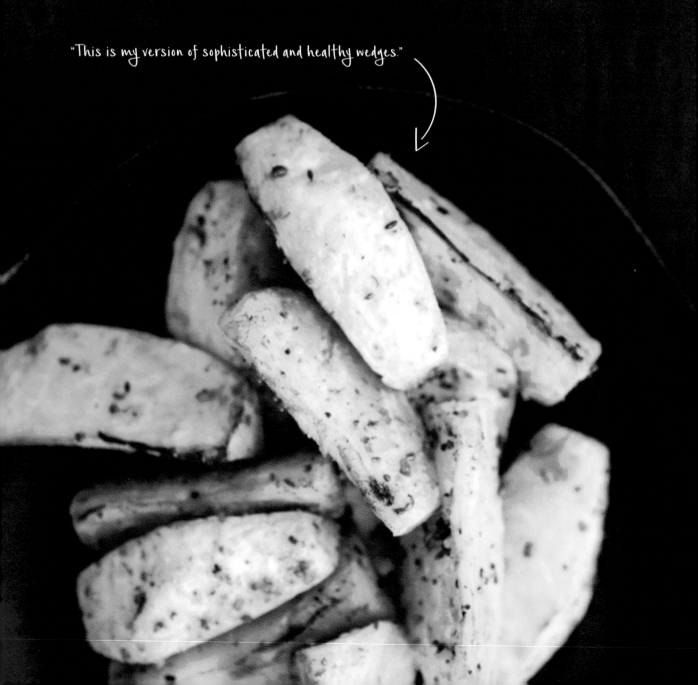

TIPS:
- Celeriac is also delicious when boiled with potato and
mashed or it can be finely shredded for salads.
- Freshly ground spices provide the best flavour!

"This is my version of sophisticated and healthy wedges."

Celeriac makes delicious oven-baked wedges! Unlike potato, these wedges won't be mushy on the inside but have a slightly crunchy texture, even when cooked. They also contain only a quarter of the carbohydrate content of potato wedges and are low in sodium. As celeriac is very hard and tricky to peel, I use a cleaver to trim off its skin, like you would with a pineapple.

SPICED CELERIAC WEDGES

PREPARATION: 10 MINUTES, COOKING: 45 MINUTES, SERVES 6

1 very large celeriac (about 1.5 kg/
   3 lb before peeling)
1 tablespoon coriander seeds
1 tablespoon fennel seeds
1 tablespoon cumin seeds
4 tablespoons extra virgin olive oil

1. Pre-heat oven to 200°C (390°F).

2. Peel celeriac and slice into 2-centimetre (1-inch) thick wedges. Place in a large baking dish.

3. Grind seeds using an electric grinder or mortar and pestle.

4. Heat oil in a small frypan and sauté seed mixture for just 30 seconds until aromatic, then remove from heat. Be careful not to burn the spices. They will continue to brown in the oven.

5. Pour spiced oil over celeriac wedges and toss to coat evenly.

6. Bake, uncovered, for 45-50 minutes until browned, turning once. Serve hot. Recipe is unsuitable for freezing.

TIP:

- Buy celeriac when in season as it can be expensive.

Per serve: energy 670 kJ (160 Cal); protein 2 g; fat 13 g; saturated fat 2 g; cholesterol 0 mg; carbohydrate 6 g; sugars 4 g; fibre 6 g; calcium 78 mg; iron 1.6 mg; sodium 25 mg

I learned the village way to make Greek salad from my Greek husband and many summer vacations visiting various parts of Greece. Perfect with some crusty bread for lunch on a hot day! You will need ripe red tomatoes and a robust extra virgin olive oil, rich in polyphenols. Although the amount of oil may initially raise your eyebrows, in the traditional Mediterranean diet, salad "swims" in olive oil! It is also customary to soak up leftover juices with chunks of good bread. The additional oregano further boosts the already high antioxidant content.

AUTHENTIC GREEK SALAD

PREPARATION: 9 MINUTES, COOKING: 0 MINUTES, SERVES 6

2 large ripe tomatoes
2 medium cucumbers
½ large red capsicum (bell pepper)
½ red onion
½ cup extra virgin olive oil
2 tablespoons lemon juice
12 kalamata or large black olives
100 g (3½ oz) feta cheese, crumbled or cut into chunks
1 teaspoon dried oregano

1. Cut tomato chunks directly into a salad bowl or platter with a lip.
2. Holding cucumber vertically, slice off alternate strips of skin and discard. (This is for appearance only). Then cut halfway down into the cucumber to make a cross and slice horizontally 1-centimetre (½-inch) chunks into bowl. Repeat with second cucumber.
3. Cut capsicum into small chunks and red onion into thin strips, and top the salad.
4. Dot with olives and feta.
5. Pour over oil followed by lemon juice and sprinkle with oregano. Serve immediately or hold the dressing and drizzle just prior to serving. Leftover salad will keep in the fridge for 24 hours.

TIPS:

- I prefer Dodoni feta, made from sheep and goats milk, containing A2 protein. It is creamy but with a bite. For a dairy-free version, swap it with Almond Cream Cheese in "feta" form (see page 224).
- Variation: Replace lemon juice with vinegar.
- Revamp leftover Greek salad by tossing through some cooked white quinoa or millet, which will soak up the juices.

Per serve: energy 1093 kJ (261 Cal); protein 5 g; fat 25 g; saturated fat 6 g; cholesterol 11 mg; carbohydrate 5 g; sugars 4 g; fibre 2 g; calcium 90 mg; iron 0.8 mg; sodium 320 mg

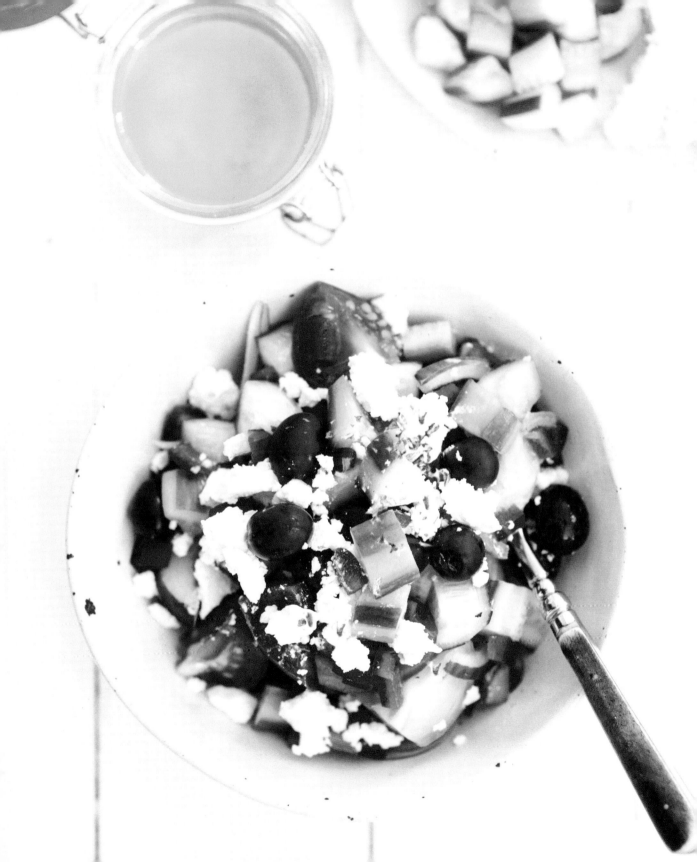

The authentic and most delicious way of making Middle Eastern tabbouleh. Unlike many versions, this tabbouleh contains only a small amount of bulgur for texture, while the bright green parsley takes centre stage. Parsley is a rich source of antioxidants and can be easily grown in a pot with minimal attention.

TABBOULEH

PREPARATION: 35 MINUTES, COOKING: 0 MINUTES, SERVES 6

¼ cup fine bulgur wheat

4 large bunches flat-leaf parsley
(providing at least 480 g/17 oz soft leaves)

1 teaspoon salt for washing parsley +
½ teaspoon for seasoning

⅓ bunch mint

5 tomatoes, finely chopped

1 Lebanese cucumber, unpeeled, washed and finely chopped

½ red capsicum (bell pepper), finely chopped

3 large shallots (scallions), finely chopped

pinch crushed black pepper

¼ teaspoon ground cumin

¼ cup extra virgin olive oil

½ cup lemon juice (about 2 juiced lemons)

1. Soak bulgur wheat in water to soften, for about 10 minutes, while preparing other ingredients. Drain in a colander, using a spoon to press out extra moisture.

2. Tear off the tender leaves and stalks from parsley bunches and place in a deep basin for washing. Discard the coarse stems and stalks. Sprinkle with 1 teaspoon of salt and cover with water. Allow to soak for a few minutes, then drain and rinse a couple of times with fresh water until the water runs clear and there is no dirt visible at the bottom of the basin. Spin dry using a salad spinner or place in small bundles on a clean tea towel (dish towel) to air-dry.

3. Similarly, pluck mint leaves from their stalks, wash then spin dry.

4. Finely chop parsley and mint leaves, and place in a large salad bowl.

5. Add remaining ingredients and toss salad to combine.
Serve as a side or for a light lunch inside Cos lettuce leaves, which can replace bread.

Per serve: energy 688 kJ (164 Cal); protein 5 g; fat 10 g; saturated fat 1 g; cholesterol 0 mg; carbohydrate 10 g; sugars 6 g; fibre 8 g; calcium 213 mg; iron 6.6 mg; sodium 260 mg

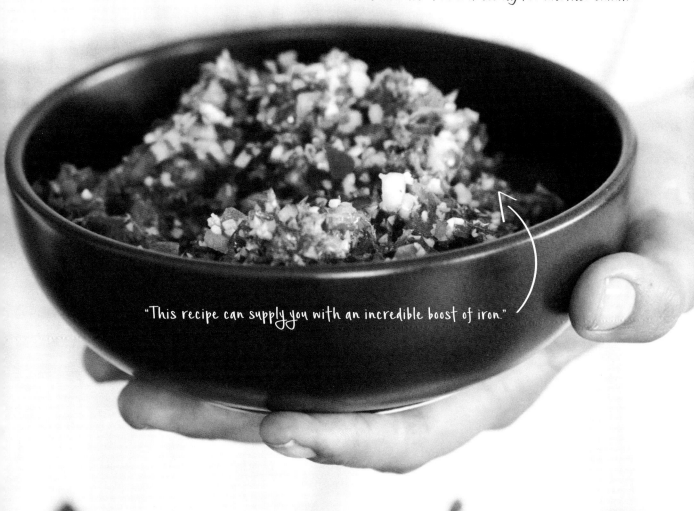

"This recipe can supply you with an incredible boost of iron."

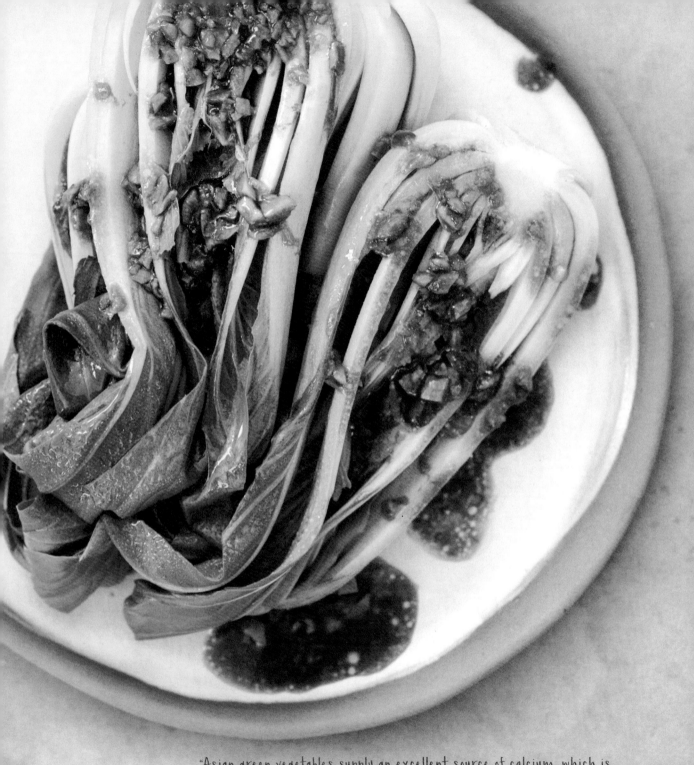

"Asian green vegetables supply an excellent source of calcium, which is readily absorbed into the body. We should all eat more of them."

A quick and delicious way to incorporate more Asian greens into your diet. Bok choy is so tender when lightly steamed, that it melts in the mouth! Being from the cruciferous family, it can provide potent anti-cancer effects.

STEAMED BABY BOK CHOY WITH GARLIC SOY SAUCE

PREPARATION: 4 MINUTES, COOKING: 7 MINUTES, SERVES 4

1 bundle baby bok choy bunches
   (about 500 g/17½ oz)
1 tablespoon extra virgin olive oil
4 cloves garlic, chopped
1 tablespoon salt-reduced soy sauce
½ teaspoon cornstarch

1. Set up a steamer on the stove while you prepare bok choy.
2. Slice bok choy bunches lengthwise, into halves or quarters (depending on size), then wash well by submerging in water. Rinse out any hard-to-get-to dirt under running water.
3. Place bok choy into steamer basket and steam for 3 minutes.
4. Meanwhile, heat oil in a small frypan and sauté garlic until just browned.
5. Stir in soy sauce, followed by cornstarch dissolved in 3 tablespoons of water and cook for 1 minute to thicken.
6. Transfer steamed bok choy onto a serving plate and drizzle with the sauce. Serve immediately. Recipe is unsuitable for freezing.

TIP:

- Use this method to prepare other Asian greens. Adjust cooking time, if required.

Per serve: energy 353 kJ (84 Cal); protein 5 g; fat 5 g; saturated fat 1 g; cholesterol 0 mg; carbohydrate 2 g; sugars 1 g; fibre 5 g; calcium 156 mg; iron 2.8 mg; sodium 281 mg

You've heard of kale in green juices and smoothies. Here's a festive-looking way to enjoy it as a salad. Massaging the leaves with lemon and salt tenderises them and the resulting flavour is reminiscent of bubble gum! Adding the avocado and olive oil boosts absorption of the carotenoid phytonutrients to fight cancer. This salad is gorgeous served with a main meal. Leftovers are great as a sandwich filling. Raw, finely shredded kale will supply ample amounts of sulforaphane—a strong anti-cancer phytonutrient.

FRESH KALE, AVOCADO AND POMEGRANATE SALAD

PREPARATION: 25 MINUTES, COOKING: 0 MINUTES, SERVES 8

300 g (10½ oz) curly kale leaves
    stripped from their stem
¼ cup lemon juice (about 1 juiced lemon)
3 tablespoons extra virgin olive oil
½ teaspoon salt
1 avocado, cut into small cubes
½ cup pomegranate seeds

1. Wash kale leaves thoroughly, in several changes of water. Press down firmly or use a salad spinner to remove excess water.
2. Roll up leaves and shred very finely, then transfer to a large salad bowl.
3. Add lemon juice, oil and salt, and massage well with a clean hand for a few minutes until kale softens. Allow to sit for at least 30 minutes for flavour to develop.
4. Prior to serving, fold in avocado and pomegranate seeds. Salad will keep in fridge for up to 2 days. Recipe is unsuitable for freezing.

TIP:

- *Clean organic kale carefully as it sometimes hides slugs, snails and aphids on the leaves. Submerge it in salted water for half an hour if required, then rinse several times.*

Per serve: energy 518 kJ (124 Cal); protein 1 g; fat 12 g; saturated fat 2 g; cholesterol 0 mg; carbohydrate 3 g; sugars 3 g; fibre 2 g; calcium 20 mg; iron 0.5 mg; sodium 153 mg

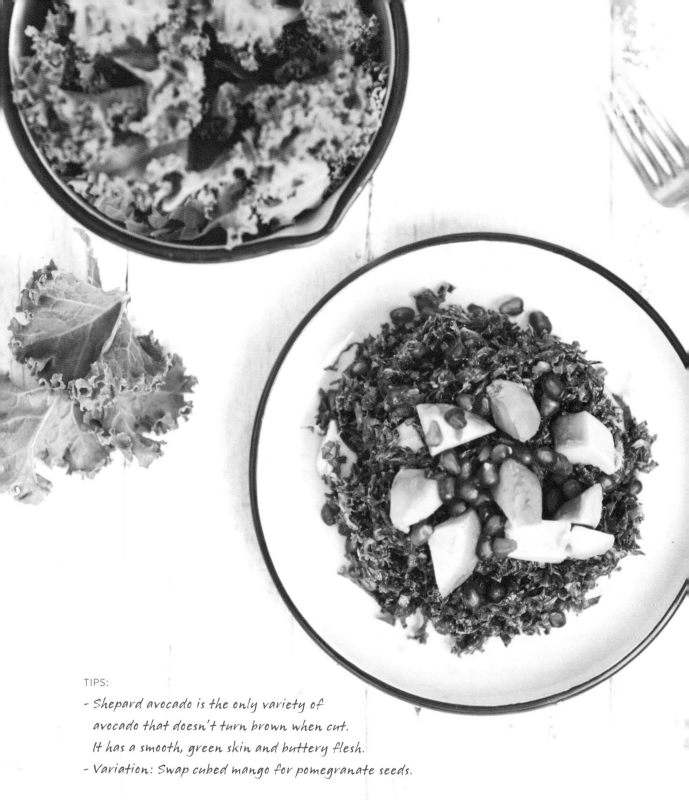

TIPS:
- Shepard avocado is the only variety of
  avocado that doesn't turn brown when cut.
  It has a smooth, green skin and buttery flesh.
- Variation: Swap cubed mango for pomegranate seeds.

Greeks enjoy eating wild and bitter dark leafy greens, which they call "horta." This version uses endive, boiled in a small amount of water, which reduces its bitterness, then dressed simply with lemon and olive oil. The combination of flavours is just wonderful! Horta is traditionally served with many main dishes.

WILTED ENDIVE LEAVES WITH LEMON AND OLIVE OIL

PREPARATION: 15 MINUTES, COOKING: 25 MINUTES, SERVES 7

1 bundle endive, approximately 1 kg (2 lb 3 oz)
½ cup extra virgin olive oil
¼ cup lemon juice (about 1 juiced lemon)

1. Place about 2.5 centimetres (1 inch) of water in a large saucepan, then cover and bring to boil.
2. Cut off the base of each endive bunch 5 centimetres (2 inches) up the stem and discard. Place leaves in kitchen sink with clean water. Swirl leaves around, then transfer them into a large bowl. Drain water from sink and rinse, then re-fill with clean water. Repeat twice until leaves are clean, pulling off any dark or old bits. Squeeze leaves firmly while tilting the bowl over the sink to remove excess water.
3. Add washed endive to boiling water, pushing it down firmly until the pot is full but you are able to just cover it with a lid. (You might need to cook the endive in 2 batches.) Bring back to boil and cook for about 10 minutes until leaves have wilted. Using tongs, transfer cooked endive to a platter or bowl, spreading it out so it doesn't clump together.
4. Repeat the process, if required, until you have cooked all the remaining leaves. You can use the same cooking water.
5. Allow endive to cool for 10-15 minutes, then drizzle with olive oil and lemon juice and serve warm. Alternatively, refrigerate and enjoy cold. Horta can last in the fridge for several days.

TIPS:

- All sorts of edible weeds were traditionally used to make horta. You can also make it with dandelion greens, beetroot leaves, chicory, nettles and any other edible dark leafy greens.
- If you are concerned about the dull colour, dunk the cooked leaves briefly into icy-cold water after cooking.

Per serve: energy 693 kJ (165 Cal); protein 2 g; fat 16 g; saturated fat 3 g; cholesterol 0 mg; carbohydrate 1 g; sugars 1 g; fibre 3 g; calcium 67 mg; iron 2.5 mg; sodium 109 mg

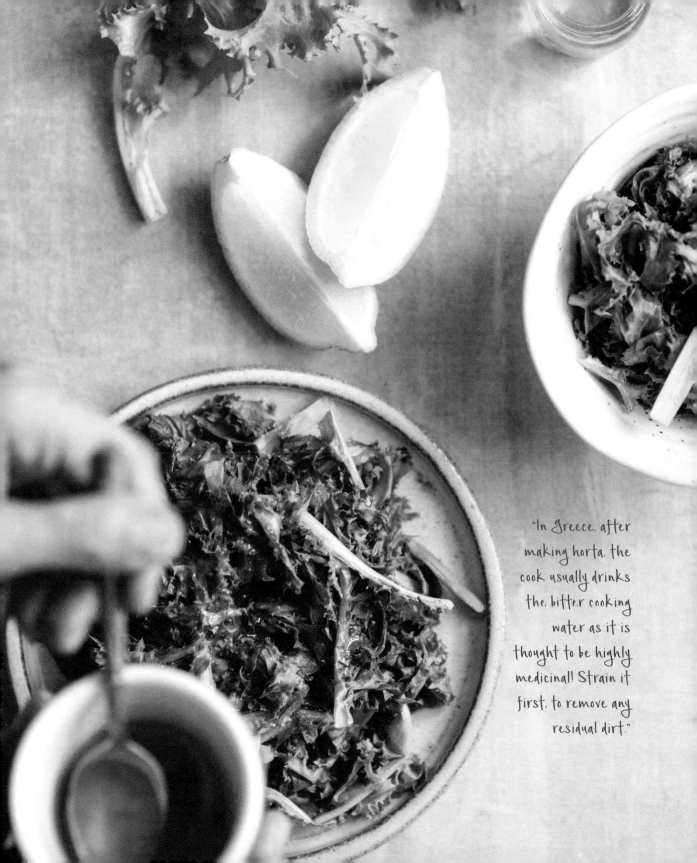

"In greece, after making horta, the cook usually drinks the bitter cooking water as it is thought to be highly medicinal! Strain it first, to remove any residual dirt."

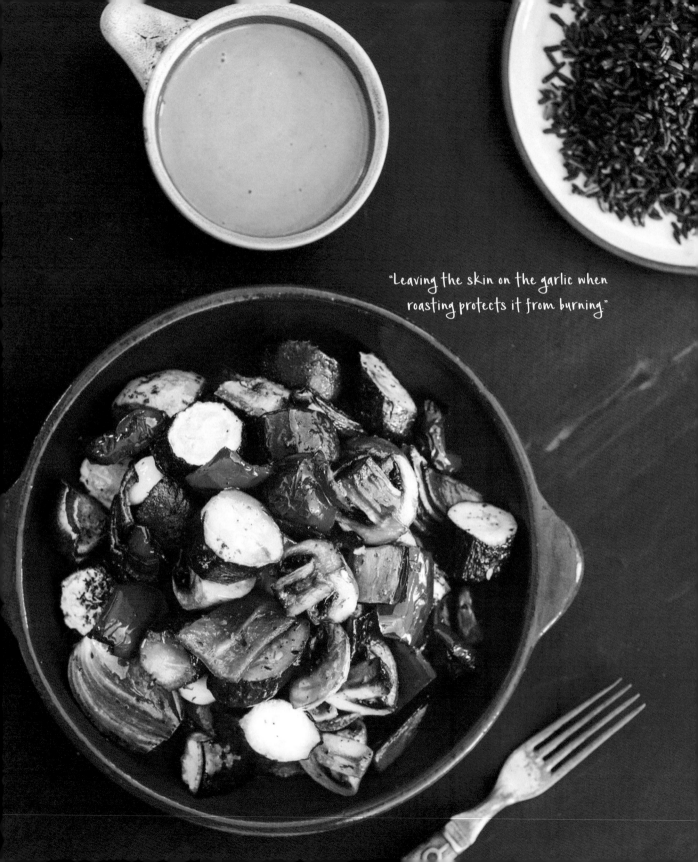

"Leaving the skin on the garlic when roasting protects it from burning."

A delicious way to eat more vegetables. The creamy dressing is an ideal swap for mayonnaise and can be used to flavour any salads and tenderly cooked grains. Tahini is made from sesame seeds and actively lowers cholesterol. Turmeric supplies the anti-inflammatory phytonutrient curcumin, which has been shown to enhance the efficacy of chemotherapy and radiotherapy in the treatment of cancers.

ROASTED VEGETABLE SALAD WITH CREAMY ORANGE TAHINI DRESSING

PREPARATION: 20 MINUTES, COOKING: 45 MINUTES, SERVES 6

4 medium zucchinis (courgettes), sliced on a slant into 2.5-centimetre (1-inch) pieces

4 large field mushrooms, chopped into large chunks

2 red Spanish onions, peeled and quartered

1 medium eggplant (aubergine), cut into large cubes

6 cloves garlic, unpeeled

1 red capsicum (bell pepper), cut into large chunks

4 sprigs dried oregano

⅓ cup extra virgin olive oil

Dressing

3 tablespoons orange juice (approximately ½ juiced orange)

1 tablespoon lemon juice

2 tablespoons tahini

2 teaspoons shiro (white) miso paste

1½ teaspoons natural maple syrup

1 small garlic clove, crushed

¼ teaspoon ground turmeric

1. Pre-heat oven to 200°C (390°F).

2. Line 2 oven trays (or baking dishes) with parchment (baking) paper and distribute prepared vegetables. Drizzle with oil, gently toss with fingers and place sprigs of oregano over the top, crushing them lightly.

3. Roast vegetables for 45–60 minutes until softened and slightly browned.

4. Meanwhile, place all dressing ingredients in a glass jar with screw-top lid and shake vigorously until blended.

5. Transfer vegetables to a serving platter and place dressing in a small jug to the side. Enjoy salad warm, as a side dish or main course on top of soft polenta or tenderly cooked grains. Dressing can be stored in the fridge for several days.

TIP:

– Variations: To vary dressing, add fresh herbs instead of turmeric and puree in a blender until smooth; substitute soy sauce for miso paste; try pomegranate syrup instead of maple syrup; or blend in some Dijon mustard.

Per serve: energy 918 kJ (219 Cal); protein 6 g; fat 17 g; saturated fat 3 g; cholesterol 0 mg; carbohydrate 8 g; sugars 6 g; fibre 5 g; calcium 60 mg; iron 1.4 mg; sodium 91 mg

This mouth-watering salad has a lovely mustardy and peppery flavour, contrasted by the sweetness of fuyu and the tang of lemon juice. Both rocket and watercress are from the cruciferous family of vegetables with important anti-cancer properties.

WATERCRESS AND ROCKET SALAD WITH FUYU FRUIT AND WALNUTS

PREPARATION: 15 MINUTES, COOKING: 0 MINUTES, SERVES 5

100 g (3½ oz) tender watercress leaves

100 g (3½ oz) rocket (arugula) leaves

2 tablespoons extra virgin olive oil

¼ cup lemon juice (about 1 juiced lemon)

freshly crushed pepper, to taste

1 fuyu fruit, sliced (should be the firm variety)

30 g (1 oz) walnuts

1. Wash leaves well in several batches of water to remove dirt and small snails, which can sometimes hide in watercress.

2. Toss leaves with oil, lemon juice and pepper in a large mixing bowl.

3. Transfer to a serving plate, and sprinkle with fuyu slices and walnuts. Serve as a starter or side salad with a main meal.

TIPS:

- Purchase a 400 g (14 oz) bunch of watercress in order to obtain about 100 g (3½ oz) of tender leaves. Juice the remaining fibrous stalks.

- Fuyu is a firm variety of persimmon. You can cut and slice fuyu as it will hold its texture well. It is deliciously sweet and does not need to be peeled.

- Variation: If fuyu is unavailable, replace with fresh mango or peach.

Per serve: energy 617 kJ (147 Cal); protein 2 g; fat 12 g; saturated fat 1 g; cholesterol 0 mg; carbohydrate 8 g; sugars 8 g; fibre 2 g; calcium 35 mg; iron 1.4 mg; sodium 8 mg

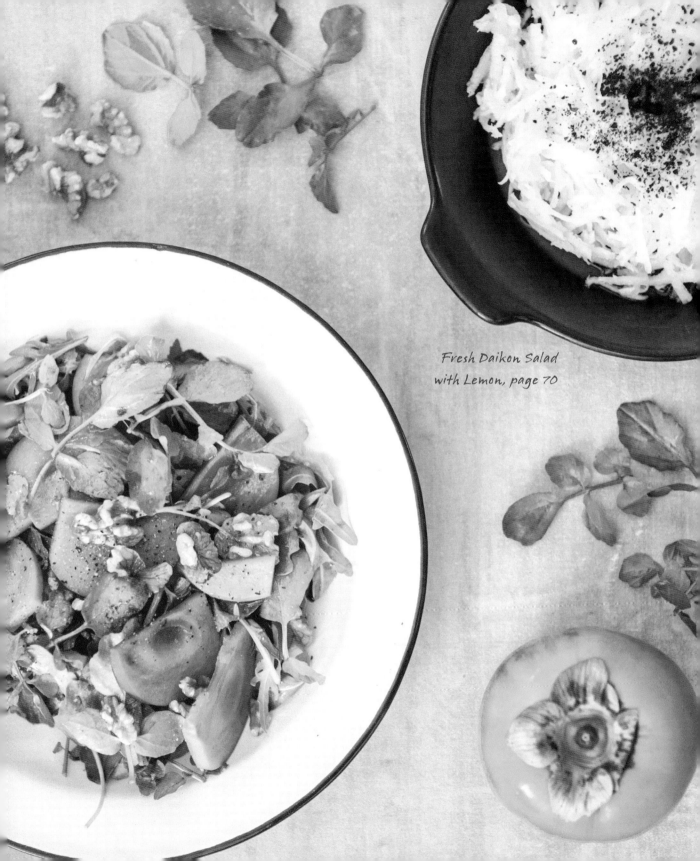

Fresh Daikon Salad
with Lemon, page 70

Daikon radish looks like an oversized white carrot! It's a favourite in Japan, often used in soups and stir-fries or pickled. As it comes from the cruciferous family, daikon has powerful anti-cancer properties, so eat it raw. Grating or chopping it results in the formation of plenty of sulforaphane. (Recipe image, page 69.)

FRESH DAIKON SALAD WITH LEMON

PREPARATION: 5 MINUTES, COOKING: 0 MINUTES, SERVES 4

1 small daikon (white Japanese radish) (about 600 g/21 oz unpeeled)
¼ cup lemon juice (about 1 juiced lemon)
2 tablespoons extra virgin olive oil
pinch sumac, for garnish

1. Peel daikon, then grate into a bowl.
2. Add lemon juice and olive oil, and toss gently to combine. Serve in salad bowl or individual plates with a sprinkle of sumac. Leftovers can be refrigerated and consumed within 2 days. The aroma will intensify as more sulforaphane is formed.

TIPS:

- Buy daikon in Asian grocery stores and at many greengrocers. Daikon comes in various sizes—some daikon can be up to 1 metre (3 feet) long!
- The Japanese generally use the top part of daikon, near the stem (with greenish skin) for salads, reserving the bottom for soups as this tends to be more bitter.
- Be sure to taste daikon first as they can vary in bitterness. Some are positively sweet throughout!
- One teaspoon of seaweed flakes sprinkled on top can supply your daily dose of essential iodine.

Per serve: energy 468 kJ (112 Cal); protein 1 g; fat 10 g; saturated fat 1 g; cholesterol 0 mg; carbohydrate 5 g; sugars 4 g; fibre 2 g; calcium 39 mg; iron 0.4 mg; sodium 35 mg

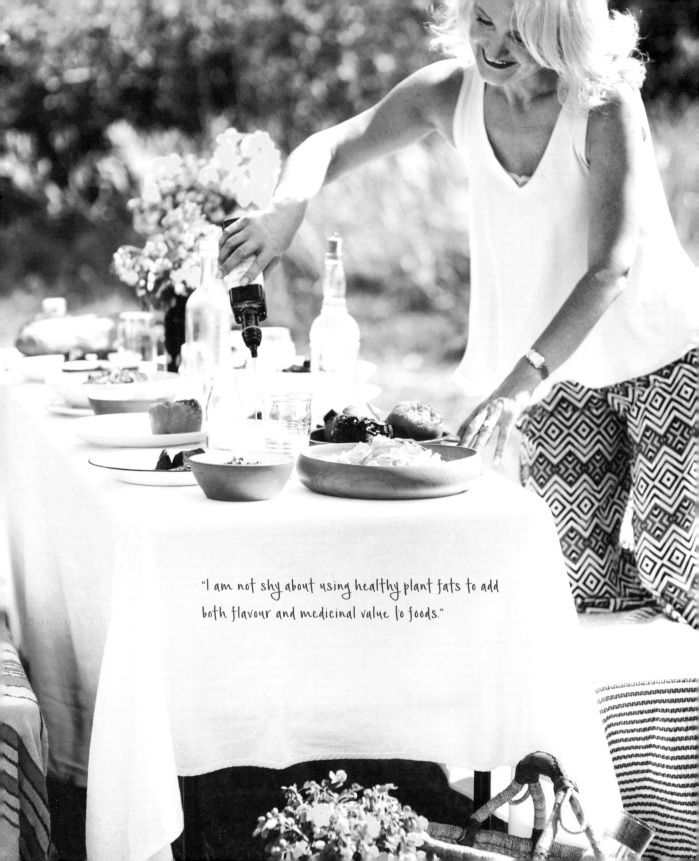

"I am not shy about using healthy plant fats to add both flavour and medicinal value to foods."

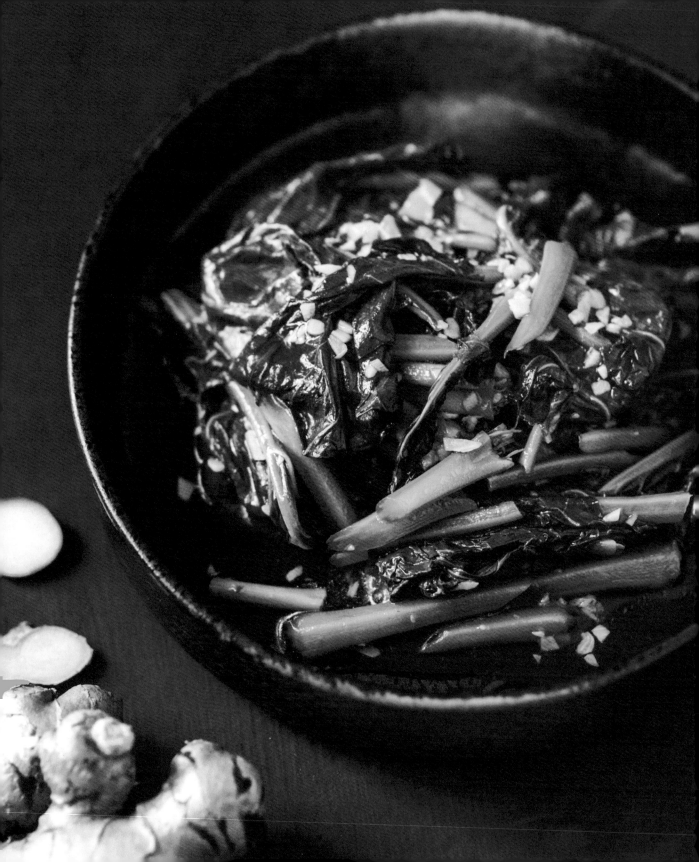

Try this simple yet delicious way to prepare Chinese broccoli, known as gai lan, slightly bitter in taste but considered a crown jewel among Asian greens. It is from the anti-cancer family of cruciferous vegetables. The succulent ginger and garlic sauce masks any bitterness.

BRAISED CHINESE BROCCOLI WITH GINGER AND GARLIC

PREPARATION: 10 MINUTES, COOKING: 10 MINUTES, SERVES 4

1 bunch (520 g/18 oz) gai lan (Chinese
   broccoli)
2 tablespoons extra virgin peanut oil
knob ginger, peeled and sliced thinly
4 cloves garlic, chopped not crushed
2 teaspoons soy sauce
2 teaspoons cornstarch

1. Separate gai lan leaves from the stems. Cut stems into 5-centimetres (2-inch) pieces on the diagonal, pulling off any side shoots and also using these. Wash gai lan well in 3 separate batches of clean water and drain or dry on a kitchen towel.

2. Warm oil in a large wok or saucepan and stir-fry ginger for a minute, followed by garlic for 30 seconds, being careful not to burn it.

3. Stir in soy sauce and ¼ cup of water. Bring to boil, then add broccoli stems and braise, covered, for 2 minutes until they turn bright green.

4. Add leaves and continue cooking with lid on for another minute, until they wilt down.

5. Dissolve cornstarch in ¼ cup of water. Pour over gai lan and mix through. Turn up heat and cook just until the sauce thickens. Transfer greens onto a serving plate and drizzle with sauce. Braised green vegetables make a great side dish to many main meals. Recipe is unsuitable for freezing.

TIPS:

- Always choose gai lan with smaller stalks and brightly coloured leaves as it will be more tender. Peel thick stems using a potato peeler.
- Variation: For extra flavour, drizzle with 1 teaspoon extra virgin sesame oil after cooking.
- Variation: Add 4 sliced Chinese mushroom caps together with the ginger.

Per serve: energy 489 kJ (117 Cal); protein 4 g; fat 10 g; saturated fat 2 g; cholesterol 0 mg; carbohydrate 2 g; sugars 1 g; fibre 4 g; calcium 110 mg; iron 2 mg; sodium 247 mg

WHOLE-GRAINS & HEALTHY CARB SIDES

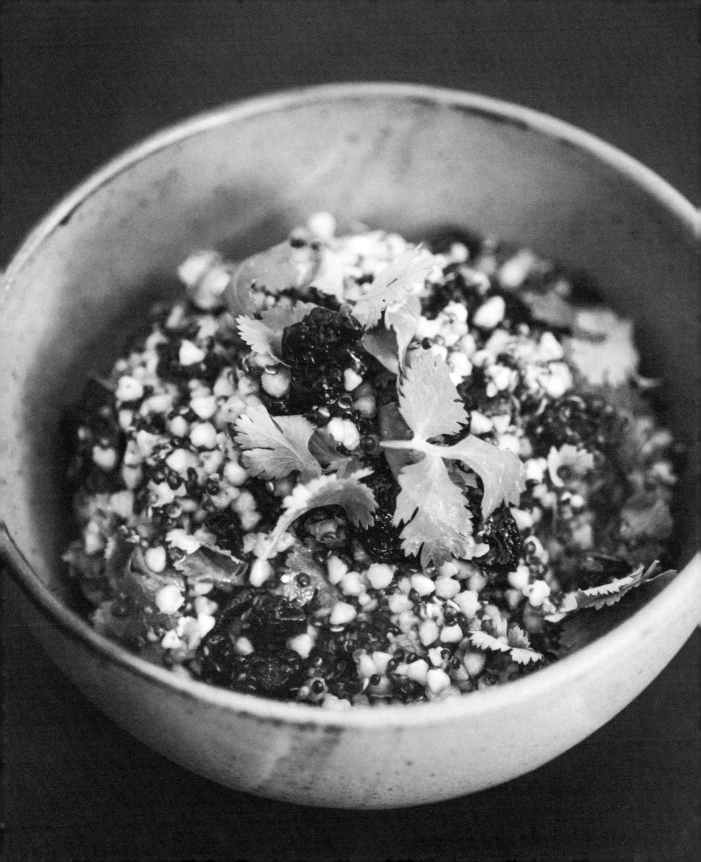

Simple Ways with Whole Grains

There are many ways to cook whole grains, such as by using the absorption method or a pressure cooker. But the easiest is using a rice cooker. Almost any combination of grains works! You can also sneak in some legumes.As various whole grains have slightly different effects in the body, it's important to get a variety over time. To reduce the blood sugar and insulin-raising effects of their carbohydrate, particularly with rice, use the minimal amount of water required, avoid pre-soaking grains (especially rice) and, like pasta, cook only until *al dente*. Slightly undercooked grains produce a smaller rise in blood sugar than mushy ones.

5 flavouring tips for whole grains
- *Stir in some ground turmeric*
- *Sprinkle in a few cardamom pods*
- *Stir in dried sliced shiitake mushrooms*
- *Mix in dried herbs*
- *Crumble in a stock cube*

8 whole-grain combos
Mix and match grains to make up 2 rice-cooker cups and add water in the rice cooker to level 2 (or more if cooking wheat or barley). Any leftovers can be frozen!
- **Brown rice + red rice**
- **Brown rice + red quinoa**
- **Brown rice + wild rice**
- **Brown rice + black-eyed beans**
- **Brown rice + puy lentils + millet**
- **Wheat berries (whole wheat) + barley**
- **Buckwheat + red rice**
- **Millet + white quinoa**

This salad includes a mix of wild and whole-grain rice, and is a great alternative to ordinary rice salads. Whole grains dampen inflammation in the body due to their fibre and phytonutrients. The gorgeous dressing gives it a surprising lift! Adding as little as 1 tablespoon of vinegar (or lemon juice) to a dressing, consumed as part of a meal, can lower blood sugar levels by as much as 30 per cent. (Recipe image, page 79.)

WILD RICE SALAD WITH WASABI DRESSING

PREPARATION: 35 MINUTES, COOKING: 45 MINUTES, SERVES 10

1 cup plain wild rice

1 cup long-grain (basmati) brown rice

2½ cups vegetable stock (made from 1 stock cube dissolved in boiling water)

1 Lebanese cucumber, chopped into 1-centimetre (½-inch) cubes

½ red capsicum (bell pepper), chopped into 1-centimetre (½-inch) cubes

¾ cup sultanas or currants

1 cup coriander (cilantro) leaves, plucked from the stem

1 cob fresh corn, use kernels only

Dressing

75 g (2½ oz) blanched almonds

⅓ cup extra virgin olive oil

1 tablespoon apple cider vinegar

2 cloves garlic, crushed

2 teaspoons wasabi paste

4 tablespoons lemon juice

1. Place both types of rice in a medium saucepan and rinse, then drain well. Add stock, cover and bring to boil. Reduce heat to a low simmer and cook for approximately 45 minutes or until all the liquid is absorbed.

2. Once cooked, remove the lid, allow rice to stand for 5 minutes, then fluff up using a fork.

3. While rice is cooking, toast almonds in a small frypan over medium-high heat until they begin to brown and become aromatic. Remove and chop roughly.

4. Place toasted almonds in a small bowl with remaining dressing ingredients and whisk until well combined.

5. In a large serving bowl, toss all the other salad ingredients together with the rice, then mix through dressing just before serving. Salad can be served warm or cold.

Per serve: energy 1385 kJ (331 Cal); protein 6 g; fat 13 g; saturated fat 2 g; cholesterol 0 mg; carbohydrate 45 g; sugars 13 g; fibre 4 g; calcium 41 mg; iron 1.6 mg; sodium 179 mg

Served cold, this light side dish is perfect for warm weather. It makes a popular appearance at buffets in Hawaii, where the cuisine is heavily influenced by Asian culture. Glass noodles are traditionally made from mung beans and have a low GI. They are also called "cellophane noodles" because of their transparent appearance when prepared. They should not be confused with rice vermicelli, which remains white in colour after cooking.

CHINESE GLASS NOODLES WITH BEAN SHOOTS

PREPARATION: 20 MINUTES, COOKING: 0 MINUTES, SERVES 8

250 g (9 oz) packet dry mung bean
   vermicelli (bean thread or glass noodles)
300 g (10½ oz) bean shoots
¼ cup mirin vinegar
2 tablespoons light soy sauce
1 tablespoon extra virgin sesame oil
1 tablespoon freshly grated ginger
1 clove garlic, crushed
1 small red chilli, finely chopped
1 shallot (scallion), finely chopped
½ bunch coriander (cilantro), chopped
1 small unpeeled cucumber, seeded,
   sliced thinly

1. Place noodles in a large bowl and cover with boiling water. Let stand for 15 minutes until softened, then place in a strainer to drain and cool. Transfer back to bowl and cut coarsely into 7.5-centimetre (3-inch) lengths with kitchen scissors.

2. In a separate bowl, cover bean shoots with boiling water for 3 minutes, then drain and cool.

3. Prepare dressing by combining vinegar, soy sauce, sesame oil, ginger, garlic and chilli in a small glass jar and shaking vigorously.

4. Toss dressing through the noodles, together with bean shoots, shallot, coriander and cucumber slices. For optimal flavour, transfer to a bowl and chill for an hour before serving. Recipe stores well in the fridge for 1-2 days but is unsuitable for freezing.

TIPS:

- Mung bean vermicelli and mirin vinegar are available at Asian grocery stores and some greengrocers. Mirin vinegar has a sweetish flavour and is only mildly acidic.
- De-seed the cucumber by slicing lengthwise and running down the middle with a metal teaspoon to scrape out seeds.
- Serve lime wedges on the side, if you'd like the noodles to taste more tart.

Per serve: energy 186 kJ (44 Cal); protein 2 g; fat 0 g; saturated fat 0 g; cholesterol 0 mg; carbohydrate 7 g; sugars 1 g; fibre 1 g; calcium 15 mg; iron 0.7 mg; sodium 185 mg

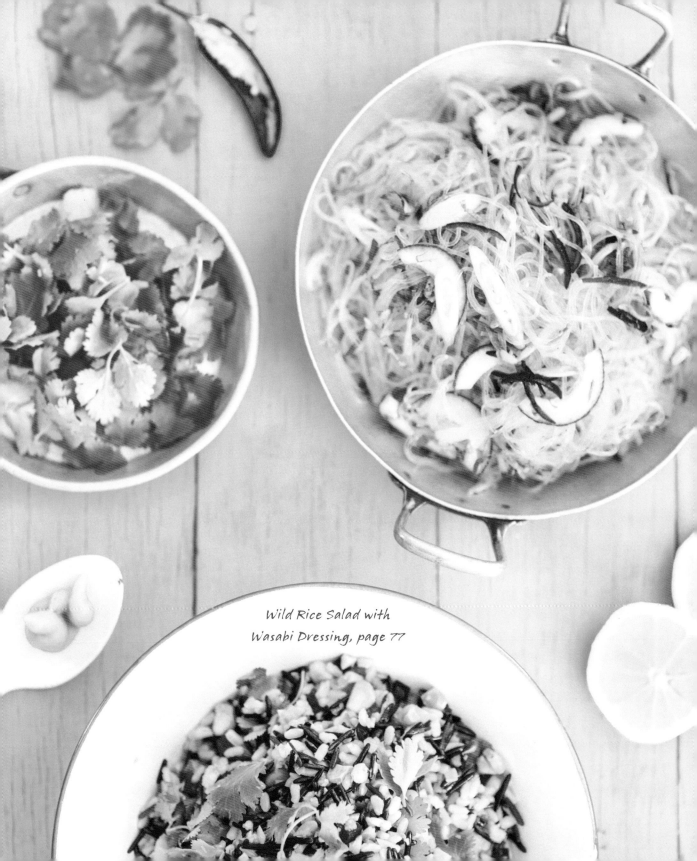

Wild Rice Salad with
Wasabi Dressing, page 77

This recipe takes a little longer to cook, but is easy to make and great for feeding large groups. Eggplant and barley are both rich in viscous fibre, which regulates blood sugar and lowers cholesterol levels. The recipe is also very high in total fibre.

OVEN-BAKED CAPSICUMS FILLED WITH EGGPLANT AND BARLEY

PREPARATION: 25 MINUTES, COOKING: 1 HOUR 55 MINUTES, SERVES 6

1 cup pearled barley
8 tablespoons extra virgin olive oil
2 medium onions, finely chopped
1 large eggplant (aubergine—620 g/22 oz),
    cubed into 1-centimetre (½-inch) pieces
1 tablespoon vegetable stock powder
2 teaspoons sweet Hungarian paprika
freshly ground black pepper
2 tablespoons chopped parsley
6 large red, yellow or orange capsicums
    (bell peppers—approximately 250 g/
    9 oz each)

TIPS:

- *Serve with a Shaved Savoy Cabbage (page 51) or Fresh Daikon Salad (page 70).*
- *For an alternative flavour, substitute smoked paprika for sweet paprika.*
- *Soak barley overnight to reduce cooking time to 30 minutes.*

1. Rinse barley and place in a medium saucepan together with 3 cups of water. Cover with lid and bring to boil, then turn down heat and simmer on low for about 50 minutes until very soft. Drain and put aside.
2. Heat 5 tablespoons of oil in a large, deep frypan and sauté onions for about 15 minutes until very soft and translucent.
3. Mix in eggplant, cover and continue cooking on low heat until eggplant becomes tender and gel-like. This can take up to 30 minutes and the eggplant will releases its juices. Stir occasionally, adding a small amount of water if eggplant starts to stick to pan.
4. Remove pan from heat and add in cooked barley, stock powder, paprika, pepper and parsley, and stir until well combined.
5. Pre-heat oven to 200°C (390°F).
6. Using the tip of a sharp knife, cut around the stem of each capsicum, being careful to create only a small hole, and discard stem. Scrape any seeds inside capsicum with a metal teaspoon and rinse out.
7. Stuff each capsicum with filling and place it on its side in a baking dish. Distribute any remaining filling between the capsicums in the baking dish, so the juice formed can thicken up. Drizzle capsicums with remaining oil and add 1½ cups of water to the base of the dish.
8. Bake for 60 minutes until the skin has completely softened. Test with a knife. Don't worry if the skin turns black: the capsicums will be more tender and you can gently remove their skin prior to serving.
9. When baked, remove capsicums from oven, cover and rest for at least 10 minutes before serving. Serve as a main, drizzling with the juices from the baking dish. Keeps for several days in the fridge.

Per serve: energy 1805 kJ (431 Cal); protein 9 g; fat 26 g; saturated fat 4 g; cholesterol 0 mg; carbohydrate 35 g; sugars 15 g; fibre 13 g; calcium 62 mg; iron 2 mg; sodium 630 mg

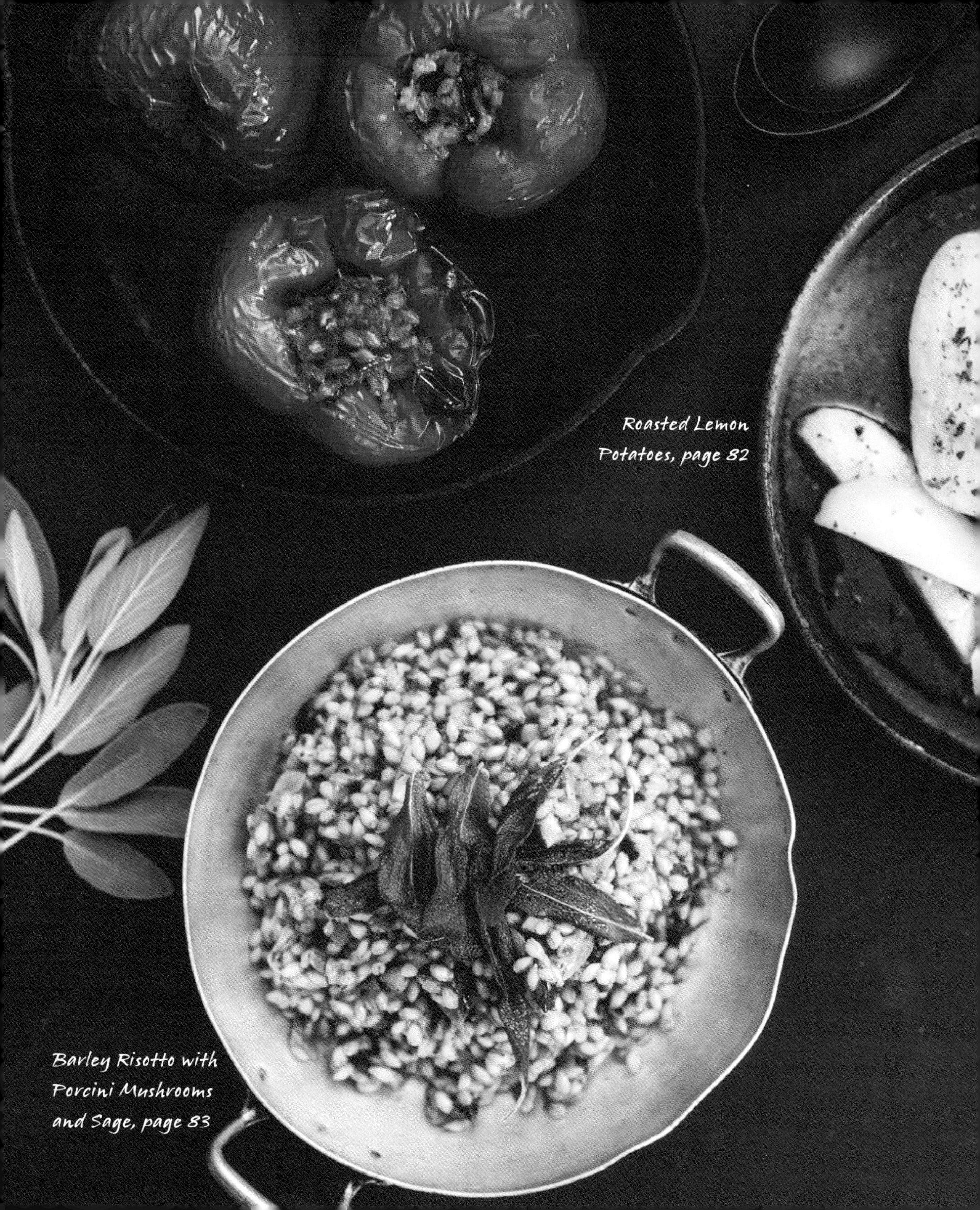

Roasted Lemon
Potatoes, page 82

Barley Risotto with
Porcini Mushrooms
and Sage, page 83

This is the classic Greek way to make the most delicious roast potatoes! The addition of lemon juice adds flavour and reduces the formation of Advanced Glycation Endproducts (AGEs) (page 380), as does the moist cooking method! Rather then being crispy, dry and browned like modern fries, the final result is tender, juicy and infused with flavour. Dutch Cream potatoes are most similar to the yellow-fleshed variety used for this summer-time dish in Greece. (Recipe image, page 81.)

ROASTED LEMON POTATOES

PREPARATION: 10 MINUTES, COOKING: 60 MINUTES, SERVES 8

1.5 kg (about 3 pounds) elongated Dutch Cream potatoes, peeled
⅓ cup lemon juice
¼ cup extra virgin olive oil
2 teaspoons dried oregano
1½ teaspoons salt

1. Pre-heat oven to 200ºC (390ºF).
2. Cut potatoes in half lengthwise, then place face down onto a board and cut each half into 3 lengths.
3. Place cut potatoes into a large baking dish and drizzle with lemon juice and olive oil, then sprinkle with oregano and salt. Using fingers, toss the potatoes until all chunks are evenly coated and spread out in the dish.
4. Drizzle 2½ cups of water around the edges so you don't wash seasoning off the potatoes but that they sit in the liquid.
5. Roast potatoes, uncovered, for 30 minutes. Remove from oven and turn over chunks, then turn down the heat to 180ºC (355ºF) and continue roasting for another 30 minutes. Serve hot or warm.

Per serve: energy 991 kJ (237 Cal); protein 6 g; fat 7 g; saturated fat 1 g; cholesterol 0 mg; carbohydrate 33 g; sugars 3 g; fibre 5 g; calcium 21 mg; iron 1.5 mg; sodium 442 mg

A delicious way to enjoy the chewy texture of barley and lower your blood cholesterol at the same time! Barley is also super low GI. The porcini mushrooms add a lovely earthy colour and flavour. (Recipe image, page 81.)

BARLEY RISOTTO WITH PORCINI MUSHROOMS AND SAGE

PREPARATION: 5 MINUTES, COOKING: 1 HOUR, SERVES 4

10 g (⅓ oz) dried porcini mushrooms
2 tablespoons extra virgin olive oil
1 medium onion, finely chopped
2 cloves garlic, crushed
1 teaspoon dried sage
¼ teaspoon salt, optional
1 cup pearled barley, rinsed and drained
2 cups stock (made with 1 x 10 g/⅓ oz
    chicken-style vegetable stock cube)
freshly ground black pepper

1. Place mushrooms in a small bowl and cover with 1 cup of boiling water. Allow to soften while preparing other ingredients, then drain, reserving the liquid, and coarsely chop them.
2. Heat oil in a casserole dish, and sauté onion and garlic until soft.
3. Stir in sage, mushrooms, salt and barley. Add stock and the reserved mushroom-soaking water and bring to boil.
4. Cover, turn down heat to simmer and cook for approximately 45 minutes, stirring occasionally to check that the liquid hasn't all been absorbed. When cooked, the barley should be *al dente* but moist. If you prefer a softer texture, add an extra ½ cup of boiling water and extend cooking time.
5. Season with black pepper and serve as a side dish in place of white rice or potato, or enjoy as a main meal with salad.

TIP:

- An easy way to cook plain barley is in a rice cooker. Measure 1 rice-cooker cup of barley and place in the cooker, adding water up to level 2, or 2½ if you prefer it softer. Cover with lid and press "Cook." The liquid will bubble up as the barley cooks and the rice cooker will switch itself off when done (in about 45-60 minutes).

Per serve: energy 1104 kJ (264 Cal); protein 6 g; fat 11 g; saturated fat 2 g; cholesterol 0 mg; carbohydrate 32 g; sugars 2 g; fibre 7 g; calcium 22 mg; iron 1.6 mg; sodium 341 mg

"Mujadara" is a simple dish loved across the Middle East. In modern times, you will see it commonly made with white rice but my version uses cracked whole wheat, which is more traditional and better for you. It can be enjoyed hot or cold as the flavour improves with refrigeration. Enjoy it as a whole-grain side dish, or simply on its own with salad or some low-fat yogurt. Lentils have a powerful anti-diabetic effect and help protect against heart disease and cancer.

BULGUR WITH BROWN LENTILS AND CARAMELISED ONION

PREPARATION: 7 MINUTES, COOKING: 45 MINUTES, SERVES 6

⅓ cup extra virgin olive oil

2 large onions, cut in half and thinly sliced

1 cup brown lentils, picked over for stones and rinsed

1 cup coarse bulgur wheat, rinsed, drained using mesh strainer

¾ teaspoon salt

crushed black pepper, to taste

1. Heat oil in a large frypan and sauté onions for approximately 25 minutes until very dark brown. Drain excess oil and reserve.

2. Meanwhile, place lentils in a large saucepan together with ¾ cup of water (just enough to submerge them). Cover and bring to boil, then turn down heat to the lowest setting and steam lentils for about 15 minutes until the water is absorbed, being careful they don't burn.

3. Add half caramelised onions, all bulgur, salt, pepper and 2 cups of water to lentils and mix to combine. Bring to boil, then turn down heat to very low and cook, covered, for approximately 20 minutes until water is absorbed. Remove lid and rest for 10 minutes.

4. Stir through reserved oil and pile onto a serving platter. Garnish with remaining caramelised onions and serve. Refrigerate or freeze leftovers.

TIP:

- If the heat source is too high, you might need to add extra boiling water to prevent lentils from burning.

Per serve: energy 1217 kJ (291 Cal); protein 11 g; fat 14 g; saturated fat 2 g; cholesterol 0 mg; carbohydrate 28 g; sugars 4 g; fibre 10 g; calcium 45 mg; iron 3.1 mg; sodium 299 mg

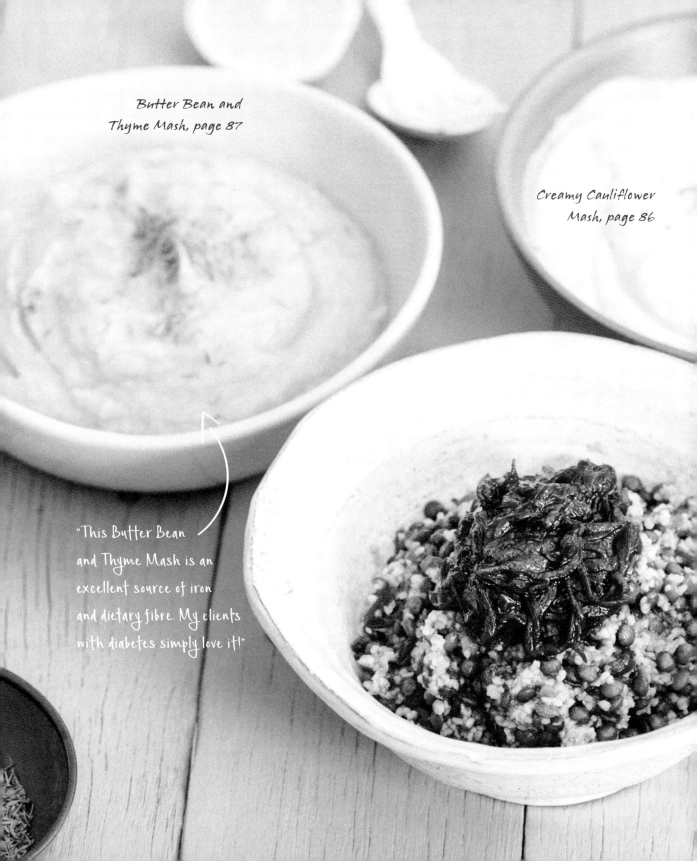

Butter Bean and
Thyme Mash, page 87

Creamy Cauliflower
Mash, page 86

"This Butter Bean
and Thyme Mash is an
excellent source of iron
and dietary fibre. My clients
with diabetes simply love it!"

"Cauliflower is nothing but cabbage with a college education," Mark Twain once said. But it has been getting a lot of attention lately. It's been roasted, fried, pickled and even turned into pizza bases! This delicious, lightly sweet mash is the ideal replacement for mashed potato as it's very low in calories and carbs. It won't cause your blood sugars to soar! (Recipe image, page 85.)

CREAMY CAULIFLOWER MASH

PREPARATION: 8 MINUTES, COOKING: 20 MINUTES, SERVES 6

1 kg (2 lb 3 oz) cauliflower (about
   1 large head)
1 tablespoon extra virgin olive oil
freshly ground pepper
pinch salt, optional

1. Wash cauliflower, then break into large florets and place in a large saucepan with 2 cups of water. Cover with lid and bring to the boil. Cook for 15 minutes until soft. Alternatively, steam the cauliflower.
2. Drain well using a colander, then place cauliflower back into the warm saucepan, with the lid on, to dry for 5 minutes.
3. Transfer cauliflower pieces into a food processor and add oil, pepper and salt, if desired. Blend for a few minutes until a smooth mash is formed. Note: Do not use a high-powered blender or it will become too runny. Serve immediately as a side. Leftovers can be refrigerated for 2 days. Unsuitable for freezing.

TIPS:

- *Cauliflower grows more optimally in cooler weather, so the cooler time of year is the best time to buy them. Select one with compact, firm curds with florets tightly pressed together. A cauliflower with a yellow tinge, brown spots or loose florets indicates over-maturity.*
- *This mash has an even lower GI than sweet potato mash, often used by people with diabetes to replace ordinary potato mash.*

Per serve: energy 278 kJ (66 Cal); protein 3 g; fat 3 g; saturated fat 0 g; cholesterol 0 mg; carbohydrate 3 g; sugars 3 g; fibre 5 g; calcium 30 mg; iron 0.8 mg; sodium 52 mg

Another delicious alternative to mashed potato, these beans (also known as Lima beans) have a buttery flavour and smooth starchy texture. They are particularly good if you have diabetes or insulin resistance to drop the GI of your entire meal and control blood sugar levels. (Recipe image, page 85.)

BUTTER BEAN AND THYME MASH

PREPARATION: 6 MINUTES + OVERNIGHT SOAKING, COOKING: 24 MINUTES INCLUDING PRESSURE COOKER, SERVES 8

500 g (17½ oz) butter beans (Lima beans), soaked overnight in plenty of water
1 tablespoon extra virgin olive oil
1 teaspoon dried thyme
1 teaspoon salt

1. Rinse and drain beans. Place beans in the base of a pressure cooker and cover with water. Secure lid and bring to high pressure then turn down heat to very low and cook under pressure for 3 minutes. Allow for natural pressure release (15 minutes) before opening lid. (Alternatively, place beans in a pot with at least 6 cups of water. Cover and bring to boil. Cook for 45–60 minutes until beans are tender, being sure to add extra boiling water, if required, so beans don't burn). Remove beans from the pressure cooker and strain in a colander.

2. Transfer beans to a food processor and add remaining ingredients and process until smooth and creamy. Note: Do not use a high-powered blender or mash will become runny. Serve immediately or chill for later use. The mash will store well in the fridge in an airtight container for several days. You can re-heat it in the microwave and stir through a small amount of boiling water, or reserved cooking water, if it has gone too thick. This mash will also soften when re-heated.

TIPS:

- For an instant version: Use 2 x 400 g (14 oz) cans of butter beans. Rinse, drain, then add remaining ingredients and 4 tablespoons of hot water from the kettle and puree until smooth.
- Use fresh herbs: 1 teaspoon dry is equal to 1 tablespoon fresh.
- Variation: Warm olive oil first and add finely chopped garlic and fresh rosemary before stirring into mash. You can also add some lemon juice.

Per serve: energy 1072 kJ (256 Cal); fat 15 g; protein 20 g; saturated fat 2 g; cholesterol 0 mg; carbohydrate 8 g; sugars 4 g; fibre 13 g; calcium 116 mg; iron 6.1 mg; sodium 290 mg

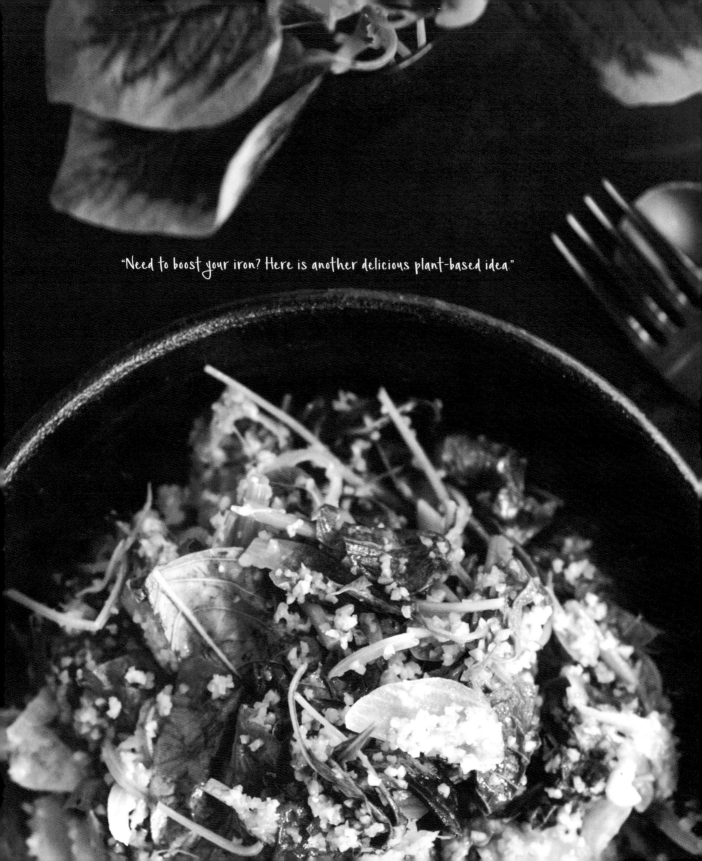
"Need to boost your iron? Here is another delicious plant-based idea."

This tangy dish, with a little heat, is eaten as a simple Middle Eastern meal or a side dish. It uses amaranth leaves, also known as en choy or Chinese spinach, easily identified by their interesting dark red and bright green colour. Amaranth has a flavour and texture similar to English spinach but it is related to beetroot. The red colour comes from antioxidants called betalains, which might colour the bulgur slightly pink during cooking. Green amaranth (called "Vlita") is a popular dish in Greece, served simply boiled and dressed with olive oil and lemon juice.

EXOTIC BULGUR WHEAT WITH AMARANTH LEAVES

PREPARATION: 15 MINUTES, COOKING: 25 MINUTES, SERVES 4

½ cup coarse bulgur wheat

1 large bunch amaranth

2 tablespoons extra virgin olive oil

1 medium brown onion, finely sliced

3 cloves garlic, sliced

1 teaspoon ground cumin

1 teaspoon Arabic seven spices

2 small fresh red chilli, finely chopped

1 lemon, quartered

1. Cover bulgur with water and allow it to hydrate for 5 minutes while preparing other ingredients. Drain using a mesh strainer.

2. Trim base from amaranth stalks and wash well, using 3 changes of water. Drain and cut into 5-centimetre (2-inch) pieces, then put aside. Note: The stalks will become tender when cooked.

3. Warm oil in a large saucepan and sauté onion slices on medium heat for approximately 7 minutes until soft. Add garlic and cook for a further minute, then stir in spices and bulgur until well combined.

4. Add amaranth pieces and drizzle with ½ cup of water. Cover with lid to build up steam, then turn down heat to very low and cook for approximately 10 minutes until the amaranth has wilted, stirring several times. If the mixture becomes too dry, add a small amount of water to prevent the bulgur from sticking to the base. The mixture should be moist but not watery or mushy.

5. Remove from heat and mix in chilli. Rest for a few minutes before serving. Serve in a bowl with lemon wedges. Recipe is unsuitable for freezing.

TIPS:

- Be sure to purchase coarse bulgur, rather than the fine variety used for tabbouleh.

- Variation: Substitute spinach or silverbeet (chard) for the amaranth.

Per serve: energy 725 kJ (173 Cal); protein 4 g; fat 10 g; saturated fat 1 g; cholesterol 0 mg; carbohydrate 13 g; sugars 3 g; fibre 9 g; calcium 171 mg; iron 8 mg; sodium 43 mg

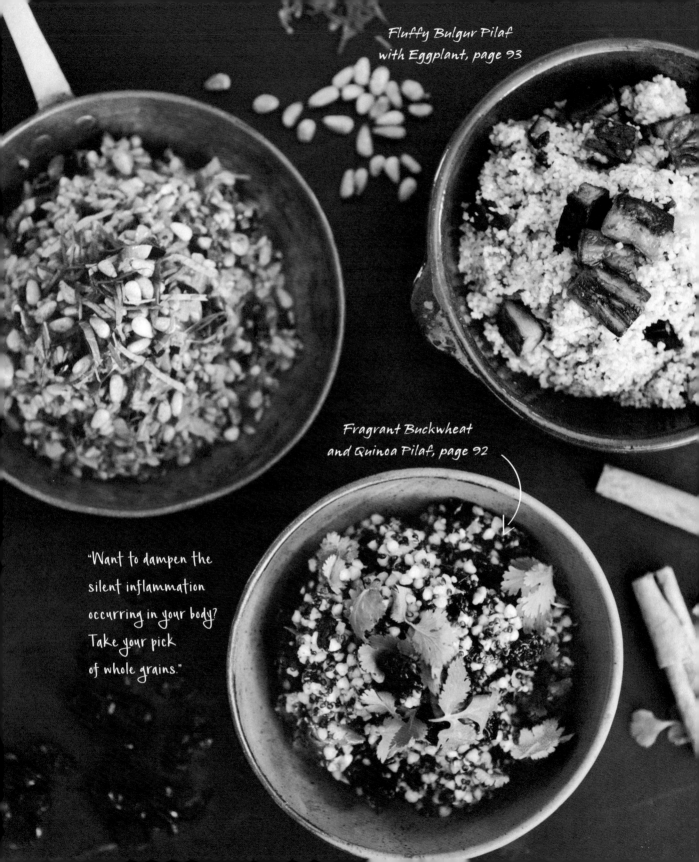

Fluffy Bulgur Pilaf
with Eggplant, page 93

Fragrant Buckwheat
and Quinoa Pilaf, page 92

"Want to dampen the
silent inflammation
occurring in your body?
Take your pick
of whole grains."

Freekeh is wheat that has been picked green, lightly roasted and cracked. It is low GI (43), high in fibre and bursting with nutrients for better bowel and heart health. This recipe shows how to dress it up Arabic style!

FREEKEH WITH AROMATIC SPICES AND PINE NUTS

PREPARATION: 10 MINUTES, COOKING: 40 MINUTES, SERVES 8

1½ cups cracked freekeh, washed and
    well drained
½ teaspoon salt
4 tablespoons extra virgin olive oil
1 onion, finely sliced
1 medium red capsicum (bell pepper),
    finely diced
4 cloves garlic, crushed
pinch cayenne pepper
1 teaspoon Arabic seven spices
1 teaspoon dried mint
¼ cup pine nuts, dry toasted
1 tablespoon finely chopped parsley

1. Place freekeh with 2½ cups of water and salt in a medium saucepan, cover and bring to boil, then cook for 1 minute. Reduce heat to simmer and continue cooking for about 20 minutes until the water is absorbed and freekeh is just cooked. Remove lid to allow excess steam to escape.
2. Meanwhile, heat oil in a frypan, and sauté onion and capsicum for about 10 minutes until very soft, adding garlic at the end of the cooking time so it doesn't burn. Remove from heat and stir in spices and mint.
3. Mix sautéed vegetables through the cooked freekeh until well combined. Transfer to a serving bowl, and sprinkle with pine nuts and parsley. Serve warm or refrigerate for later use. Recipe will store in the fridge for up to 5 days.

TIPS:
- Buy freekeh from a health-food store or large supermarket.
- For extra flavour, sprinkle the dish with a little crumbled feta before serving.

Per serve: energy 1101 kJ (263 Cal); protein 7 g; fat 14 g; saturated fat 2 g; cholesterol 0 mg; carbohydrate 24 g; sugars 3 g; fibre 6 g; calcium 24 mg; iron 1.7 mg; sodium 148 mg

A gluten-free, whole-grain side dish to replace potato, white rice or pasta at main meals. Cinnamon, fenugreek, coriander and ginger are some of the most effective spices to help lower blood sugar levels in people with diabetes. (Recipe image, page 90).

FRAGRANT BUCKWHEAT AND QUINOA PILAF

PREPARATION: 15 MINUTES, COOKING: 25 MINUTES, SERVES 6

2 tablespoons extra virgin olive oil
2 teaspoons fresh ginger, grated
4 cardamom pods, bruised
2 small cinnamon sticks, snapped in two
2 teaspoons black mustard seeds
1 teaspoon ground cumin
1 teaspoon fenugreek seeds
½ cup buckwheat
½ cup red quinoa
2 cups vegetable stock
¼ cup lemon juice (about 1 juiced lemon)
½ cup dried cranberries
1 cup loosely packed fresh coriander
    (cilantro) leaves

1. Heat oil in a large frypan. Add ginger, cardamom, cinnamon, mustard seeds, cumin and fenugreek seeds, and cook over medium heat for 1 minute or until aromatic. Ensure heat is not too high to prevent burning the spices.
2. Add buckwheat and quinoa, and stir to coat with spice mixture.
3. Add stock, cover and bring to boil. Reduce heat slightly and simmer for approximately 20 minutes or until the liquid is absorbed, stirring occasionally.
4. Stir in lemon juice and cook, uncovered, for a few more minutes until most of the moisture is absorbed. Fold in cranberries and coriander, and transfer to a serving dish. Enjoy warm or refrigerate for later use.

TIPS:

- Quinoa comes in a variety of colours, including white, red and black. The darker colours have more intense flavours.
- Bruise cardamom pods with a mortar and pestle.
- Variation: Fold through roasted vegetables, such as capsicum (bell pepper), zucchini (courgette) and eggplant (aubergine) prior to serving.

Per serve: energy 899 kJ (214 Cal); protein 5 g; fat 8 g; saturated fat 1 g; cholesterol 0 mg; carbohydrate 29 g; sugars 10 g; fibre 4 g; calcium 45 mg; iron 4 mg; sodium 329 mg

A lovely pilaf using an easy whole grain and the allure of Arabic seven spices, also known as "baharat." Baharat is a blend of aromatic spices, including paprika, cumin, coriander, nutmeg, cloves, cinnamon and black pepper. Spices can lift foods from ordinary to extraordinary, and pack a punch with phytonutrients. Enjoy this dish hot or cold. (Recipe image, page 90.)

FLUFFY BULGUR PILAF WITH EGGPLANT

PREPARATION: 10 MINUTES, COOKING: 35 MINUTES, SERVES 6

250 g (9 oz) coarse bulgur wheat
6 tablespoons extra virgin olive oil
1 small onion, finely chopped
1 large ripe tomato, finely chopped
1 teaspoon tomato paste
1 teaspoon brown sugar
1 teaspoon Arabic seven spices
½ teaspoon salt, optional
freshly crushed pepper, to taste
1 medium eggplant (aubergine), cut into
    2.5-centimetre (1-inch) cubes

1. Rinse bulgur with running water using a fine-mesh strainer. Drain while preparing other ingredients.
2. Heat 3 tablespoons of oil in a deep pot and sauté onion until very soft.
3. Stir in bulgur, chopped tomatoes, tomato paste, sugar and seasonings, and ½ cup of water. Cover with lid and turn down heat to very low, then cook for 15 minutes, stirring occasionally to ensure pilaf doesn't stick to bottom of pan. If mixture appears too dry, add a little more water.
4. Remove from stove and rest pilaf, covered, for 10 minutes until the grain is tender.
5. Meanwhile, heat remainder of oil in a large pan and fry eggplant cubes for 10 minutes until golden. Eggplant will release its juices as it softens.
6. Fold fried eggplant through the pilaf and serve immediately or refrigerate for later use.

TIP:

- Buy coarse bulgur wheat from Middle Eastern grocery stores. It is different to the fine bulgur used to make tabbouleh, which would go soggy in this recipe.

Per serve: energy 1338 kJ (320 Cal); protein 5 g; fat 19 g; saturated fat 3 g; cholesterol 0 mg; carbohydrate 27 g; sugars 4 g; fibre 10 g; calcium 34 mg; iron 1.3 mg; sodium 19 mg

The secret to potato salad is to cook the potatoes the day before. Cooked and cooled potatoes have a lower GI, meaning they will raise your blood sugar less than potatoes served steaming hot or mashed. Instead of mayonnaise, take inspiration from the Greeks and dress your salad simply with lemon juice and olive oil. This will further bring down the GI, and add flavour and antioxidants to your table. Greek potato salad also includes raw onions (a prebiotic) and parsley, which provide additional antioxidant and anti-inflammatory benefits.

GREEK POTATO SALAD

PREPARATION: 15 MINUTES, COOKING: 35 MINUTES, SERVES 6

1.2 kg (2½ lb) potatoes (about 6), scrubbed well
1 small onion, sliced thinly
½ cup loosely packed chopped parsley
¼ cup extra virgin olive oil
¼ cup lemon juice (about 1 juiced lemon)
1 teaspoon salt

1. Place potatoes in a large saucepan and cover with cold water. Bring to boil and cook for about 20 minutes until tender, testing with a fork. Drain and allow potatoes to cool in the saucepan with the lid on.
2. Peel potatoes, cut into chunks, and place together with onion and parsley in a salad bowl. Add remaining ingredients and toss gently until the flavours combine. Serve immediately or refrigerate and enjoy over several days.

TIPS:

- You can use Carisma, Nicola, Nadine or Kipfler potatoes (about 12 Kipflers, depending on size). Despite their odd finger-like shape, Kipfler potatoes are easy to peel once cooked and don't fall apart even if overcooked. Carisma and Nicola potatoes are low-GI varieties.
- Variation: Vinegar can be substituted for lemon juice.

Per serve: energy 911 kJ (218 Cal); protein 5 g; fat 10 g; saturated fat 2 g; cholesterol 0 mg; carbohydrate 25 g; sugars 3 g; fibre 4 g; calcium 23 mg; iron 1.3 mg; sodium 394 mg

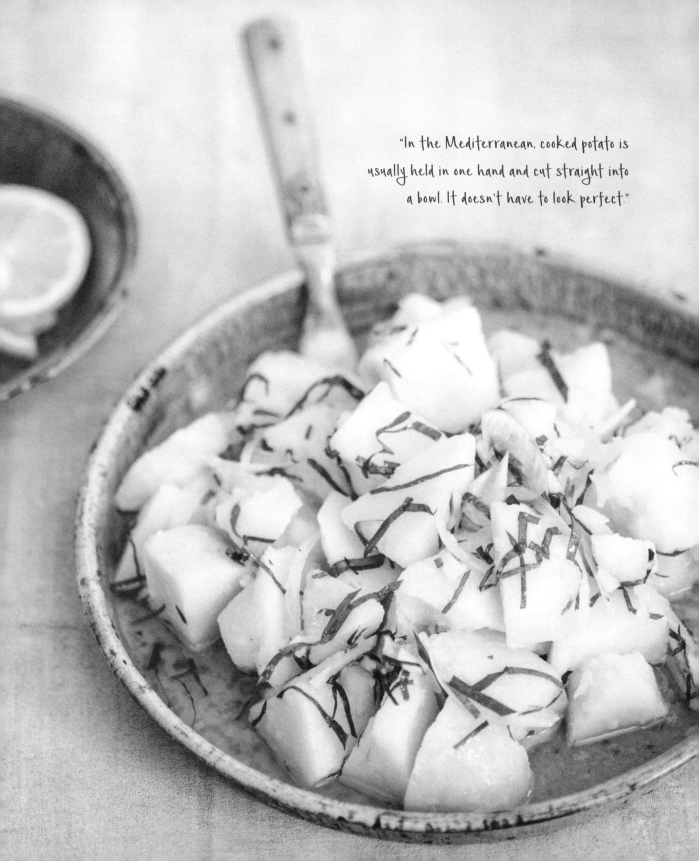

"In the Mediterranean, cooked potato is usually held in one hand and cut straight into a bowl. It doesn't have to look perfect."

LIGHTER PLATES

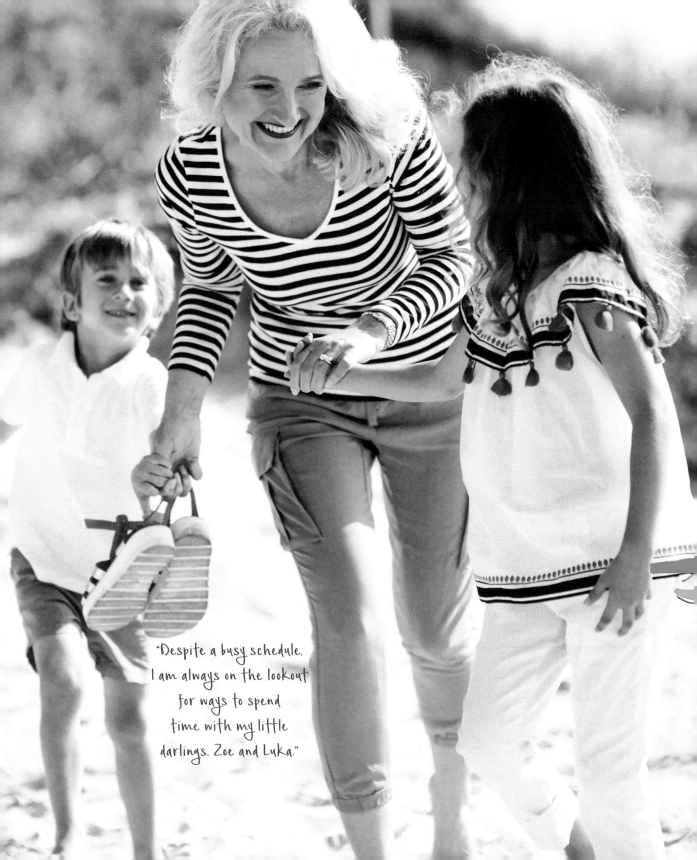

"Despite a busy schedule, I am always on the lookout for ways to spend time with my little darlings, Zoe and Luka."

A delicious fresh curry you can enjoy with my Raw Yellow Rice. The sauce features fresh herbs and spices with their myriad of healing phytonutrients. Get ready for some serious crunch!

RAW THAI GREEN CURRY

PREPARATION: 30 MINUTES + 15 MINUTES MARINATING, COOKING: O MINUTES, SERVES 6

Sauce

1 bunch coriander (cilantro) + 6 sprigs for
   garnish
2 sticks lemongrass (white part only),
   coarsely chopped
2.5-centimetre (1-inch) piece ginger, peeled
3 cloves garlic
1 spring onion bulb
1 birdseye chilli, deseeded
½ teaspoon salt
6 tablespoons lime juice (about 2 juiced
   limes)
¼ cup almond meal
2 teaspoons raw agave syrup
1½ cups coconut milk

Vegetables

½ large carrot, finely julienned
8 baby sweetcorn, cut into 2.5-centimetre
   (1-inch) pieces
10 button mushrooms, wiped, sliced
80 g (3 oz) green beans, cut into
   2.5-centimetre (1-inch) pieces
2 kaffir lime leaves, finely shredded

1. Place all ingredients for curry sauce into a high-powered blender and process for 1 minute until smooth.
2. Combine vegetables in a medium bowl and mix through approximately 1 cup of the curry sauce. Place vegetables aside for at least 15 minutes to marinate.
3. Divide marinated vegetables between 6 serves. Plate up each serve alongside some Raw Yellow Rice (page 100) or Kelp Noodles (page 101). Drizzle with remaining sauce and garnish with kaffir lime and a sprig of coriander.

TIP:

*- Cherry tomatoes can be substituted for carrots. Simply slice in half, allowing
   2 tomatoes per serve.*

Per serve: energy 712 kJ (170 Cal); protein 5 g; fat 13 g; saturated fat 9 g; cholesterol 0 mg; carbohydrate 6 g; sugars 5 g; fibre 4 g; calcium 55 mg; iron 3 mg; sodium 310 mg

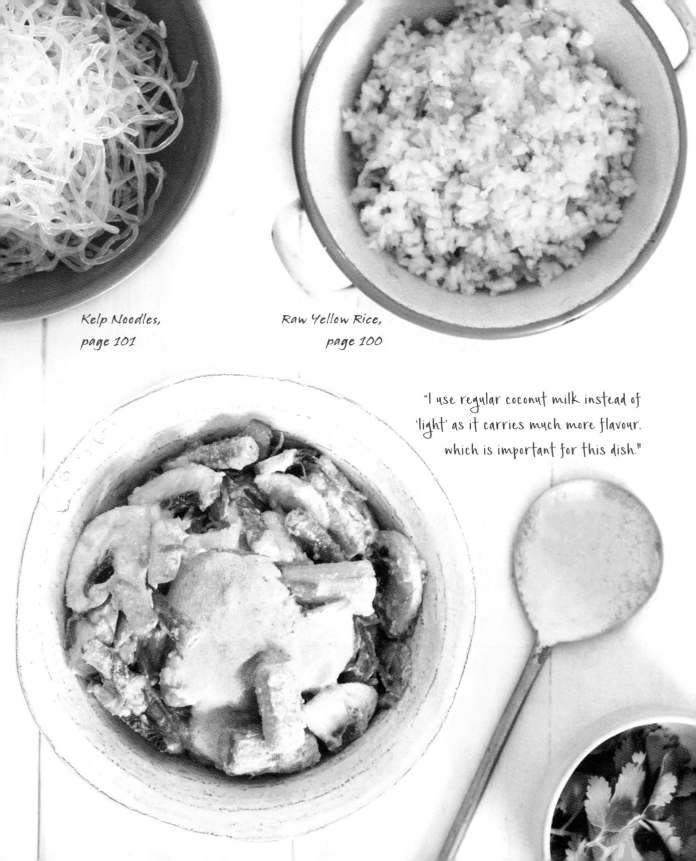

Kelp Noodles,
page 101

Raw Yellow Rice,
page 100

"I use regular coconut milk instead of
'light' as it carries much more flavour,
which is important for this dish."

This sweetish "raw rice" goes well with Raw Thai Green Curry (page 98). Rutabaga (also know as swede) is an inexpensive and underappreciated root vegetable from the cruciferous family. In addition to being very low in calories, it can boost your internal detox mechanisms to reduce cancer risk, including bladder cancer, especially if consumed raw. (Recipe image, page 99.)

RAW YELLOW RICE

PREPARATION: 7 MINUTES, COOKING: 0 MINUTES, SERVES 6

2 large rutabaga (swedes)
(approximately 750 g/26½ oz total),
peeled and roughly chopped
1 tablespoon extra virgin olive oil
1 tablespoon finely chopped coriander
(cilantro)
¼ teaspoon salt

1. Place rutabaga in a food processor and pulse for 15-30 seconds until very fine and texture resembles rice.
2. Transfer to a large bowl and mix through remaining ingredients. Serve immediately as a side dish in place of common carbohydrate foods such as rice and pasta. Recipe stores well in the fridge for 2 days but is unsuitable for freezing.

TIPS:

- Turnips (also from the cruciferous family) look similar to swedes on the outside, with purplish skin. But turnips have a white smooth flesh and can taste spicy, like radish, whereas swedes, which originate from Sweden, taste sweeter and milder and have a cream-coloured flesh.
- Variation: You can also make raw rice from fresh cauliflower.
- Enjoy raw yellow rice with any plant-based "raw chilli" or "raw bolognaise" and other raw toppings and sauces.

Per serve: energy 230 kJ (55 Cal); protein 1 g; fat 3 g; saturated fat 0 g; cholesterol 0 mg; carbohydrate 5 g; sugars 4 g; fibre 3 g; calcium 28 mg; iron 0.4 mg; sodium 111 mg

Raw foodists use kelp noodles as they require no cooking. Kelp noodles are made from edible brown seaweed, so are rich in iodine. They're also fat-free, gluten-free, low-carb and provide only 6 calories per serve! With a neutral taste and slightly crunchy texture that softens with soaking, they mop up flavours extremely well, so the longer you leave them marinating in a sauce, the better they'll taste! (Recipe image, page 99.)

KELP NOODLES

PREPARATION: 5 MINUTES, COOKING: 0 MINUTES, SERVES 4

454 g (16 oz) packet kelp noodles
¼ cup lemon juice (about 1 juiced lemon)

1. Loosen and rinse kelp noodles to remove the salty liquid from package.
2. Using kitchen scissors, cut noodles roughly into 7.5-centimetre (3-inch) lengths if you intend to use them for broths, salads and stir-fries or leave whole for long "spaghetti."
3. Place in a medium bowl, cover with lemon juice and water, and allow to soak for at least 10 minutes to soften noodles.
4. Rinse and drain noodles. They are now ready to use as a healthy side dish. Kelp noodles are unsuitable for freezing.

TIPS:

- Purchase kelp noodles from health-food stores, specialty food stores or online.
- Kelp noodles will store in your pantry for 6 months, if unopened.
- Top with tomato-based sauces, creamy nut/seed sauces or pesto and marinate for at least 4 hours (the best is 24-48 hours).
- Limit your intake of iodine-rich seaweed products to 3-4 serves per week to ensure you don't take in too much iodine.

Per serve: energy 25 kJ (6 Cal); protein 0 g; fat 0 g; saturated fat 0 g; cholesterol 0 mg; carbohydrate 1 g; sugars 0 g; fibre 1 g; calcium 150 mg; iron 0.7 mg; sodium 35 mg

Black beans and rice are a classic Mexican combination and these gluten-free burgers bring these traditional flavours together for the whole family to enjoy! Diets with black beans improve biomarkers of colonic health and reduce inflammation during colitis. Legumes, in general, are crucially important to help prevent inflammatory bowel disease. Serve burgers on lightly toasted buns topped with the fresh salsa, or form into falafel-sized balls for wraps.

BLACK BEAN BURGERS WITH FRESH SALSA

PREPARATION: 20 MINUTES, COOKING: 28 MINUTES, SERVES 8

2 tablespoons chia seeds
5 tablespoons extra virgin olive oil
1 medium onion, finely chopped
1 clove garlic, crushed
400 g (14 oz) soft cooked black beans
1½ cups cooked medium-grain brown rice
⅓ cup brown rice flour
1½ teaspoons cumin
3 tablespoons fresh coriander (cilantro)
1 teaspoon salt
pepper to taste

Salsa
1 large, firm tomato, finely diced
½ medium Lebanese cucumber, peeled and
  finely diced
¼ red Spanish onion, peeled and finely diced
½ medium avocado, peeled and finely diced
2 tablespoons chopped fresh coriander
  (cilantro)
½ small red chilli, deseeded, finely chopped
2 tablespoons lemon juice
1 tablespoon extra virgin olive oil

1. Place chia seeds in a small bowl and stir in 6 tablespoons of water to make "chia egg." Allow to swell and thicken for 15–30 minutes, stirring frequently to prevent clumps.
2. Heat 1 tablespoon of oil in a large frypan. Sauté onion until translucent. Add garlic and stir for another 30 seconds. Set aside.
3. Meanwhile, prepare salsa by combining all ingredients. Set aside. Makes approximately 2 cups.
4. Mash beans coarsely in a medium bowl with a fork. Add rice, rice flour, cumin, coriander, salt, pepper, "chia egg" and onion mixture. Stir until well combined, then divide mixture into 8. Using moistened hands, form 8 round balls, then flatten into burgers.
5. Heat remaining oil in the frypan and cook burgers in 2 batches on medium-high for approximately 3 minutes on each side, or until golden. Serve immediately with burger buns of your choice or freeze burgers for up to 3 months and reheat in oven.

Per serve: energy 1206 kJ (288 Cal); protein 8 g; fat 18 g; saturated fat 3 g; cholesterol 0 mg; carbohydrate 21 g; sugars 3 g; fibre 8 g; calcium 47 mg; iron 2.2 mg; sodium 298 mg

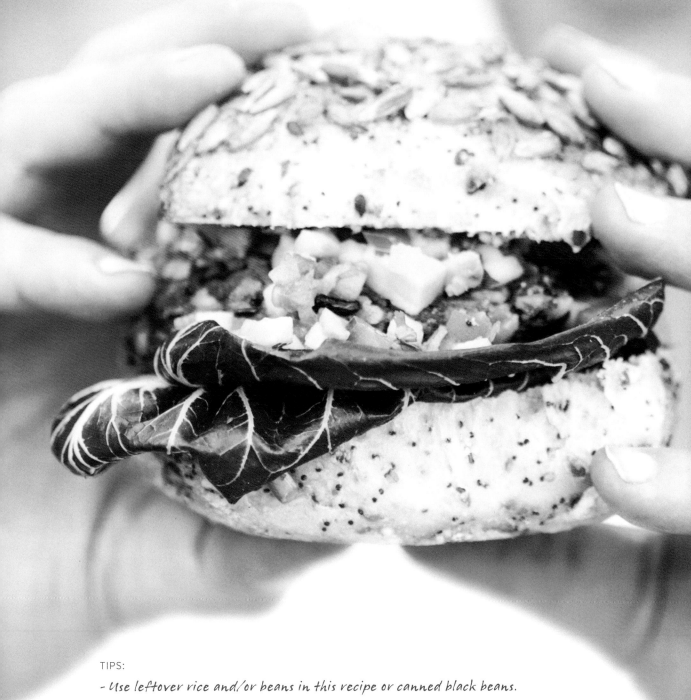

TIPS:

- Use leftover rice and/or beans in this recipe or canned black beans. Home-cooked beans are usually softer and taste better!
- Timings to cook dry black beans using a pressure cooker: 5 minutes if pre-soaked or 20 minutes if unsoaked, allowing for natural pressure release.
- Variation: Swap brown rice flour with lupin flour or besan (chickpea) flour.

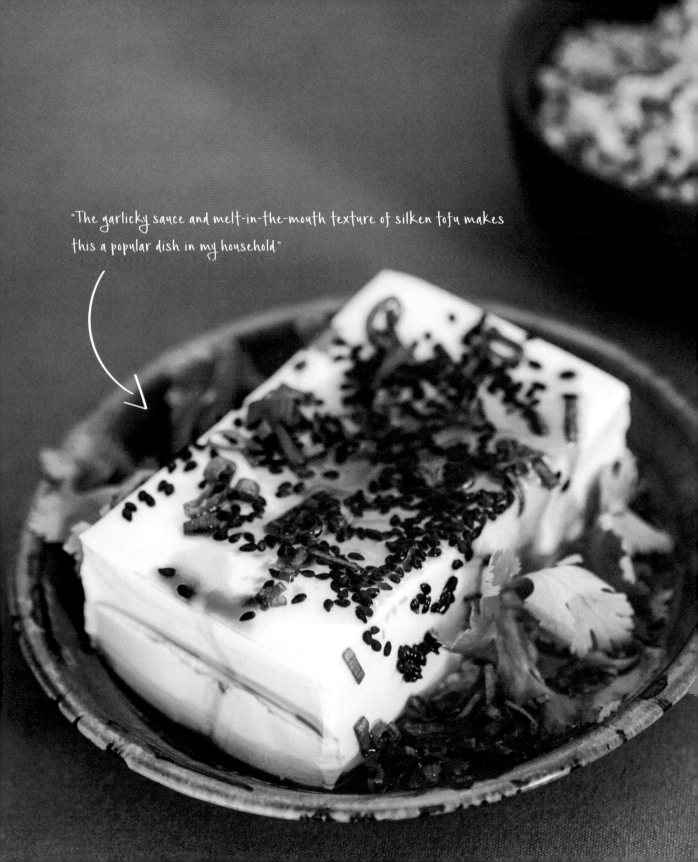

"The garlicky sauce and melt-in-the-mouth texture of silken tofu makes this a popular dish in my household."

An easy and delicious idea to enjoy more tofu, which provides plant protein. Tofu is made from soybeans and contains a high level of isoflavones. Frequent use of tofu is associated with a reduced risk of breast and prostate cancers, as well as other chronic diseases. The most recent research also suggests breast cancer survivors who consume soy foods regularly have a lower risk of cancer recurrence and live longer!

STEAMED SILKEN TOFU WITH GARLICKY SOY SAUCE

PREPARATION: 5 MINUTES, COOKING: 10 MINUTES, SERVES 4

600 g (21 oz) silken firm tofu in one block
¼ cup extra virgin olive oil
8 cloves garlic, chopped (not crushed)
1 tablespoon light soy sauce
1 shallot (scallion), green part only,
    finely chopped
few sprigs coriander (cilantro)
1 teaspoon black sesame seeds

1. Invert tofu block into a steamer or large plate with a lip and place in a steamer for 7 minutes.
2. Meanwhile, warm oil gently and lightly sauté garlic until golden, being careful not to burn it. Stir in soy sauce.
3. Invert tofu block onto a serving plate with a lip (or drain the steaming plate of any surplus water if you wish to serve on that), being careful to keep it in one piece.
4. Drizzle with garlicky soy sauce and sprinkle with shallot, coriander and sesame seeds. Serve hot with a large spoon for helpings. Tofu goes well with steamed multigrain rice and Asian greens.

TIP:
- If you need to avoid added salt, omit soy sauce and add 1 red chilli, chopped.

Per serve: energy 1390 kJ (332 Cal); protein 19 g; fat 26 g; saturated fat 4 g; carbohydrate 1 g; sugars 0 g; fibre 12 g; cholesterol 0 mg; calcium 486 mg; iron 4.8 mg; sodium 237 mg

A lovely Greek recipe, known as "ara-ka", highlighting the central role of tenderly cooked vegetables as the main meal in traditional Mediterranean diets. Don't worry if the onions make you cry! Strong, pungent onions have a higher antioxidant activity. Their potency can be up to seven times greater than that of mild onions. Serve stew with whole-grain rice or bread and a dollop of low-fat Greek-style yogurt or feta cheese.

GREEK-STYLE PEA STEW WITH MINT

PREPARATION: 10 MINUTES, COOKING: 27 MINUTES INCLUDING PRESSURE COOKER, SERVES 6

6 tablespoons extra virgin olive oil

2 medium onions, chopped

2 tablespoons ground paprika

140 g (5 oz) tomato paste

1 kg (2 pounds) packet frozen peas

1 medium carrot, finely chopped

3 cloves garlic, crushed

1 teaspoon salt

leaves stripped from 1 bunch fresh mint
(20 g/¾ oz)

1. Heat oil in the base of a pressure cooker and sauté onions for about 5 minutes until softened, then stir in paprika and tomato paste.
2. Add peas, carrot, garlic, salt, mint and 1½ cups of water, and stir well. Cover securely with the pressure cooker lid and heat until the cooker reaches full pressure.
3. Turn down heat to very low and cook for 2 minutes on high pressure. Remove from stove and allow for natural pressure release before opening lid. Serve hot or cold.

TIPS:

- *Variation: Swap mint with fresh dill.*
- *To cook conventionally, use a large saucepan and increase water to 2 cups. When contents come to boil, turn down heat and simmer, covered, for about 50 minutes or until peas are very tender.*
- *Use Homemade Soy Yogurt (page 294) or Almond Cream Cheese in "feta" form (see page 224) for dairy-free accompaniments.*

Per serve: energy 1338 kJ (320 Cal); protein 12 g; fat 19 g; saturated fat 3 g; cholesterol 0 mg; carbohydrate 17 g; sugars 9 g; fibre 16 g; calcium 81 mg; iron 4 mg; sodium 545 mg

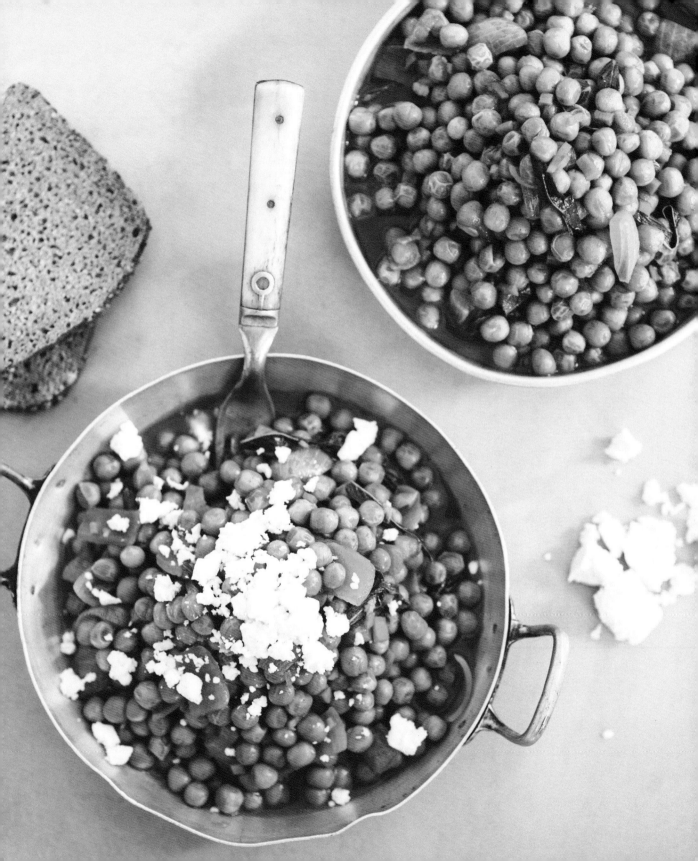

A delicious garlicky peasant Italian meal with a hint of bitterness and heat. Eat it on its own or with a side salad. This recipe is ideal to make when fresh borlotti beans are in season, but you can also cook it throughout the year using dried borlotti beans. Known as "cicoria" in Italian, like legumes, chicory contains a high amount of prebiotics for intestinal health.

FRESH BORLOTTI BEANS WITH CHICORY

PREPARATION: 15 MINUTES, COOKING: 40 MINUTES, SERVES 4

1 kg (2 lb 3 oz) fresh borlotti beans
   in their pods
1 large bunch chicory, chopped into
   2.5-centimetre (1-inch) pieces
½ cup extra virgin olive oil
4 large cloves garlic, finely sliced
1 hot chilli, finely sliced
1 teaspoon salt
lemon wedges, for serving

1. Shell beans and place in a medium saucepan, then cover with plenty of water and bring to boil. Turn down heat and simmer for approximately 30 minutes until very soft. Drain and put aside, reserving 1 cup of the cooking water.
2. Meanwhile, wash chicory pieces in 3 changes of water to ensure all dirt is removed. Steam in a large pot for 10-15 minutes until tender. Tip: Give the firmer stems a head start before adding the leaves.
3. Heat oil in a large pot, and sauté garlic and chilli for 1 minute.
4. Stir in salt, then toss through cooked beans and cook for a few minutes until flavours combine.
5. Fold in chicory and add a little of the reserved cooking water to moisten, if the mixture appears a little dry. Cover and remove from heat. Rest for a few minutes before serving. Serve hot or cold with a squeeze of lemon. Recipe stores well in the fridge for several days.

TIPS:

- Chicory bunches can vary; adjust seasonings accordingly.
- Chicory can be replaced with other dark green leafy vegetables, like endive.
- To reduce bitterness, boil chicory in 2.5 centimetres (1 inch) of water, as they do in Italy, instead of steaming it.

Per serve: energy 1928 kJ (461 Cal); protein 14 g; fat 30 g; saturated fat 5 g; cholesterol 0 mg; carbohydrate 35 g; sugars 3 g; fibre 8 g; calcium 140 mg; iron 6 mg, sodium 635 mg

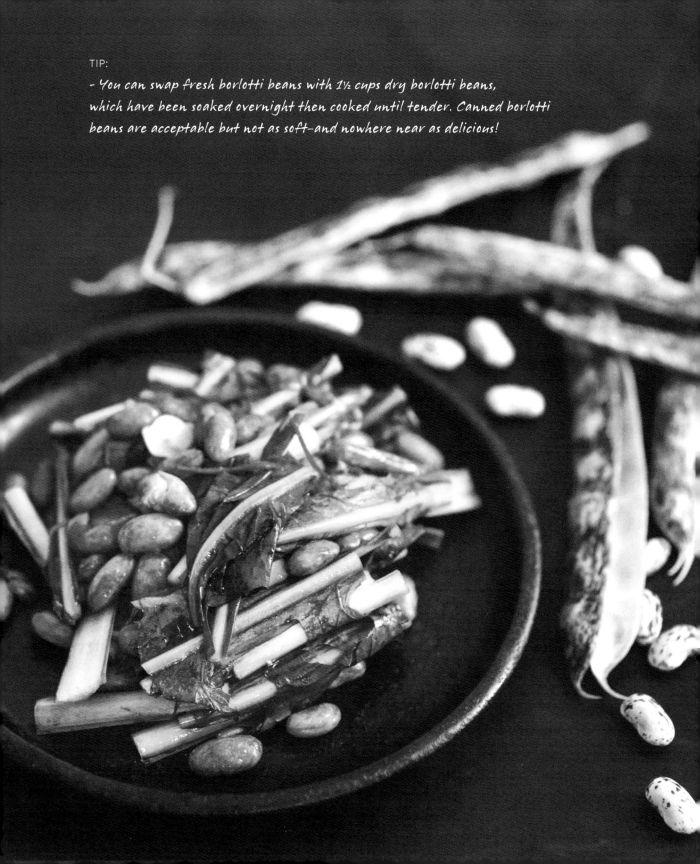

TIP:

- You can swap fresh borlotti beans with 1½ cups dry borlotti beans, which have been soaked overnight then cooked until tender. Canned borlotti beans are acceptable but not as soft—and nowhere near as delicious!

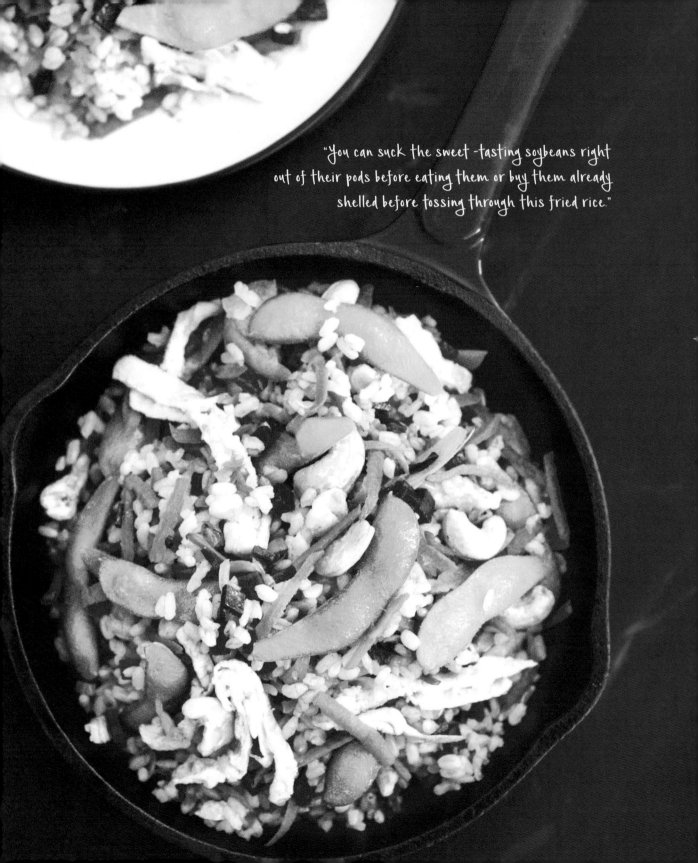

"You can suck the sweet-tasting soybeans right out of their pods before eating them or buy them already shelled before tossing through this fried rice."

Make this flavoursome dish whenever you have leftover brown rice. Apart from being a healthy whole-grain, brown rice is ideal to use as the grains don't stick together. The recipe is perfect for a light meal with a green salad or you can serve it as a side dish.

CASHEW FRIED RICE

PREPARATION: 7 MINUTES, COOKING: 13 MINUTES, SERVES 4

2½ cups cooked medium-grain brown rice

1 egg, optional

2 tablespoons extra virgin olive oil +
    1 teaspoon

1 small onion, finely chopped

½–1 small red chilli, deseeded,
    finely chopped

1 clove garlic, crushed

4 rashers imitation (soy) bacon,
    chopped into small pieces

1 medium carrot, peeled and grated

½ cup frozen shelled edamame

¼ cup cashews

2 teaspoons salt-reduced soy sauce

2 teaspoons extra virgin sesame oil

1. If using egg, make an omelette by whisking egg with a fork and pouring into a hot pan or wok to which you have added 1 teaspoon of oil. Cook omelette on both sides. Remove from the pan and slice into thin strips. Set aside.

2. Heat oil in the same pan, and sauté onion, chilli and garlic. Add imitation bacon and cook until bacon becomes slightly crispy. Add carrot and edamame, and cook for a further few minutes.

3. Toss in cooked brown rice, cashews, soy sauce, sesame oil and strips of omelette. Lightly fry until flavours combine. Serve hot or refrigerate and use within a few days.

TIPS:

- If you don't have leftover rice in the fridge or freezer, cook 1 cup of rice using a rice cooker or the absorption method. Spread on a tray and cool in the fridge before using. Rice blends–combinations of red, brown and black rice–also work well.

- Raw cauliflower rice can be substituted for cooked rice. Simply pulse cauliflower in a food processor until it resembles rice grains.

- Imitation bacon is made from soy protein and available from supermarkets.

- Edamame are green (immature) soybeans available from the freezer in Asian supermarkets.

Per serve: energy 1654 kJ (395 Cal); protein 10 g; fat 20 g; saturated fat 3 g; cholesterol 1 mg; carbohydrate 41 g; sugars 3 g; fibre 5 g; calcium 32 mg; iron 2.1 mg; sodium 226 mg

Try this simple and tasty dish for long-lasting energy! Chickpeas are loaded with fibre to fill you up and provide low GI, slow-release carbs. They encourage the growth of healthy gut bacteria.

SPICED CHICKPEAS WITH SILVERBEET AND LEMON

PREPARATION: 12 MINUTES, COOKING: 25 MINUTES, SERVES 6

1 kg (2 lb 3 oz) bunch of silverbeet (chard), trimmed then chopped into 5-centimetre (2-inch) pieces
4 tablespoons extra virgin olive oil
1 large onion, sliced into rings
4 cloves garlic, crushed
1 tablespoon cumin seeds
1 tablespoon coriander seeds
½ tablespoon fennel seeds
1 cassia stick
½ teaspoon salt
freshly crushed black pepper, to taste
3 cups cooked chickpeas (garbanzos)
⅓ cup lemon juice

1. Wash silverbeet, then steam for about 10 minutes or until tender.
2. Heat oil in a large pan and sauté onion until translucent. Add garlic and cook for another 30 seconds.
3. Add spices and continue frying for 1 minute, until they just begin to pop and release their aroma, being careful not to burn them.
4. Mix in chickpeas until they are well coated with the spices.
5. Toss in steamed silverbeet and turn up heat, stirring until the flavours have combined. Drizzle with lemon juice. Serve immediately with a salad. Recipe can be refrigerated for several days.

TIP:

- 2 x 400 g (14 oz) cans of chickpeas, drained, provide around 3 cups of chickpeas. If cooking from scratch, pre-soak 1 cup of chickpeas overnight, then boil for 50 minutes until tender.

Per serve: energy 1125 kJ (269 Cal); protein 12 g; fat 19 g; saturated fat 3 g; cholesterol 0 mg; carbohydrate 9 g; sugars 7 g; fibre 10 g; calcium 187 mg; iron 7 mg; sodium 258 mg

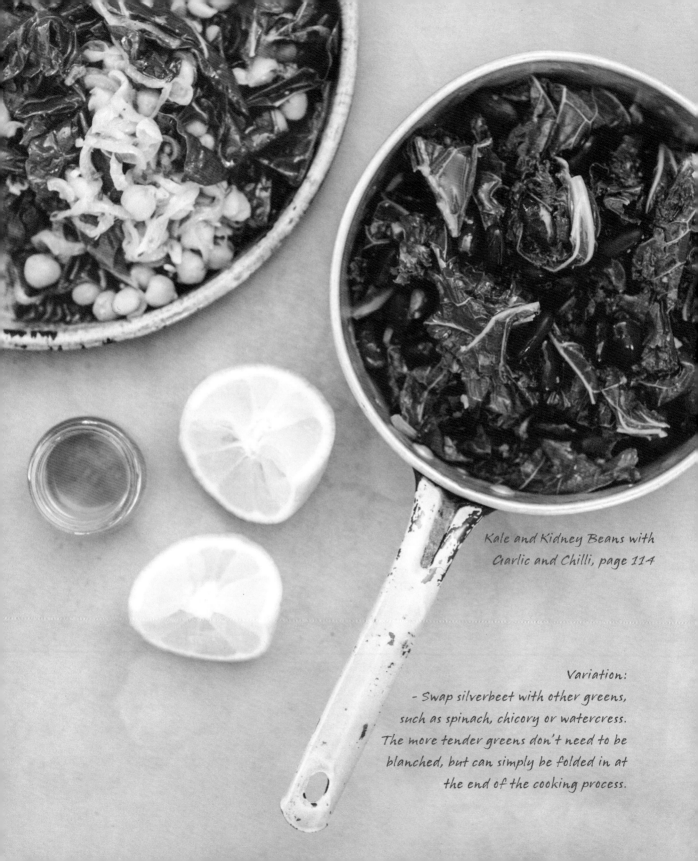

Kale and Kidney Beans with
Garlic and Chilli, page 114

Variation:
- Swap silverbeet with other greens,
such as spinach, chicory or watercress.
The more tender greens don't need to be
blanched, but can simply be folded in at
the end of the cooking process.

Kidney beans are low GI and kale is one of the most nutrient-dense greens you can eat. In order to form the anti-cancer phytonutrient called sulforaphane, kale must be chopped or chewed first so its myrosinase enzyme can get to the precursor phytonutrients, which are separated by the plant cell walls. As blanching and extended cooking progressively destroy myrosinase, it's best to chop kale (and other cruciferous family vegetables) at least 40 minutes prior to cooking. Once formed, sulforaphane is heat resistant! (Recipe image, page 113.)

KALE AND KIDNEY BEANS WITH GARLIC AND CHILLI

PREPARATION: 15 MINUTES + OVERNIGHT SOAKING, COOKING: 40 MINUTES INCLUDING PRESSURE COOKER, SERVES 6

1½ cups kidney beans, soaked overnight

400 g (14 oz) kale leaves (from 1 large bunch), chopped into 2.5-centimetre (1-inch) pieces

¾ cup extra virgin olive oil

4 very large cloves garlic, crushed

1 hot red chilli, finely chopped

¾ teaspoon salt

4 lemon wedges, for serving

1. Drain and rinse kidney beans, and place in a pressure cooker with 6 cups of water. Secure lid and bring to pressure. Cook at high pressure for 6 minutes, allowing for natural pressure release (about 15 minutes) before opening lid. Drain beans, reserving 1 cup of the cooking water.

2. Meanwhile, prepare and cook kale in a large steamer for approximately 8 minutes until tender.

3. Heat oil in a large pan, and sauté garlic and chilli on medium heat for 30 seconds until fragrant, being careful not to burn them.

4. Stir in salt and fold in the cooked beans. Cook for one minute until flavours combine then add ½–1 cup of the bean cooking water to create a thin sauce.

5. Toss through the kale and continue cooking for a few minutes until ingredients are combined. Cover dish with a lid and let sit for a few minutes before serving with lemon wedges. Recipe stores well in the fridge for several days.

TIPS:

- Buy a large bunch of kale so you can remove fibrous stems (add them to the juicer) and only use the tender leaves for this recipe. Wash well as kale can hide dirt and bugs!

- You can also use 2 x 420 g (15 oz) cans of kidney beans, which provide about 3 cups of cooked beans. But they will not be as tender, nor the flavour as delicious as cooking the beans yourself.

- Top with a dollop of tangy soy or dairy yogurt before serving, if desired.

Per serve: energy 1883 kJ (450 Cal); protein 16 g; fat 38 g; saturated fat 6 g; cholesterol 0 mg; carbohydrate 8 g; sugars 5 g; fibre 12 g; calcium 112 mg; iron 4.9 mg; sodium 305 mg

Here's a fast and healthier way to enjoy pizza, using Greek pita bread. These pizzas will emerge with a crispy thin base and a sweetish, lightly spiced zucchini topping. Traditional feta cheese is made from sheep and goats milk, which contains A2 protein but this can also be substituted with Almond Cream Cheese in "feta" form (see page 224) for a dairy-free version. (Recipe image, page 117.)

ZUCCHINI, CHILLI AND FETA PIZZAS

PREPARATION: 12 MINUTES, COOKING: 13 MINUTES, SERVES 4

4 Greek pita breads
4 tablespoons tomato pasta sauce
4 medium zucchinis (courgettes),
  sliced thinly lengthwise
120 g (4 oz) feta cheese, crumbled
1 teaspoon chilli flakes
120 g (4 oz) baby rocket (arugula) leaves
2 tablespoons extra virgin olive oil
4 teaspoons lemon juice

1. Pre-heat oven to 180°C (350°F).
2. Place pita breads on 2 large oven trays and spread with pasta sauce.
3. Lay zucchini slices on top, side by side, until you have covered the surface, and sprinkle with the feta and chilli flakes.
4. Place trays into oven and bake for about 13 minutes until the pita becomes crisp. Note: Raw zucchinis won't brown much.
5. Remove from oven and transfer pizzas onto dinner plates. Top with fresh rocket, and drizzle with olive oil and lemon juice. Serve immediately.

TIPS:

- Use a mandoline to thinly, evenly and quickly slice zucchinis.
- Variation: Replace raw zucchini with chargrilled zucchini slices purchased from the deli or make your own by spraying thin slices of zucchini with olive oil and cooking on a cast-iron grill pan or placing under a griller for about 5 minutes until golden. This brings out the sweetness in zucchinis and can be done in advance. Store cooked zucchinis in an airtight container in the fridge until required.
- Wholemeal Lebanese bread can also be substituted, as can a gluten-free base. Unfortunately, Greek pita does not come in a wholemeal variety.
- Cut uncooked pizza into bite-size pieces before baking if you intend to serve it as an appetiser.

Per serve: energy 1811 kJ (433 Cal); protein 15 g; fat 18 g; saturated fat 6 g; cholesterol 20 mg; carbohydrate 50 g; sugars 8 g; fibre 4 g; calcium 151 mg; iron 2.4 mg; sodium 1117 mg

This dish is called "nasu [meaning eggplant/aubergine] dengaku" in Japanese. It is tenderly cooked eggplant topped with a sweet miso sauce. While the eggplant is traditionally fried, I bake it before applying the miso topping. The Japanese love sweet things and usually use a lot more sugar, which helps with the caramelisation of the topping. Dengaku can also be made with other vegetables, mushrooms and even grilled konnyaku balls threaded onto skewers. Eggplant is rich in viscous fibre, which lowers elevated cholesterol.

SWEET MISO GLAZED EGGPLANT ROUNDS

PREPARATION: 10 MINUTES, COOKING: 45 MINUTES, SERVES 4

2 medium eggplants (aubergines)
3 tablespoons extra virgin olive oil
2 tablespoons verjuice
3 tablespoons sweet miso, light in sodium
1 tablespoon honey
2 teaspoons black sesame seeds

TIPS:

- *Japanese eggplant is smaller, narrower and less watery than globe eggplant, but is more difficult to source.*
- *Verjuice is pressed from unripened grapes. It has a delicate acidity and is available from good delicatessens.*

1. Pre-heat oven to 180°C (350°F) and line 2 trays with parchment (baking) paper.
2. Slice eggplants into 2-centimetre (1-inch) rounds and place on the trays, then brush with olive oil. Bake for 35 minutes until softened and golden.
3. Meanwhile, place verjuice and miso in a small saucepan over a medium heat and stir to dissolve. Blend in honey and 3 tablespoons of water, then reduce heat to low and continue cooking for about 5 minutes until the glaze thickens and becomes shiny. (Alternatively, place all ingredients in a small glass bowl and heat for 1 minute in microwave, then stir). Cover and set aside until eggplant is cooked.
4. Remove eggplant rounds from the oven and brush each surface thickly with the miso paste, using the brush from the oil.
5. Place eggplant back in the oven for a further 10 minutes until the topping starts to bubble and brown. Turn up the heat to 250°C (480°F) for the final 5 minutes—or use a chef's torch to achieve the same result.
6. Sprinkle each round with sesame seeds and serve with a healthy carb side dish and Asian greens. Recipe is unsuitable for freezing but leftovers can be refrigerated and consumed over a couple of days.

Per serve: energy 997 kJ (238 Cal); protein 4 g; fat 16 g; saturated fat 2 g; cholesterol 0 mg; carbohydrate 18 g; sugars 17 g; fibre 6 g; calcium 56 mg; iron 0.9 mg; sodium 461 mg

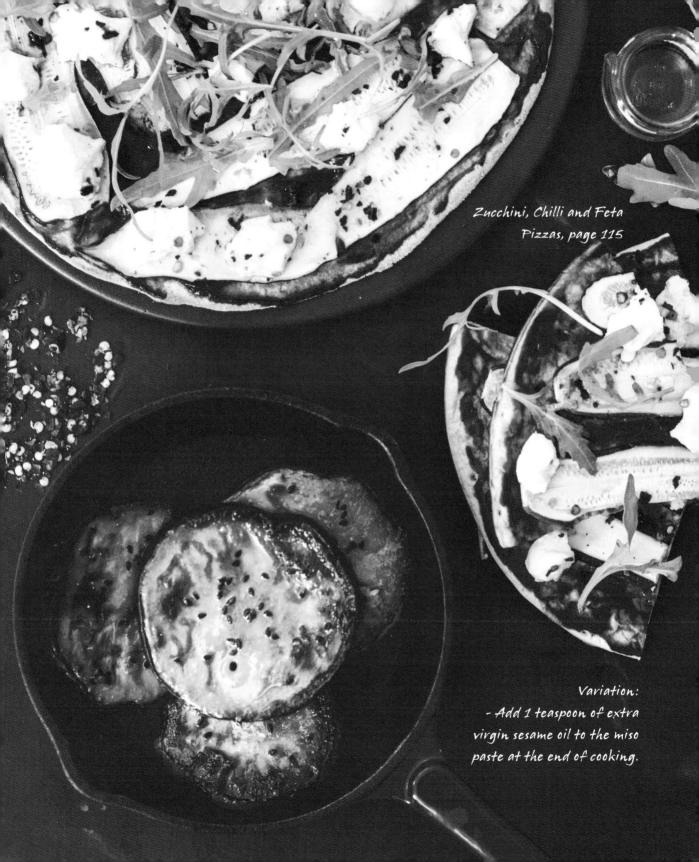

Zucchini, Chilli and Feta
Pizzas, page 115

Variation:
- Add 1 teaspoon of extra
virgin sesame oil to the miso
paste at the end of cooking.

Make this tangy Middle Eastern salad using warmed canned fava beans (broad beans) and enjoy as a simple meal, or serve as a side dish. If you prepare it a day ahead, the flavour is even better.

WARM FAVA BEAN SALAD

PREPARATION: 15 MINUTES, COOKING: 8 MINUTES, SERVES 5

1 x 825 g (29 oz) can fava beans
1 large clove garlic, crushed
3 tomatoes, finely chopped
½ Spanish onion, finely chopped
1 bunch parsley, finely chopped
mint leaves from a few stalks, chopped
½ teaspoon ground cumin
½ teaspoon Arabic seven spices
pinch freshly ground black pepper, optional
2 tablespoons extra virgin olive oil
¼ cup lemon juice (about 1 juiced lemon)

1. Remove fava beans from can and warm gently in a saucepan. Drain and place in a salad bowl together with all the other prepared ingredients.
2. Toss salad gently to combine. The salad should taste tangy and glisten.
3. Serve in bowls with Lebanese or Turkish bread on the side, or pile on top of light toast like bruschetta.

TIPS:

- Canned fava beans are available from Arabic supermarkets.
- Variation: Substitute 4 finely chopped shallots (scallions) for the Spanish onion.

Per serve: energy 894 kJ (214 Cal); protein 14 g; fat 8 g; saturated fat 1 g; cholesterol 0 mg; carbohydrate 13 g; sugars 5 g; fibre 15 g; calcium 88 mg; iron 4.9 mg; sodium 27 mg

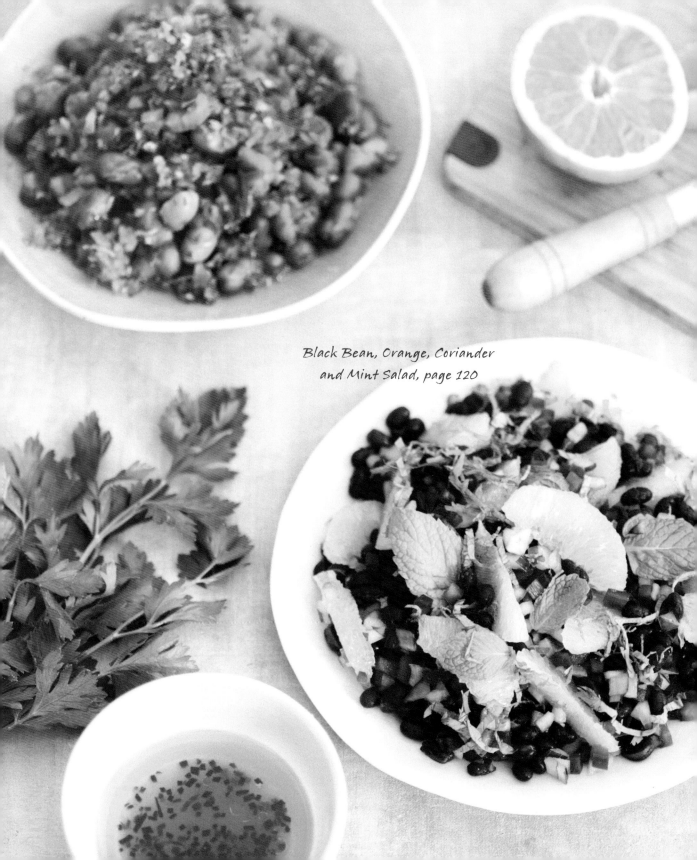

Black Bean, Orange, Coriander
and Mint Salad, page 120

This brightly coloured salad is very refreshing on a hot day. It's easy to make, and packed full of flavour and fibre. Eat it as a main or serve alongside other foods. The antioxidant content of black beans (also known as turtle beans) and other dark-coloured legumes, per serve, exceeds many fruits and vegetables! (Recipe image, page 119.)

BLACK BEAN, ORANGE, CORIANDER AND MINT SALAD

PREPARATION: 20 MINUTES, COOKING: 0 MINUTES, SERVES 6

2 x 440 g (16 oz) cans black beans, rinsed
   and drained
1 small red onion, finely chopped
½ large red capsicum (bell pepper),
   finely diced
2 large oranges, peeled, segmented
   and diced
1 bunch fresh coriander (cilantro), chopped
1 bunch fresh mint, chopped

Dressing
¼ cup extra virgin olive oil
¼ cup lemon juice (about 1 juiced lemon)
1 small hot chilli, deseeded, finely chopped

1. Place beans, onion, capsicum, oranges and herbs in a large salad bowl.
2. Add dressing ingredients to a glass jar and shake vigorously to emulsify. Pour over the salad ingredients and toss gently until well combined.
3. Serve immediately or store in the fridge for 1-2 days. Recipe is unsuitable for freezing.

TIPS:
- This salad looks great served on a bed of rocket or baby lettuce.
- Be careful not to touch your eyes for several hours after chopping chilli!
- Swap canned beans with 3 cups of cooked beans.

Per serve: energy 1288 kJ (308 Cal); protein 15 g; fat 10 g; saturated fat 2 g; cholesterol 0 mg; carbohydrate 30 g; sugars 9 g; fibre 16 g; calcium 94 mg; iron 4 mg; sodium 11 mg

Loved by many people in Asia, the flavour of bitter melon (also known as bitter gourd) can challenge Western palates. However, it is worth pursuing for its excellent blood sugar-lowering effects. This recipe uses warm spices to balance the bitterness. Enjoy the fritters with a tangy yogurt dipping sauce, which further masks any remaining bitterness. (Recipe image, page 122.)

BITTER MELON FRITTERS

PREPARATION: 15 MINUTES + 30 MINUTES DRAINING, COOKING: 18 MINUTES, MAKES 6 LARGE FRITTERS

2 bitter melons, washed
1½ teaspoons salt
½ cup chickpea (besan) flour
2 tablespoons brown rice flour
½ teaspoon turmeric
½ teaspoon cumin
½ teaspoon garam masala
½ teaspoon ground ginger
1 clove garlic, crushed
3 tablespoons extra virgin olive oil

1. Slice bitter melons in half, lengthwise. Remove seeds using a metal spoon and coarsely grate melons. Place grated melons into a colander and mix in 1 teaspoon of salt. Sit colander over a bowl for 30-60 minutes to extract some of the bitter juices. Discard the juice, as it will be too salty to drink.

2. Prepare batter by mixing remainder of salt, flours and spices in a bowl. Set aside.

3. Squeeze excess moisture from the grated bitter melon in the colander, then rinse melon by holding the colander under running tap. Take handfuls of grated melon, squeeze out the moisture, then add to the dry batter mixture.

4. Add garlic to the mixture and gradually combine everything, drizzling in ¼ to ½ cup of water until mixture forms a thick paste. Note: The amount of water required will depend on the size of the bitter melons and how much moisture has been extracted from them.

5. Heat oil in a medium frypan. Divide mixture into 6, form round patties and slide each into the pan. Flatten slightly, then cook until golden brown, turning over once. Alternatively, make 24 mini-fritters.

6. Place cooked fritters on paper towelling to absorb excess oil. Serve hot as part of a main meal or in a burger bun. Fritters can be stored in the fridge for several days.

TIPS:

- Salt helps extract some of the bitterness.
- Variation: Substitute cold-pressed mustard seed oil, which has a nutty flavour and is traditionally used in northern India.

Per serve: energy 541 kJ (129 Cal); protein 3 g; fat 10 g; saturated fat 2 g; cholesterol 0 mg; carbohydrate 5 g; sugars 0 g; fibre 3 g; calcium 22 mg; iron 1.2 mg; sodium 582 mg

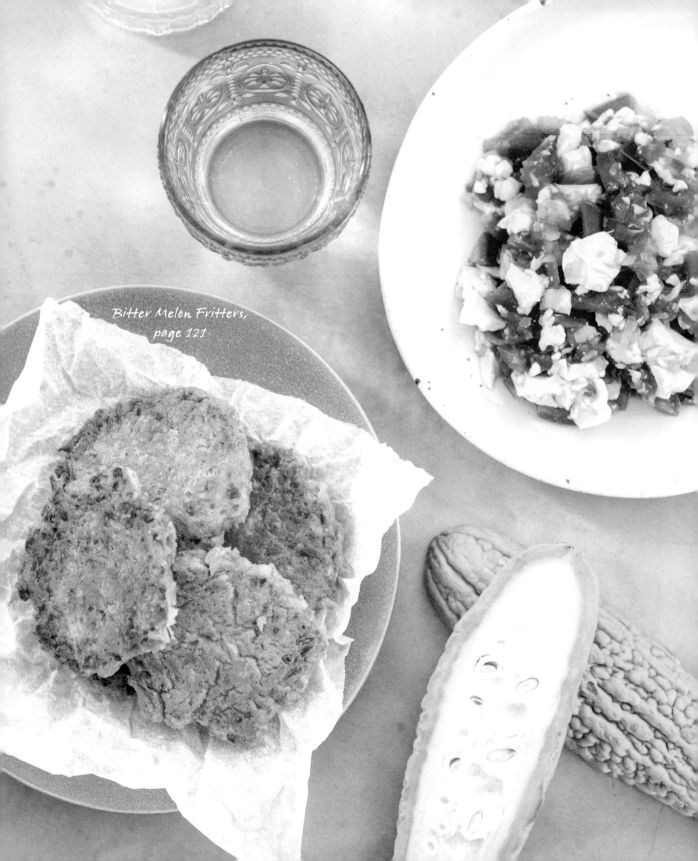

Bitter Melon Fritters,
page 121

This is an Asian twist to a Greek idea, usually made with eggs and tomatoes. The tofu and turmeric combination makes this dish reminiscent of soft scrambled eggs, yet it's much healthier and delicious! Serve for breakfast or a light dinner with grainy bread and any sides of your choice, such as pan-seared mushrooms or wilted spinach.

SCRAMBLED TOFU WITH TOMATO

PREPARATION: 4 MINUTES, COOKING: 15 MINUTES, SERVES 3

600 g (21 oz) classic or regular
   (medium texture) tofu
3 tablespoons extra virgin olive oil
1 small onion, finely chopped
1 soft medium tomato, coarsely chopped
¼ teaspoon turmeric
½ teaspoon salt
coarsely ground pepper, to taste

1. Drain tofu pieces, then place on a board and wrap in kitchen towelling to absorb excess moisture. Allow to sit while preparing other ingredients.
2. Heat oil in a pan and sauté onion on medium heat for about 5 minutes until golden.
3. Add tomato and continue cooking for a further 5 minutes until tomato softens. Stir in seasonings.
4. Break up tofu with your hands and add to pan, stirring gently to incorporate the flavours. Continue cooking on low heat for a further 5 minutes until the tofu is heated through. Serve immediately. Note: If liquid starts to separate from the tofu, simply stir again before serving.

TIP:

- For flavour variations, add garlic, herbs or sprinkle with some seaweed from a shaker.

Per serve: energy 1255 kJ (300 Cal); protein 17 g; fat 26 g; saturated fat 4 g; cholesterol 0 mg; carbohydrate 3 g; sugars 3 g; fibre 7 g; calcium 112 mg; iron 4 mg; sodium 397 mg

Here's a healthy party food for kids—made with the goodness of walnuts. Walnuts provide plant protein and healthy fats. Serve with your favourite dipping sauce and, if using for a meal, round off with some colourful raw vegetable sticks.

MINI SAUSAGE ROLLS

PREPARATION: 40 MINUTES, COOKING: 30 MINUTES, SERVES 10

1 tablespoon chia seeds

½ cup rolled oats

1 cup walnuts

1 teaspoon ground cumin

1 teaspoon dried oregano

generous amount of freshly ground pepper

1 very large onion, quartered

4 cloves garlic

2 tablespoons light soy sauce

2 teaspoons dark soy sauce

2 cups multigrain breadcrumbs

10 sheets fillo pastry

¼ cup extra virgin olive oil

2 teaspoons black sesame seeds

Per serve: energy 1305 kJ (312 Cal); protein 8 g; fat 17 g; saturated fat 2 g; cholesterol 0 mg; carbohydrate 30 g; sugars 3 g; fibre 4 g; calcium 45 mg; iron 1.6 mg; sodium 585 mg

1. Place chia seeds in a small bowl and cover with 6 tablespoons of water to make "chia egg." Allow to sit for 10-15 minutes until chia swells and thickens, stirring frequently to prevent clumps forming.

2. Pre-heat oven to 180°C (350°F).

3. Place oats, walnuts and spices into a food processor, and process until fine. Add onion and garlic, and continue blending until smooth.

4. While the motor is running, pour in soy sauces through the chute, followed by the "chia egg," then gradually drizzle in breadcrumbs until you achieve a thick consistency that comes together. Transfer mixture to a bowl.

5. Place 2 fillo sheets vertically in front of you on a clean bench. Brush one with olive oil and lay the other on top until it sticks.

6. Divide walnut mixture into 5 portions. Moistening your hands with water, take half of each portion and roll into a sausage, about 2 centimetres (almost 1 inch) wide. Place this on the fillo near the edge closest to you, starting from the left edge finishing in the middle. Repeat with the other half of the portion and continue the sausage from the middle to the right edge. Join the 2 sausages in the middle so there is no break.

7. Roll fillo tightly, brushing the end with oil to seal it. Transfer to a large sheet of parchment (baking) paper and, using a wet serrated knife, cut the roll into 4 equal pieces, wiping the knife between each cut. Press down the 2 ends of each mini roll like a pillow, as they will rise with baking.

8. Repeat with remaining fillo and 4 portions of walnut mixture, then gently slide the parchment paper with the mini rolls onto a large baking tray. Brush top of each roll with some oily water (add water to the oil container) and sprinkle with the sesame seeds.

9. Bake for 30 minutes until golden, basting half way with some more water so the rolls don't dry out and crack. Serve hot. Makes 20 mini-rolls.

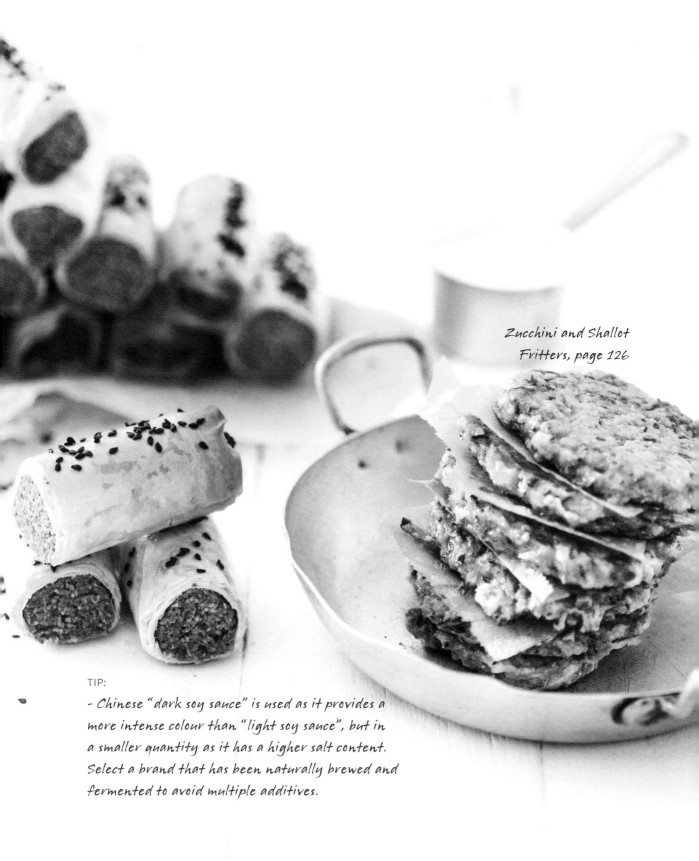

Zucchini and Shallot
Fritters, page 126

TIP:
- Chinese "dark soy sauce" is used as it provides a
more intense colour than "light soy sauce", but in
a smaller quantity as it has a higher salt content.
Select a brand that has been naturally brewed and
fermented to avoid multiple additives.

In Greece, these are called "kolokithokeftedes," meaning zucchini meatballs. They are popular with children due to their slightly sweet taste. Once prepared, store in the fridge and use over several days. Zucchini fritters are great in sandwiches, for picnics, as meze or just on their own with salad and bread as a meal. (Recipe image, page 125.)

ZUCCHINI AND SHALLOT FRITTERS

PREPARATION: 15 MINUTES, COOKING: 40 MINUTES, SERVES 6

1 kg (2 lb 3 oz) zucchinis (courgettes), unpeeled
1 teaspoon salt + ½ teaspoon
1 tablespoon chia seeds
freshly ground black pepper, to taste
1 teaspoon dried oregano
½ teaspoon sweet Hungarian paprika
2 cloves garlic, crushed
2 tablespoons freshly chopped dill
2 shallots (scallions), finely sliced (use both green and white parts)
1 cup plain wholemeal flour
½ cup extra virgin olive oil

1. Grate zucchinis and place in a colander over a bowl. Rub in 1 teaspoon of salt and sit for 10-30 minutes to extract moisture. Before using, take up handfuls and squeeze out juice.
2. Meanwhile, place chia seeds in a small bowl and stir in 5 tablespoons of water to make "chia egg." Allow this to swell and thicken for about 10 minutes, stirring frequently to prevent clumps.
3. In a large bowl, place the "chia egg" and stir in remaining salt, pepper, oregano, paprika, garlic, dill, shallots and zucchini.
4. Fold in flour until you achieve the consistency of a thick batter. Add a little more flour if the batter seems runny as the fritters won't bind and will soak up more oil.
5. Heat oil in a large frypan until rippling, then drop spoonfuls of the mixture and flatten slightly to form fritters. Cook each side for about 4 minutes until golden brown, turning once. When crisp, remove from the oil and place on paper towelling to drain. Serve immediately or refrigerate for later. Makes 24 fritters or 48 mini fritters.

TIPS:

- Use the wide holes of a food processor grating disc to grate zucchinis.
- Lupin or besan (chickpea) flour can be substituted for the wholemeal flour.
- Serve with Greek-style Yogurt Dip with Cucumber and Mint (page 222), or plain dairy or soy yogurt on the side.

Per serve: energy 1171 kJ (280 Cal); protein 4 g; fat 21 g; saturated fat 3 g; cholesterol 0 mg; carbohydrate 16 g sugars 3 g; fibre 6 g; calcium 51 mg; iron 1.9 mg; sodium 579 mg

A simple Greek-style salad, ideal for lunch, a picnic or as a side to a main meal. My family and friends around the world love it and make it repeatedly! Black-eyed beans are easy to prepare as they do not require soaking and cook quickly. They contain plant protein and the perfect carbohydrates to regulate blood sugar levels. (Recipe image, page 128.)

BLACK-EYED BEAN SALAD WITH LEMON AND SHALLOTS

PREPARATION: 8 MINUTES, COOKING: 20 MINUTES INCLUDING PRESSURE COOKER, SERVES 6

2 cups black-eyed beans

4 shallots (scallions), sliced into 1-centimetre (½-inch) lengths (use both green and white parts)

1 teaspoon dried oregano

⅓ cup extra virgin olive oil

⅓ cup lemon juice

1 teaspoon salt

1. Place beans into a pressure cooker with 6 cups of water. Cover with lid and bring to pressure, then turn down heat to very low and cook under pressure for 5 minutes. Remove from heat and run cold water on lid, over the sink, to rapidly bring down the pressure to stop the cooking process, then open lid. (For conventional cooking: Place beans in a large saucepan and cover with about 12 cups of water. Bring to boil and cook, half covered, for approximately 45 minutes or until beans are tender but not mushy.)

2. Drain and rinse beans with cold water.

3. Transfer beans to a large salad bowl and add remaining ingredients. Mix with a large metal spoon until well combined. Serve immediately or store in the fridge for several days and enjoy chilled. Recipe is unsuitable for freezing as it contains fresh shallots.

TIPS:

- You can find dry black-eyed beans at Asian and Indian grocery stores or subsitute with canned black-eyed beans from supermarkets.
- Use a fresh extra virgin olive oil (check labels). This is important for the overall flavour and health properties.
- To release more flavour, split the white portion of the shallots lengthwise before slicing them.
- To make a delicious spread for toast, add chopped raw onion to leftovers and puree in a blender until smooth.

Per serve: energy 1540 kJ (368 Cal); protein 21 g; fat 26 g; saturated fat 4 g; cholesterol 0 mg; carbohydrate 9 g; sugars 5 g; fibre 14 g; calcium 133 mg; iron 6.6 mg; sodium 775 mg

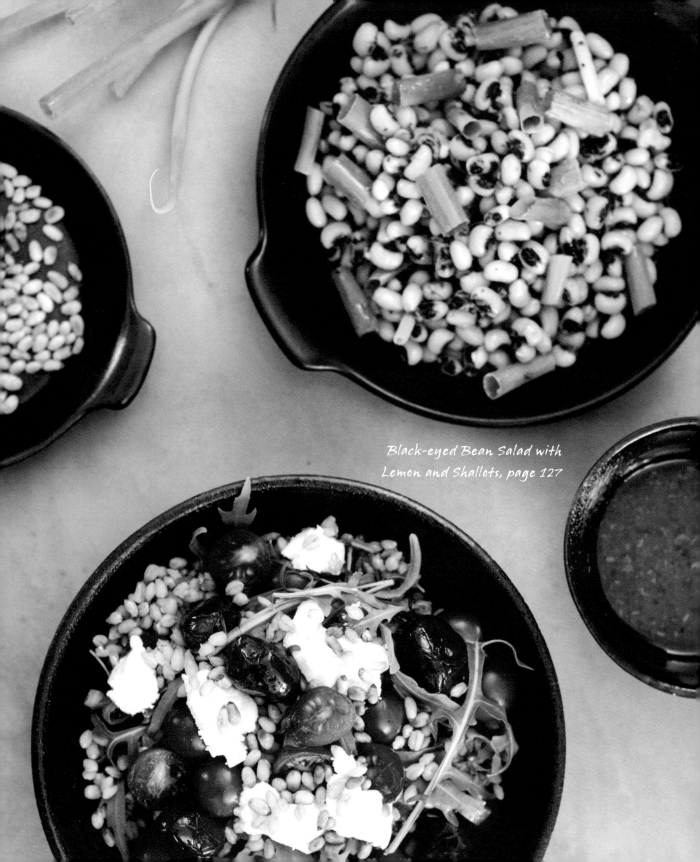

Black-eyed Bean Salad with
Lemon and Shallots, page 127

This summer salad is excellent for a healthy lunch or picnic. To prevent the rocket from wilting, fold it in just before eating. Leftovers are wonderful, as the flavours continue to improve. Barley is full of viscous fibre and will help lower your cholesterol and blood sugar levels, if elevated.

BARLEY SALAD WITH CHERRY TOMATOES, FETA AND PINE NUTS

PREPARATION: 12 MINUTES, COOKING: 40 MINUTES, SERVES 6

Salad
1 cup pearled barley
⅓ cup pine nuts
⅓ cup chopped fresh herbs (examples: basil, mint)
12 whole black olives
250 g (9 oz) punnet cherry tomatoes
100 g (3½ oz) rocket (arugula)
100 g (3½ oz) feta, crumbled

Dressing
¼ cup extra virgin olive oil
3 tablespoons lemon juice
1 clove garlic, crushed

1. Place barley in a medium saucepan and rinse with water, then drain. Add 6 cups of water, cover and bring to boil. Turn down heat and simmer for approximately 30 minutes or until the barley is just tender. Rinse under cold water to stop the cooking process, then drain.
2. Meanwhile, dry toast pine nuts for a few minutes in a small pan until golden.
3. Place all dressing ingredients in a screw-top jar and shake well.
4. Transfer barley into a large mixing bowl with herbs and stir through dressing. Add toasted pine nuts, olives, tomatoes (cut some in half to create more juice), rocket and feta cheese, and toss gently to combine. Serve with freshly ground black pepper, if desired. Salad will store in the fridge for several days but is unsuitable for freezing.

TIPS:

- Save time and energy using a pressure cooker. Add 3 cups of water to the barley and cook under pressure for 5 minutes.
- If eating dairy-free, swap dairy feta with Almond Cream Cheese in "feta" form (see page 224).

Per serve: energy 1399 kJ (334 Cal); protein 8 g; fat 23 g; saturated fat 5 g; cholesterol 11 mg; carbohydrate 22 g; sugars 2 g; fibre 5 g; calcium 78 mg; iron 1.8 mg; sodium 315 mg

Soba noodle salad is usually served cold in Japan. Here is a quick version you can make in your kitchen.

JAPANESE SOBA NOODLE AND MUSHROOM SALAD

PREPARATION: 13 MINUTES, COOKING: 9 MINUTES, SERVES 2

Dressing

1½ tablespoons salt-reduced tamari

2 teaspoons extra virgin sesame oil

1 teaspoon lime juice

1 teaspoon apple cider vinegar

1 teaspoon honey

1 clove garlic, crushed

Salad

½ carrot, finely julienned

50 g (1½ oz) fresh shiitake mushrooms, finely sliced

100 g (3½ oz) medium firm tofu, cut into 1.5-centimetre (½-inch) cubes

125 g (4½ oz) 100% buckwheat soba noodles (half a packet)

1 shallot (scallion), finely sliced

1 teaspoon black sesame seeds

1. Place dressing ingredients in a medium bowl and stir to combine.
2. Add prepared carrot, mushrooms and tofu to the bowl. Toss and allow to marinate while cooking noodles.
3. Cook noodles in boiling water for 4 minutes or according to instructions. Drain, then rinse with cold water to stop the cooking process and drain again.
4. Add noodles to vegetable mixture and toss gently to ensure everything is evenly distributed and dressing coats noodles.
5. Divide soba between 2 bowls. Sprinkle with shallot and sesame seeds and serve. Noodle salad can be refrigerated for a day but is unsuitable for freezing.

TIPS:

- If fresh shiitake mushrooms are unavailable, use the same amount of dried shiitake. Cover with boiling water and leave for 5 minutes to rehydrate, then squeeze out excess moisture and slice. You can also use enoki mushrooms—just trim them at the bottom.
- Variation: Garnish with fried wakame, cut up nori sheets or a sprinkling of seaweed from a shaker.

Per serve: energy 816 kJ (195 Cal); protein 9 g; fat 8 g; saturated fat 1 g; cholesterol 0 mg; carbohydrate 19 g; sugars 5 g; fibre 6 g; calcium 53 mg; iron 2.6 mg; sodium 540 mg

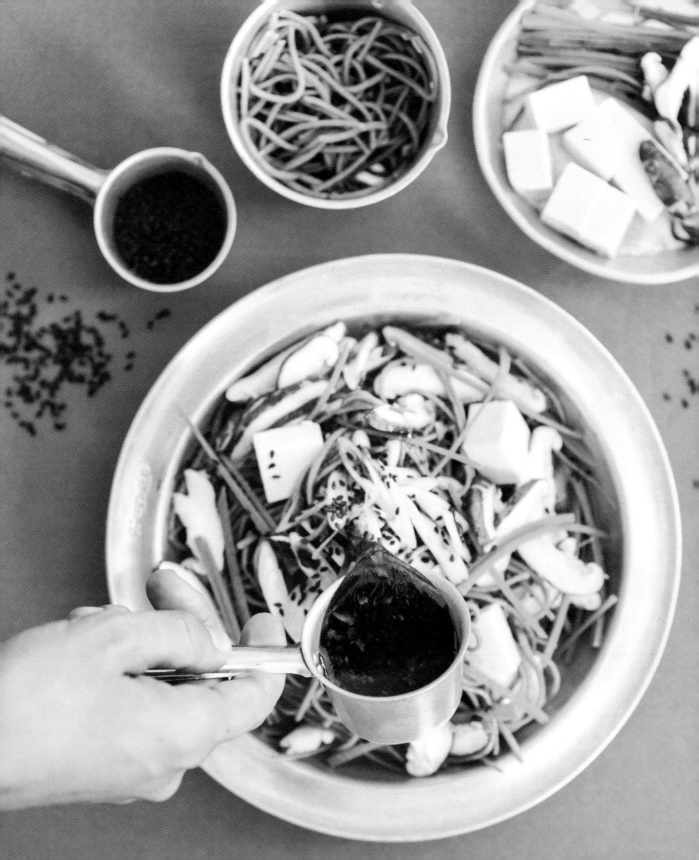

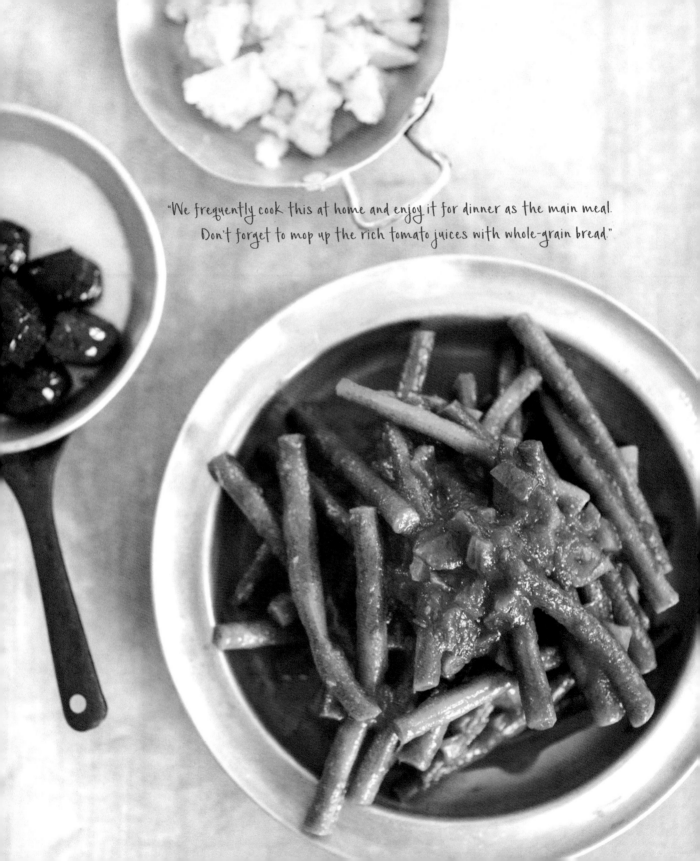

"We frequently cook this at home and enjoy it for dinner as the main meal. Don't forget to mop up the rich tomato juices with whole-grain bread."

This is a wonderful tomato-based meal when French beans are in season. Unlike a stir-fry, the beans are soft cooked and juicy, which is the traditional Mediterranean way. Tomato is rich in a powerful antioxidant called lycopene that protects against prostate cancer and macular degeneration.

MEDITERRANEAN BRAISED GREEN BEANS WITH TOMATO

PREPARATION: 15 MINUTES, COOKING: 20 MINUTES INCLUDING PRESSURE COOKER, SERVES 4

1 kg (2 lb 3 oz) green (French) beans,
  ends trimmed
4 tablespoons extra virgin olive oil
1 large onion, coarsely chopped
2 cloves garlic, sliced
½ teaspoon salt
freshly crushed black pepper, to taste
3 tablespoons tomato paste
400 g (14 oz) tomato pasta sauce

1. Warm oil in the base of a large pressure cooker and sauté onion for a few minutes, adding salt and pepper. Stir in garlic and cook for another 30 seconds, followed by tomato paste.
2. Rinse beans in a colander and add them to the cooker, together with tomato pasta sauce. Wash out the jar with about ½ cup of water and add this also before mixing. Secure the lid on the pressure cooker and turn up heat. Wait until the cooker reaches full pressure, then reduce heat to the lowest level and cook beans for 3 minutes. (If cooking beans using a regular pot, add a further 1 cup of water. Bring covered beans to boil, then turn down heat and simmer for 40-45 minutes until very soft.)
3. Remove pressure cooker from stove and place in the sink. Run cold water over lid until the pressure is released so you can open the lid immediately. Serve beans in individual bowls, hot or cold. In Greece, feta cheese and some olives are also commonly served as condiments to this dish.

TIPS:
- Variation: Add some carrot pieces or baby zucchini.
- Variation: Tomato pasta sauce can be replaced with 400 g (14 oz) ripe fresh tomatoes, which you have chopped, or canned diced tomatoes.
- Garnish with freshly chopped dill.

Per serve: energy 1341 kJ (320 Cal); protein 9 g; fat 20 g; saturated fat 3 g; cholesterol 0 mg; carbohydrate 19 g; sugars 14 g; fibre 12 g; calcium 173 mg; iron 3.9 mg; sodium 771 mg

Tofu burgers make an excellent instant lunch, dinner or quick snack. Unlike minced meat burgers, which can promote heart disease and cancer, regular consumption of tofu, from an early age, has been repeatedly linked with lower rates of these diseases. Did I mention these burgers are also super delicious?

TOFU BURGERS WITH GINGER, CHILLI AND GARLIC

PREPARATION: 5 MINUTES, COOKING: 10 MINUTES, SERVES 2

200 g (7 oz) firm tofu
2 teaspoons extra virgin olive oil
1 teaspoon ginger, minced
½ red chilli, deseeded, finely chopped
1 clove garlic, crushed
1 tablespoon soy sauce

1. Cut the tofu into 4 slices, approximately 1 centimetre (½ inch) thick (each slice should cover a burger bun). Place the tofu on absorbent kitchen paper to soak up excess moisture.
2. Heat half of oil in a frypan and brown tofu slices for a few minutes, turning once so both sides are golden. Remove and put aside.
3. Place remaining oil in pan, add ginger, chilli and garlic, and fry for about 10 seconds.
4. Dilute soy sauce with 4 tablespoons of water, and pour over ginger, chilli and garlic in the pan. You will hear a hissing sound. Keep the windows open as the chilli might make you cough.
5. Toss tofu slices back into the pan for 1 minute, allowing them to absorb some of the juices.
6. Serve tofu burgers on a grainy bun with your favourite vegetables, such as baby spinach, sliced tomatoes, char-grilled eggplant (aubergine) and alfalfa. Drizzle remaining sauce from the pan on top of the burgers. Makes 4 burgers.

TIPS:

- Firm tofu is an excellent source of calcium if set with calcium sulphate. Check the ingredients list.
- Store unused tofu submerged in cold water in a container in the fridge. Change the water daily and the tofu will stay fresh for 1 week.

Per serve: energy 734 kJ (175 Cal); protein 13 g; fat 12 g; saturated fat 2 g; cholesterol 0 mg; carbohydrate 1 g; sugars 0 g; fibre 8 g; calcium 323 mg; iron 3.1 mg; sodium 729 mg

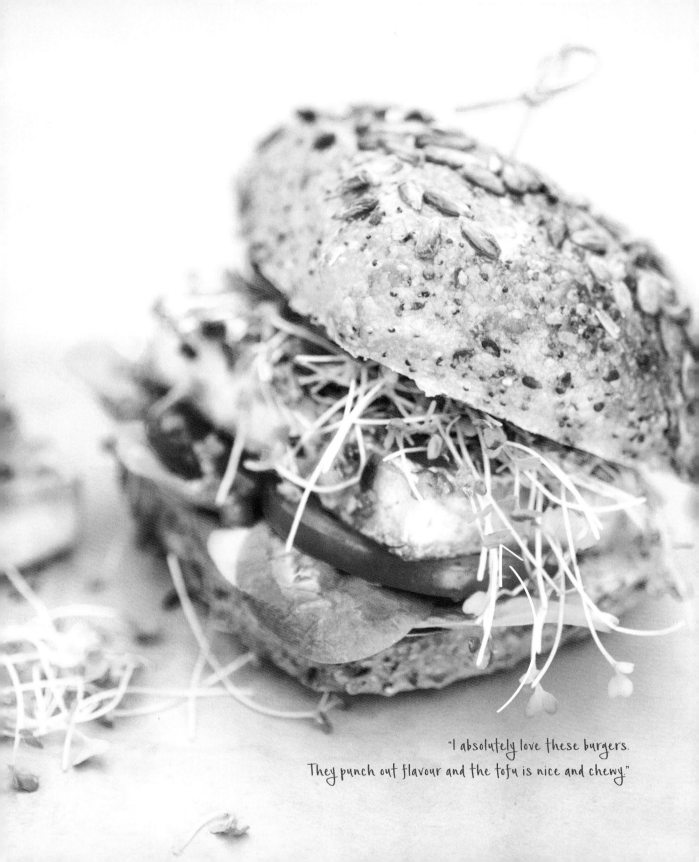

"I absolutely love these burgers.
They punch out flavour and the tofu is nice and chewy."

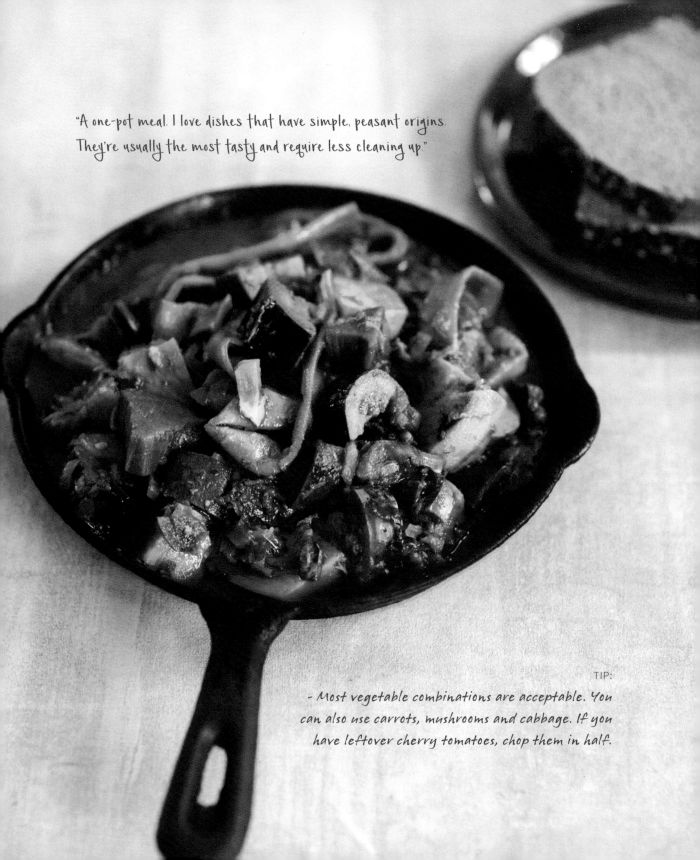

"A one-pot meal. I love dishes that have simple, peasant origins. They're usually the most tasty and require less cleaning up."

TIP:
- Most vegetable combinations are acceptable. You can also use carrots, mushrooms and cabbage. If you have leftover cherry tomatoes, chop them in half.

The beauty of this simple, tasty Turkish dish is that it cooks in one pot. It's also a smart way to use up leftover vegetables from the bottom of the fridge! Almost any combination works. It's called "turlu", meaning "mix" in Turkish, so this is equivalent to a Turkish ratatouille. The olive oil not only brings everything together but provides significant polyphenols with anti-inflammatory properties.

VILLAGE-STYLE VEGETABLE STEW

PREPARATION: 15 MINUTES, COOKING: 16 MINUTES INCLUDING PRESSURE COOKER, SERVES 4

1 medium eggplant (aubergine), cut into
  large chunks
100 g (3½ oz) flat green beans, topped
  and tailed
1 large zucchini (courgette), cut into large
  chunks
1 large potato, peeled and cut into chunks
1 large red onion, coarsely chopped
2 cloves garlic, coarsely chopped
300 g (10½ oz) fresh soft tomato, coarsely
  chopped or grated
freshly ground pepper, to taste
1 tablespoon ground paprika
1 x 10 g (⅓ oz) chicken-style vegetable
  stock cube, dissolved in ¼ cup
  boiling water
½ cup extra virgin olive oil
2 tablespoons parsley, coarsely chopped

1. Prepare vegetables and place in pressure cooker.

2. Add remaining ingredients and stir until combined. Cover with lid and bring to pressure (takes about 15 minutes), then turn down heat to very low and cook for just 1 minute under pressure. Allow for natural pressure release before opening lid. (If cooking conventionally, bring to boil then turn down heat and simmer, covered, for about 1 hour until very tender. You will also need to add 2 cups of water so the dish does not burn.)

3. Serve stew hot or cold with crusty whole-grain bread for mopping up the juices. Stew can be stored in the fridge for several days but is unsuitable for freezing.

TIPS:

- If your stew seems too watery (depending on the water content of the vegetables), drain the excess liquid and place in a small saucepan, then bring to boil to reduce the volume, before adding back to the stew.
- You can swap parsley with fresh coriander (cilantro).

Per serve: energy 1509 kJ (360 Cal); protein 5 g; fat 30 g; saturated fat 5 g; cholesterol 0 mg; carbohydrate 15 g; sugars 8 g; fibre 8 g; calcium 73 mg; iron 2 mg; sodium 208 mg

MAIN PLATES

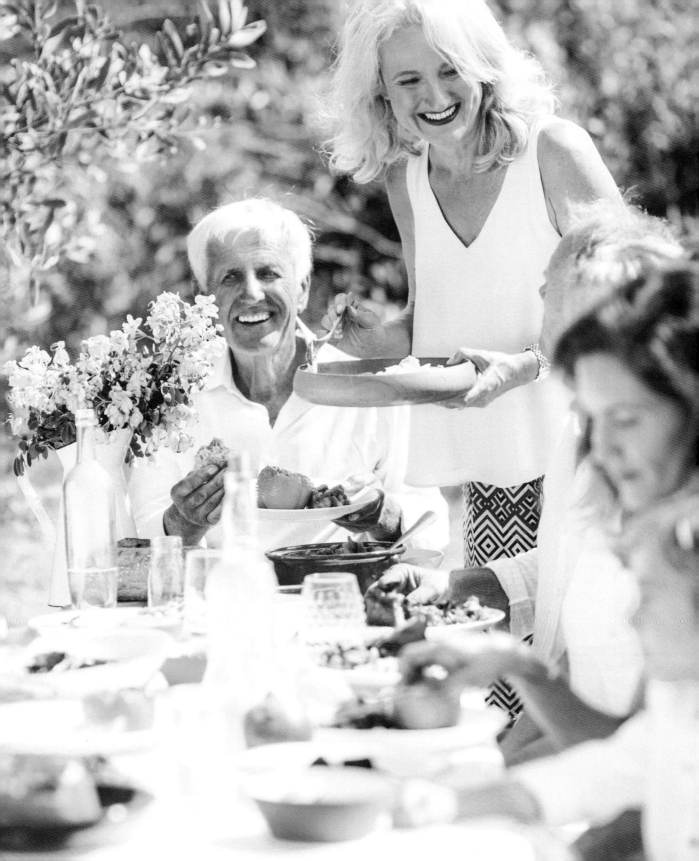

This Moroccan-style dish will impress with its vibrant colours and fragrant dressing. Adding liberal amounts of herbs and spices can significantly boost both the flavour and antioxidant content of your meal.

ROASTED VEGETABLES ON COUSCOUS WITH MOROCCAN DRESSING

PREPARATION: 20 MINUTES, COOKING: 45 MINUTES, SERVES 6

Roasted Vegetables

2 small Spanish onions, peeled and quartered

2 medium Desiree potatoes, scrubbed well and quartered

500 g (17½ oz) butternut pumpkin (butternut squash), peeled and cut into 2.5-centimetre (1-inch) chunks

1 small sweet potato, peeled and cut into 2.5-centimetre (1-inch) chunks

1 tablespoon extra virgin olive oil

1½ cups whole wheat couscous

Dressing

½ cup extra virgin olive oil

½ teaspoon hot paprika

1 tablespoon ground cumin

1 tablespoon ground coriander

2 tablespoons coriander (cilantro) leaves, chopped

2 tablespoons passata (tomato puree)

5 tablespoons lemon juice

Salad Topping

80 g (3 oz) mixed green leaves, washed and drained

100 g (3½ oz) feta cheese, crumbled

2 tablespoons pepitas (pumpkin seeds)

1. Pre-heat the oven to 200ºC (390ºF).

2. Prepare vegetables and spread on 2 oven trays lined with parchment (baking) paper. Brush with olive oil.

3. Place trays in hot oven and roast vegetables for 45 minutes, removing onions after about 30 minutes or when browned.

4. Place couscous in a glass bowl and pour over 1½ cups of boiling water. Cover and let stand for 10 minutes, then fluff up with a fork.

5. Prepare dressing by combining all ingredients and mixing well. Set aside.

6. Pile up ingredients on a serving platter in the following order: couscous, roasted vegetables, green leaves, crumbled feta, pepitas. Pour over the salad dressing. Serve immediately. Leftovers can be stored in the fridge for several days.

TIPS:

- For a dairy-free version, use Almond Cream Cheese in "feta" form (see page 224).

- Variation: Substitute the couscous (which is an instant type of pasta) with cooked white quinoa, which is a pseudograin and much more nutritious.

Per serve: 1786 kJ (427 Cal); protein 10 g; fat 29 g; saturated fat 6 g; cholesterol 11 mg; carbohydrate 31 g; sugars 9 g; fibre 6 g; calcium 102 mg; iron 1.6 mg; sodium 231 mg

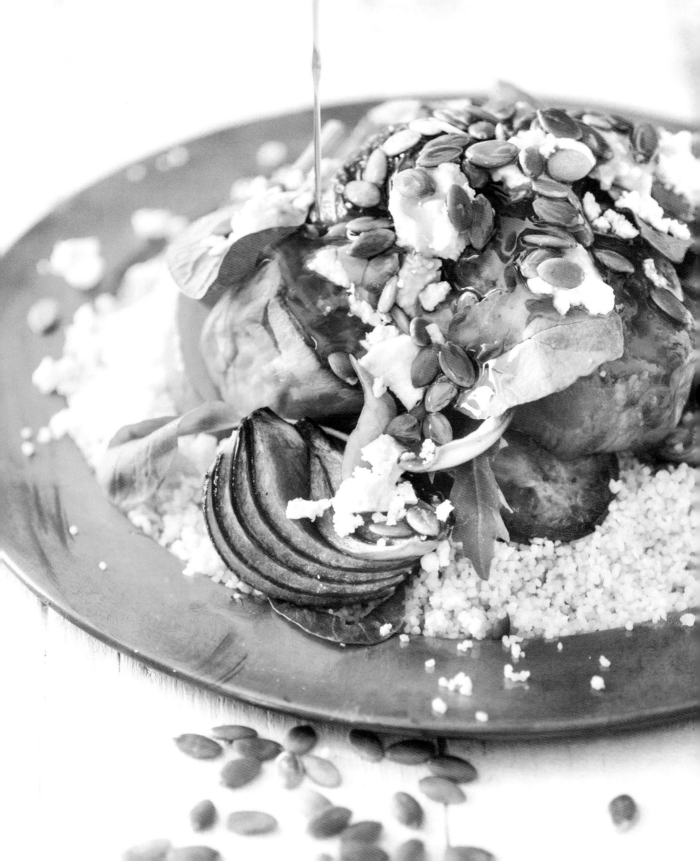

You will love making this easy curry with its slightly sweet and spicy flavour. Chickpeas are low GI and ideal if you are trying to lose weight and better manage your blood sugar.

CHICKPEA CURRY WITH PUMPKIN AND BABY SPINACH

PREPARATION: 10 MINUTES, COOKING: 30 MINUTES, SERVES 4

2 tablespoons extra virgin olive oil

1 medium onion, finely chopped

2 cloves garlic, crushed

1 teaspoon chilli powder

1 teaspoon ground coriander

2 teaspoons ground cumin

500 g (17½ oz) plain tomato pasta sauce

1½ cups cooked chickpeas (garbanzos)

320 g (11 oz) peeled pumpkin (butternut squash), chopped into small pieces

pinch salt, optional

120 g (4 oz) baby spinach leaves

2 teaspoons freshly chopped coriander (cilantro)

1. Heat oil in a large saucepan and sauté onion for about 5 minutes until soft. Stir in garlic and cook for 30 seconds.

2. Mix in chilli powder, coriander, cumin, tomato pasta sauce and ½ cup of water. Stir well.

3. Add chickpeas and pumpkin pieces, and bring to boil. Adjust flavour with extra salt, if desired.

4. Reduce heat and simmer for around 15 minutes or until pumpkin is tender.

5. Stir through baby spinach leaves until they start to wilt, followed by coriander, and serve immediately. Curry goes well with steamed whole-grain and red rice. Garnish with extra coriander leaves, if desired. Store curry in the fridge for several days or freeze individual portions on top of leftover rice.

TIPS:

- One 400 g (14 oz) can of chickpeas supplies around 1½ cups when drained. If using this, rinse chickpeas well.

- If you find this curry a little hot, try some plain dairy or soy yogurt on the side.

Per serve: energy 1203 kJ (287 Cal); protein 9 g; fat 13 g; saturated fat 2 g; cholesterol 0 mg; carbohydrate 29 g; sugars 15 g; fibre 10 g; calcium 118 mg; iron 4.1 mg; sodium 639 mg

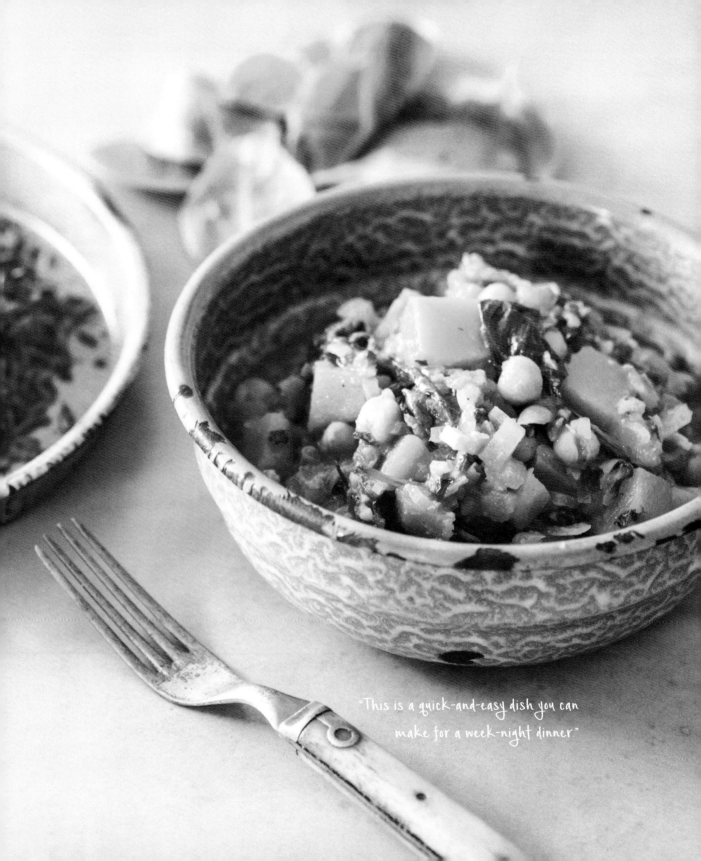

"This is a quick-and-easy dish you can make for a week-night dinner."

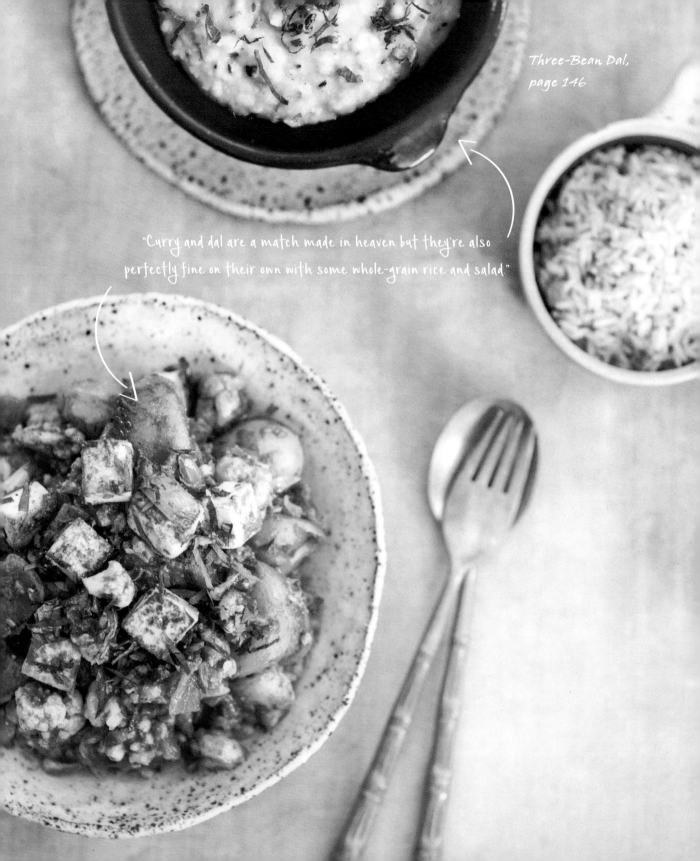

Three-Bean Dal,
page 146

"Curry and dal are a match made in heaven but they're also
perfectly fine on their own with some whole-grain rice and salad"

Tofu is an excellent replacement for chicken and provides beneficial plant protein and isoflavones to guard against chronic disease. Crisping up the tofu before adding to the curry gives it a chewier texture.

INDIAN POTATO, CAULIFLOWER AND TOFU CURRY

PREPARATION: 8 MINUTES, COOKING: 35 MINUTES, SERVES 5

600 g (21 oz) baby potatoes

3 tablespoons extra virgin peanut oil

200 g (7 oz) firm tofu, cut into
    small cubes

2 onions, coarsely chopped

small bunch fresh coriander (cilantro),
    chopped

2 tablespoons Korma curry paste (mild
    or medium hot)

280 g (10 oz) fresh cauliflower, pulled
    apart into small florets

1. Steam potatoes for about 15 minutes until tender, then remove from heat and allow to cool. If the baby potatoes are a little large, halve them.

2. Heat oil in a large saucepan and fry tofu cubes until golden. Remove from pan and place on absorbent paper.

3. Reduce heat, add onions to the remaining oil and sauté until translucent.

4. Dissolve curry paste with ½ cup of water and add to onions.

5. Add cauliflower and 1 cup of boiling water. Cover and simmer for about 15 minutes until the cauliflower becomes tender.

6. Fold in potato, coriander and tofu cubes until the flavours have combined. Add an additional ½ cup of boiling water at this stage if you want more sauce, then heat through and serve. Serve curry with steamed whole-grain rice and some dal for an impressive meal. Curry stores well in the fridge for 2 days but is unsuitable for freezing.

TIPS:

- Be sure to remove excess moisture from the tofu with kitchen towelling to prevent spitting when you add it to the oil.
- Serve my Three-Bean Dal (page 146) or Pakistani-style Dal with Green Chilli (page 175) with this curry.

Per serve: energy 974 kJ (233 Cal); protein 5 g; fat 14 g; saturated fat 2 g; cholesterol 0 mg; carbohydrate 19 g; sugars 5 g; fibre 5 g; calcium 46 mg; iron 2.2 mg; sodium 239 mg

This special dal combines the flavours and textures of three different types of beans—a tip I picked up from Indian chefs in London! Ideal to spoon over tenderly cooked whole-grains and serve with a salad. (Recipe image, page 144.)

THREE-BEAN DAL

PREPARATION: 10 MINUTES, COOKING: 35 MINUTES, SERVES 6

½ cup red lentils

½ cup channa dal (split and skinned desi chickpeas)

½ cup moong dal (split and skinned mung beans)

1 large onion, finely chopped

1 teaspoon salt

½ teaspoon turmeric

1 tablespoon extra virgin olive oil

1 teaspoon cumin seeds

1 teaspoon chilli flakes

3 cloves garlic, crushed

3 tablespoons fresh coriander (cilantro), chopped

1. Pick over and rinse lentils and dal. Place in a large pot with onion, salt, turmeric and 5 cups of water, and bring to boil. Reduce heat and simmer, half-covered, for 15-20 minutes until soft, stirring frequently so lentils and dal don't stick to the bottom of the pot.

2. Heat oil in a frypan. Add cumin seeds and fry for about 1 minute until they start to pop. Add dried chilli and continue frying for another 5 seconds. Add garlic, removing pan from heat as soon as garlic begins to turn golden so it doesn't burn.

3. Stir hot oil mixture through lentils and dal, and place in a serving dish. Garnish with chopped coriander. Recipe stores well in the fridge for several days and will thicken upon storage. It also freezes well.

TIPS:

- Omit chilli if you prefer a less spicy flavour.
- Use yellow split peas if you can't find channa dal, but split peas are firmer so best soaked first, as they take a little longer to cook.

Per serve: energy 755 kJ (180 Cal); protein 12 g; fat 4 g; saturated fat 1 g; cholesterol 0 mg; carbohydrate 21 g; sugars 3 g; fibre 7 g; calcium 48 mg; iron 3.3 mg; sodium 392 mg

Split peas are the characterising ingredient of this tangy Persian curry, which is both low GI and very high fibre. Traditionally known as "lape khoresht", this delicacy commonly includes a few baby potatoes or even some green peas. It is also made with lamb, but this meat-free version is much healthier. (Recipe image, page 149.)

PERSIAN SPLIT PEA, LIME AND TOMATO CURRY

PREPARATION: 10 MINUTES, COOKING: 55 MINUTES, SERVES 6

2 tablespoons extra virgin olive oil

1 large onion, chopped

2 cloves garlic, crushed

1½ teaspoons turmeric

1½ teaspoons curry powder

½ teaspoon hot paprika

2 cups passata (tomato puree)

1 x 10 g (⅓ oz) chicken-style vegetable stock cube

2 cups yellow split peas, washed and drained

2 dried Persian limes

½ bunch fresh coriander (cilantro), chopped

1. Heat oil in a deep saucepan, and sauté onion and garlic until soft.

2. Mix in spices, passata and stock cube, dissolved in 2 cups of boiling water.

3. Add split peas and bring to boil. Turn down heat and simmer, covered, for approximately 50 minutes or until the peas are very soft. Stir regularly so peas do not stick to the bottom of the pan, gradually adding an extra 2½ cups or more of boiling water as the mixture thickens and peas absorb the water.

4. Crush limes into halves with your hands and add to curry. Continue cooking for another 10 minutes so the flavour permeates curry. Allow to rest for at least 20 minutes and remove limes before serving. Serve with steamed whole-grain rice and garnish with freshly chopped coriander. Recipe freezes well.

TIPS:

- Buy dehydrated limes at a Persian grocery store or use lime juice, to taste.
- If desired, add baby potatoes and a little more water halfway through the cooking process.
- The longer you leave in limes, the more sour the flavour that will develop. You can leave limes in curry overnight and remove them the next day before serving.

Per serve: energy 831 kJ (198 Cal); protein 10 g; fat 8 g; saturated fat 1 g; cholesterol 0 mg; carbohydrate 24 g; sugars 9 g; fibre 6 g; calcium 34 mg; iron 2.1 mg; sodium 234 mg

Known as "ghormeh sabzi", this popular Persian dish is traditionally made with kidney beans, lamb and lots of herbs, including fenugreek leaves. Variations include this lighter, meat-free version with black-eyed beans and the more readily available herbs. While it will take some time, this dish can be made in advance and is perfect for leftovers. The extraordinary amount of herbs and the lemon juice come together to create a unique flavour, rich in antioxidants and low GI.

PERSIAN HERB STEW WITH BLACK-EYED BEANS

PREPARATION: 20 MINUTES, COOKING: 1 HOUR 15 MINUTES, SERVES 6

2 cups black-eyed beans
3 tablespoons extra virgin olive oil
1 large onion, chopped
2 cloves garlic, minced
½ teaspoon salt
1 teaspoon turmeric
2 teaspoons curry powder
1½ teaspoons paprika
2 bunches flat parsley
2 bunches dill
2 bunches coriander (cilantro)
3 cups stock made with 1 x 10 g (⅓ oz) chicken-style vegetable stock cube
½ cup lemon juice (about 2 juiced lemons)

1. Add beans to a medium saucepan and cover with double the amount of water. Bring to boil and cook for approximately 15 minutes until they are three-quarters cooked. Drain and put aside.
2. Meanwhile, thoroughly wash herbs and spin dry using a salad spinner, then chop finely.
3. Heat oil in a large saucepan, and sauté onions and garlic until soft.
4. Stir in salt and spices, being careful not to burn them.
5. Add chopped herbs and sauté gently for about 5 minutes, stirring frequently, until they start to turn dark green.
6. Mix in parboiled beans and stock. Cover and bring to boil, then turn down heat and simmer for approximately 20 minutes until beans are soft. Tip: The stew should be soupy but not too runny once cooked. It will thicken further on standing.
7. Stir through lemon juice and cook for a few more minutes to amalgamate the flavours. Serve hot over whole-grain rice or polenta. A dollop of yogurt makes a nice accompaniment. Recipe is suitable for freezing.

TIP:

- *To save time, pulse herbs in a blender rather than chopping with a knife. You can also pre-chop batches of herbs and freeze for later use.*

Per serve: energy 1470 kJ (351 Cal); protein 22 g; fat 22 g; saturated fat 3 g; cholesterol 0 mg; carbohydrate 12 g; sugars 8 g; fibre 16 g; calcium 212 mg; iron 9.8 mg; sodium 444 mg

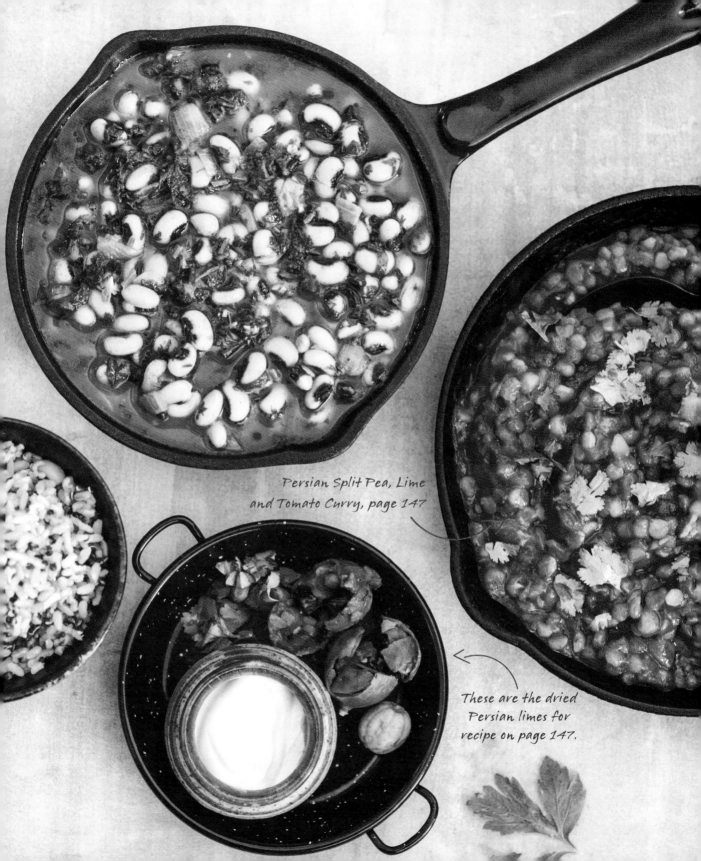

Persian Split Pea, Lime and Tomato Curry, page 147

These are the dried Persian limes for recipe on page 147.

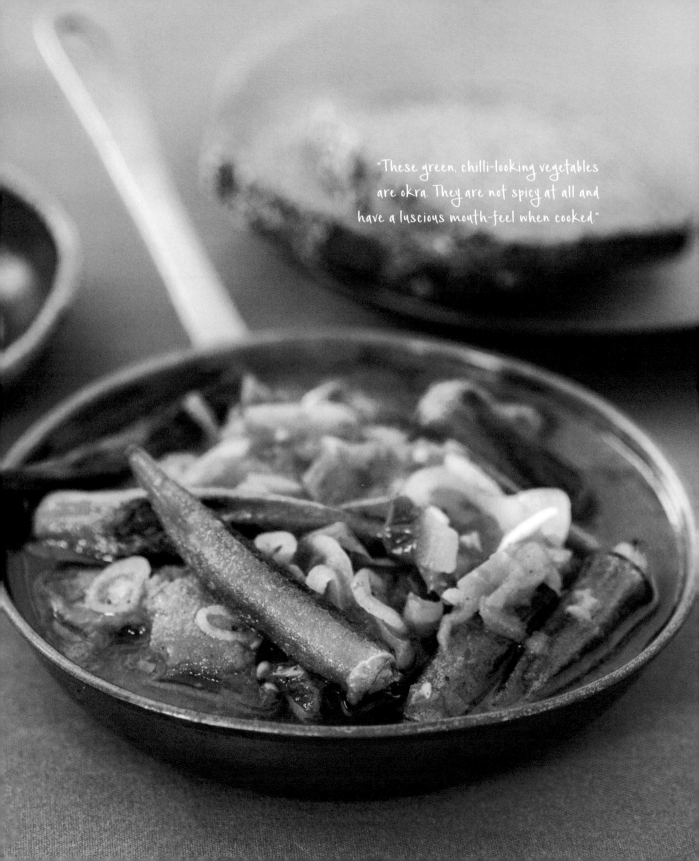

"These green, chilli-looking vegetables are okra. They are not spicy at all and have a luscious mouth-feel when cooked."

Originally from Africa, okra is prized in Indian, Caribbean, Mediterranean and Middle Eastern cookery. Called "bemi" in Lebanon, and also known as "ladies fingers" or "bhindi" in India, this is a tasty way to cook okra—a potent cholesterol-lowering vegetable due to its high content of viscous fibres. It will also help regulate your blood sugar and insulin levels.

OKRA IN FRAGRANT TOMATO SAUCE

PREPARATION: 5 MINUTES, COOKING: 35 MINUTES, SERVES 4

3 tablespoons extra virgin olive oil
1 onion, sliced thinly into rings
3 cloves garlic, crushed
2 soft medium-sized tomatoes, sliced
1 teaspoon allspice or Arabic seven spices
1 teaspoon ground cumin
1 teaspoon salt
pepper, to taste
400 g (14 oz) okra, washed and dried

1. Heat 2 tablespoons of the oil in a medium saucepan, and sauté onion and garlic until translucent. Stir in tomato, spices, salt and pepper. Cook, covered, for a few minutes until tomato dissolves.
2. Add 2 cups of water and bring to boil, then turn down heat and simmer, covered, for approximately 10 minutes.
3. Meanwhile, heat remaining oil in a non-stick pan and sauté okra over medium heat until it begins to brown, approximately 10 minutes. This step helps reduce the excessive "lusciousness" of okra (due to high content of soluble fibre) when you eat it.
4. Add browned okra to tomato mixture and continue to simmer, covered, for a further 15 minutes or until the okra is soft without falling apart. Serve with whole-grain bread or wholemeal Lebanese bread plus some plain yogurt or soy yogurt on the side.

TIPS:

- Look for firm, small green okra (no longer than 8 centimetres/3 inches) as these are most tender. A brownish tinge indicates they are stale. Avoid any that appear shrivelled or feel very soft when gently squeezed.
- You can also buy frozen, sliced okra from Indian grocery stores, but it will ooze more "lusciousness."
- Okra is used in curries, vegetable stews and soups.

Per serve: energy 753 kJ (180 Cal); protein 4 g; fat 14 g; saturated fat 2 g; cholesterol 0 mg; carbohydrate 7 g; sugars 7 g; fibre 5 g; calcium 106 mg; iron 2 mg; sodium 587 mg

The way the eggplant is prepared in this dish is delicious—perfect for sandwiches or as part of a simple meal with bread and salad. Eggplants (aubergines) are rich in viscous fibre, which lowers elevated cholesterol and regulates blood sugar levels. They should be used regularly as part of any healthy diet.

CRISPY EGGPLANT CUTLETS WITH PAPRIKA AND GARLIC SAUCE

PREPARATION: 15 MINUTES, COOKING: 45 MINUTES, SERVES 8

1 kg (2 lb 3 oz) eggplant (aubergine) (about 2 medium)

⅓ cup plain wholemeal flour

¾ cup extra virgin olive oil

½ teaspoon salt + ¼ teaspoon

2 teaspoons sweet paprika

1 teaspoon dried oregano

freshly crushed black pepper, to taste

4 cloves garlic

2 slices wholemeal/whole-grain bread

2 tablespoons lemon juice

1. Pre-heat oven to 200°C (390°F). Prepare 2 baking trays by drizzling with ¼ cup of olive oil.

2. Trim stalks and base of eggplants and slice lengthwise into 1-centimetre (½-inch) thick cutlets.

3. Place flour onto a plate with a lip and dust eggplant cutlets so they are coated on both sides. Lay cutlets on baking trays, slightly overlapping each other.

4. Drizzle cutlets with the remaining oil and 2 tablespoons of water, then season with ½ teaspoon of salt followed by paprika, oregano and pepper, and place in oven. Bake for 30 minutes or until golden.

5. Meanwhile, puree garlic cloves with bread (first softened in ¼ cup of water), lemon juice, the remaining salt and ¾ cup of additional water in blender until a smooth and runny sauce is formed.

6. Remove eggplant from oven and pour the garlic sauce over it. Return to oven for another 15-20 minutes, until sauce is absorbed and eggplant is crisp.

7. Cut into squares or pull off pieces and serve hot or cold. Recipe stores well in the fridge for several days.

TIP:

- Avoid layering eggplant cutlets right up to the edge of the trays to prevent burning.

Per serve: energy 1113 kJ (266 Cal); protein 4 g; fat 22 g; saturated fat 3 g; cholesterol 0 mg; carbohydrate 11 g; sugars 4 g; fibre 5 g; calcium 61 mg; iron 0.9 mg; sodium 269 mg

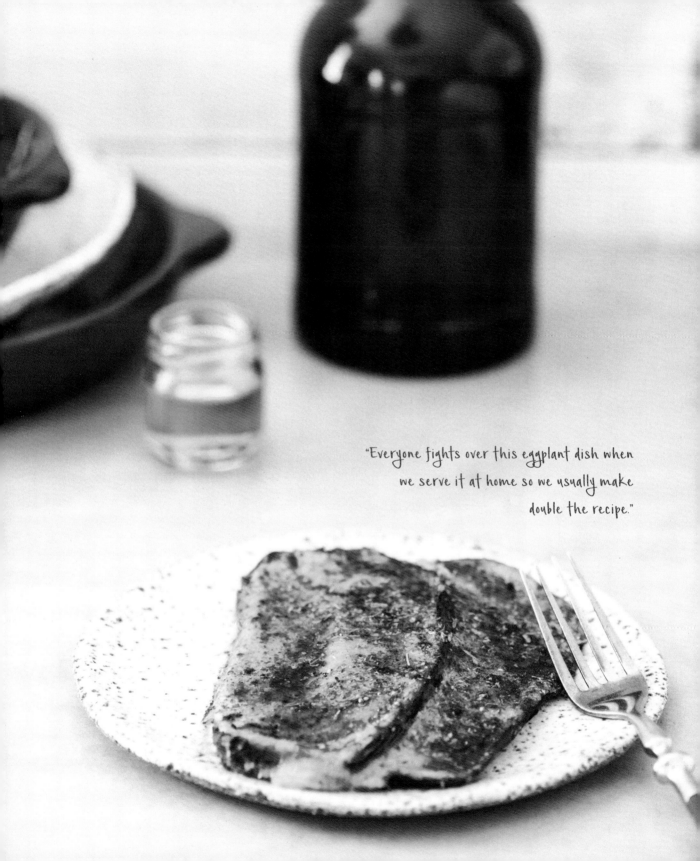

"Everyone fights over this eggplant dish when
we serve it at home so we usually make
double the recipe."

This great-tasting sauce with Mediterranean flavours is perfect for pasta or rice—and you can get it on the table fast! Lentils are ideal to replace red meat, particularly mince, and are loved by kids due to their soft texture. They are a good source of protein and minerals, such as iron, and promote intestinal health.

LENTIL, OLIVE AND SEMI-DRIED TOMATO PASTA SAUCE

PREPARATION: 5 MINUTES, COOKING: 20 MINUTES, SERVES 4

2 tablespoons extra virgin olive oil
1 large onion, finely chopped
2 cloves garlic, crushed
½ teaspoon ground coriander
½ teaspoon ground cumin
400 g (14 oz) can brown lentils
500 g (17½ oz) tomato pasta sauce
12 small pieces semi-dried tomatoes
12 pitted kalamata olives
2 tablespoons fresh dill, chopped

1. Heat oil in a medium saucepan and sauté onion for a few minutes until soft. Stir in garlic for another 30 seconds and then spices, being careful not to burn.
2. Add lentils, tomato pasta sauce, semi-dried tomatoes and olives, and bring to boil, then turn down heat and simmer, stirring occasionally, for 10 minutes. Add dill and serve hot on top of whole-grain pasta or rice.

TIPS:

- You can buy organic brown lentils in BPA-free cans from some greengrocers and health-food stores. Or cook your own lentils and freeze in 1½-cup portions to replace 1 can.
- Chop leftover dill immediately and freeze for later use to avoid waste.

Per serve: energy 1265 kJ (302 Cal); protein 11 g; fat 15 g; saturated fat 2 g; cholesterol 0 mg; carbohydrate 25 g; sugars 14 g; fibre 10 g; calcium 87 mg; iron 4 mg; sodium 758 mg

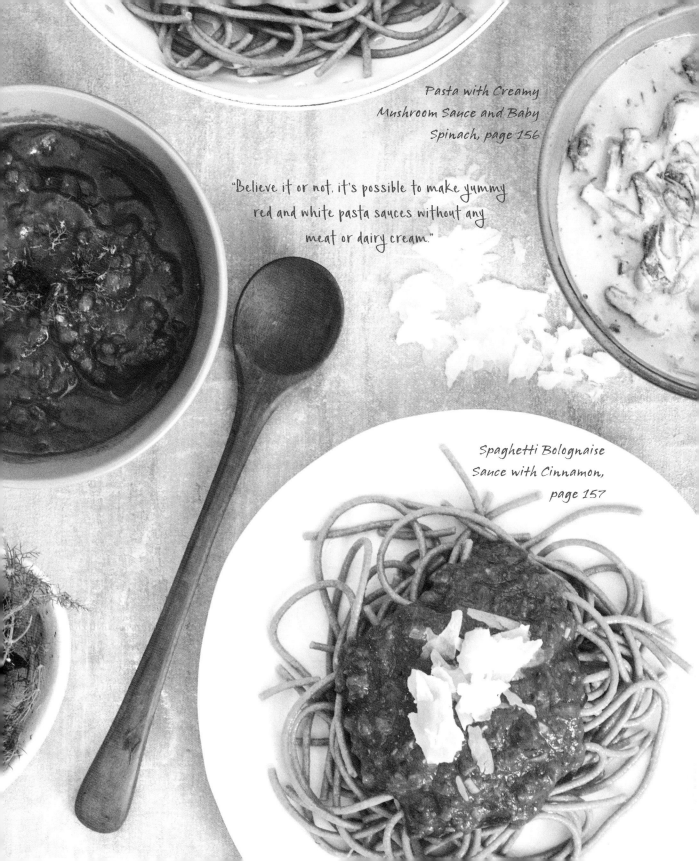

Pasta with Creamy
Mushroom Sauce and Baby
Spinach, page 156

"Believe it or not, it's possible to make yummy
red and white pasta sauces without any
meat or dairy cream."

Spaghetti Bolognaise
Sauce with Cinnamon,
page 157

Love a creamy sauce but don't want all that artery-clogging dairy fat? Here is my lovely version based on tahini, which is cholesterol-free and low in saturated fat. Mushrooms are anti-inflammatory and important for immunity. "Vitamin D mushrooms" also provide a good source of this vital nutrient, which promotes calcium absorption into the body for strong bones. (Recipe image, page 155.)

PASTA WITH CREAMY MUSHROOM SAUCE AND BABY SPINACH

PREPARATION: 15 MINUTES, COOKING: 20 MINUTES, SERVES 6

400 g (14 oz) dry penne pasta

1 tablespoon extra virgin olive oil

400 g (14 oz) vitamin D button
  mushrooms, wiped over and sliced

1 teaspoon salt

¼ teaspoon chilli flakes

3 cloves garlic, crushed

handful of coriander (cilantro), chopped

¾ cup tahini

¼ cup lemon juice (about 1 juiced lemon)

100 g (3½ oz) baby spinach leaves,
  lightly chopped

1. Cook pasta for 7 minutes or until *al dente*. Drain.

2. Meanwhile, heat olive oil in a large, deep frypan and sauté mushrooms for 5-7 minutes, until they release their juices and start turning golden brown.

3. Season with salt and chilli flakes, then stir in garlic and coriander, and cook for 1 minute.

4. In a small jug, blend tahini, 1½ cups of water and lemon juice—the mixture will look curdled at this stage—then pour over mushrooms and bring to boil. Cook for 1 minute, stirring constantly, until sauce just starts to thicken, and becomes smooth and creamy.

5. Stir in spinach and cook for 30 seconds until it just starts to wilt. Add drained pasta and serve immediately. A fresh leaf-and-tomato salad makes a nice accompaniment.

TIPS:

- Tahini is made by grinding sesame seeds into a thin paste. Buy it from Middle Eastern grocery stores and health-food stores.
- You can also use ordinary button mushrooms. "Vitamin D mushrooms" are available from specialty grocers. Make your own by exposing mushrooms to sunlight. Leaving them in the midday summer sun for just 10-15 minutes will generate enough vitamin D for your daily needs in just one serve (100 g or 3 button mushrooms).

Per serve: energy 2089 kJ (499 Cal); protein 17 g; fat 24 g; saturated fat 3 g; cholesterol 0 mg; carbohydrate 49 g; sugars 1 g; fibre 8 g; calcium 136 mg; iron 3.4 mg; sodium 421 mg

This is a really easy meat-free bolognaise, based on textured vegetable protein (TVP), an extruded product made from soybean flour. TVP is inexpensive and, as it's dehydrated, has a long shelf life in the pantry. The recipe packs in the flavour, while providing a good source of soy protein and isoflavones to keep your cholesterol in check. A perfect meal for the whole family. (Recipe image, page 155.)

SPAGHETTI BOLOGNAISE SAUCE WITH CINNAMON

PREPARATION: 4 MINUTES, COOKING: 25 MINUTES, SERVES 6

1 cup dehydrated textured vegetable protein (TVP)
3 tablespoons extra virgin olive oil
1 medium onion, peeled and finely chopped
2 cloves garlic, crushed
½ teaspoon salt
2 teaspoons dried sweet basil
pinch ground hot paprika
2 tablespoons tomato paste
1 cinnamon stick
500 g (17½ oz) tomato pasta sauce

1. Place TVP in a small bowl and cover with ⅔ cup of boiling water. Set aside and allow to rehydrate while preparing other ingredients.
2. Heat oil in a medium saucepan, and sauté onion and garlic until soft and translucent.
3. Stir in salt, basil, paprika, tomato paste, cinnamon stick, hydrated TVP, tomato pasta sauce and 1½ cups of boiling water, which you have used to wash out the tomato pasta sauce bottle.
4. Cover saucepan and bring to boil, then turn down heat and simmer for 15 minutes, half-covered, stirring occasionally. Serve hot on top of spaghetti with a sprinkle of parmesan cheese or nutritional yeast seasoning (dairy-free alternative). Sauce will store well in the fridge for 4 days and freezes well.

TIPS:

- For an alternative meat-free "mince," replace TVP with frozen Quorn (mycoprotein) from the supermarket.
- Wholemeal spaghetti will boost the fibre content of your meal.
- Substitute regular pasta with konnyaku (konjac) spaghetti to lower the carb and calorie content.

Per serve: energy 805 kJ (192 Cal); protein 9 g; fat 12 g; saturated fat 2 g; cholesterol 0 mg; carbohydrate 12 g; sugars 7 g; fibre 7 g; calcium 66 mg; iron 1.6 mg; sodium 557 mg

This sauce is stunningly different but easy to make. It is reminiscent of exotic Persian flavours combining eggplant, currants and cumin. Like okra, eggplant is rich in viscous fibres, which absorb water many times their own weight to form a gel that binds bile acids (the body's building blocks for cholesterol). Viscous fibre is also fermented in the colon to form short-chain fatty acids, which promote intestinal health and slow down the liver's production of cholesterol.

PASTA SAUCE WITH EGGPLANT, RED CAPSICUM AND CURRANTS

PREPARATION: 5 MINUTES, COOKING: 30 MINUTES, SERVES 4

2 tablespoons extra virgin olive oil
½ medium red capsicum (bell pepper), chopped into small pieces
1 medium eggplant (aubergine), sliced into chips
½ tablespoon ground cumin
2 cloves garlic, crushed
500 g (17½ oz) tomato pasta sauce
¼ cup currants
pinch salt
pinch hot paprika
12 pitted kalamata olives
2 tablespoons chopped coriander (cilantro)

1. Heat oil in a medium saucepan and sauté capsicum until soft.
2. Add eggplant chips and mix with capsicum. Cover pan and sauté on medium heat for about 10 minutes, until eggplant softens and starts turning golden brown. Stir occasionally, so eggplant doesn't burn. It will release some juices.
3. Add cumin and garlic, and fry for 1 minute. Mix in tomato pasta sauce, currants, salt, hot paprika and an extra ½ cup of water. Allow sauce to simmer, half-covered, for another 10 minutes, until flavours combine.
4. Toss in olives and coriander, and serve sauce hot on top of cooked whole-grain pasta. Both spirali and penne work well.

TIP:

- Use a mandoline to slice the eggplant with the blade designed for cutting chips/French fries.

Per serve: energy 1065 kJ (254 Cal); protein 5 g; fat 15 g; saturated fat 2 g; cholesterol 0 mg; carbohydrate 22 g; sugars 18 g; fibre 7 g; calcium 86 mg; iron 2.9 mg; sodium 957 mg

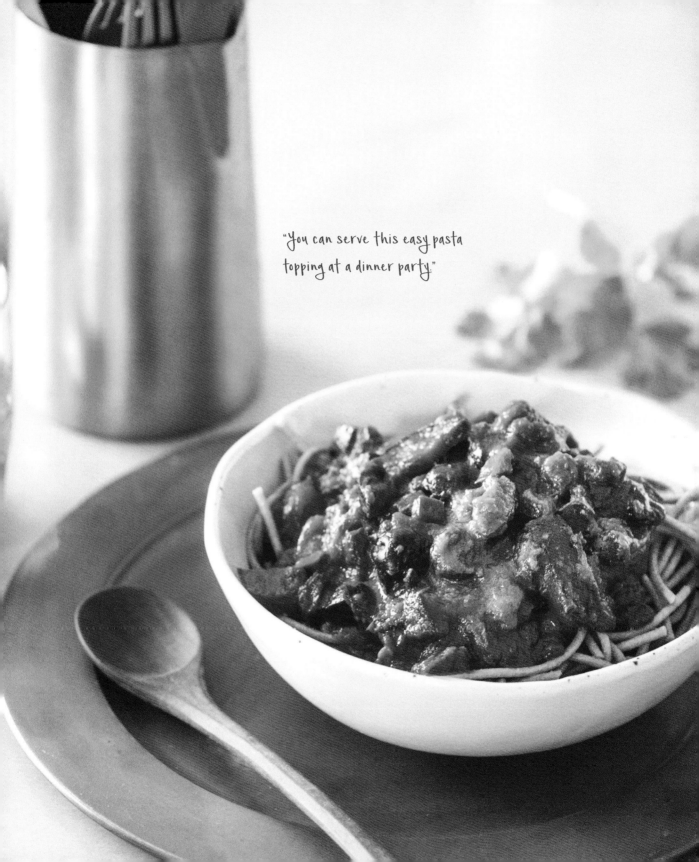

"You can serve this easy pasta topping at a dinner party."

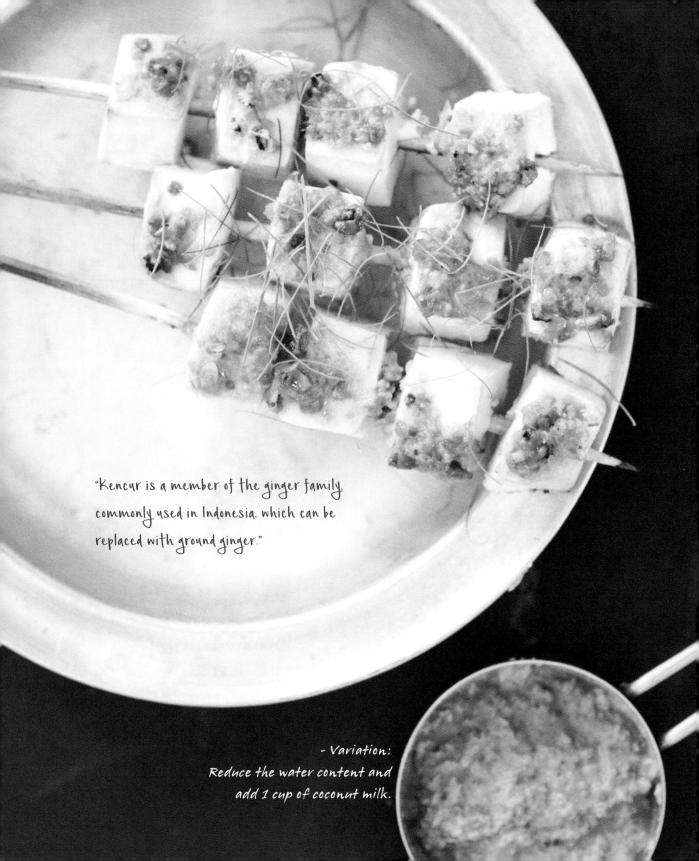

"Kencur is a member of the ginger family, commonly used in Indonesia, which can be replaced with ground ginger."

- Variation:
Reduce the water content and add 1 cup of coconut milk.

A delicious replacement for chicken or beef satay! The sauce can also be enjoyed over steamed vegetables. Tofu is made from soybeans, traditionally recognised in Asia as "meat from the soil." Peanuts are also a legume and can help regulate blood sugar levels. This recipe is rich in calcium and iron.

TOFU SKEWERS WITH INDONESIAN SATAY SAUCE

PREPARATION: 15 MINUTES, COOKING: 35 MINUTES, SERVES 6

12 wooden skewers, pre-soaked in water for 30 minutes
250 g (9 oz) roasted, unsalted peanuts
1 tablespoon brown sugar
1 tablespoon light soy sauce
1 tablespoon dark soy sauce
3 kaffir lime leaves for cooking + 1 leaf for garnish, finely sliced
½ teaspoon ground kencur
½ teaspoon ground hot chilli
2 tablespoons lemon juice
600 g (21 oz) firm tofu

1. Grind peanuts in a food processor for less than 1 minute, until they resemble the texture of coarse sand with some small pieces, then transfer to a medium saucepan.

2. Add sugar, soy sauces, kaffir lime leaves, kencur, hot chilli and 2 cups of water. Mix well and bring to boil. Turn down heat slightly and simmer for about 10 minutes until sauce starts to thicken, stirring frequently so it doesn't burn. Remove from heat and mix in lemon juice. Remove kaffir lime leaves.

3. Meanwhile, cut tofu into 48 cubes and thread 4 onto each skewer. Place skewers on a baking tray and brush tofu with some of the satay sauce. Grill for 10-15 minutes until warmed through or heat on a barbecue.

4. Serve skewers on a platter and drizzle with remaining satay sauce or serve on the side in a small bowl. Garnish with kaffir lime.

TIPS:

- The combination of light and dark soy sauces is vital to achieve the desired colour.

- Cook sauce in advance and refrigerate for up to 1 week or freeze for 2 months. Sauce will thicken on standing, and can be thinned down with a little boiling water before serving.

- Swap brown sugar with palm sugar, which is made from the sap of palm trees and has a more caramel flavour. Buy it in blocks from Asian grocery stores and grate required amount.

Per serve: energy 1604 kJ (383 Cal); protein 23 g; fat 27 g; saturated fat 4 g; cholesterol 0 mg; carbohydrate 8 g; sugars 5 g; fibre 11 g; calcium 348 mg; iron 4 mg; sodium 421 mg

A delicious slow-cooked Mediterranean dish to enjoy over several days. These giant white beans, called "gigantes" in Greece, are buttery and tender. They can be prepared without soaking and are first boiled, then cooked in the oven with herbs and spices. Lima beans are a terrific protein source, as well as being low GI and high in viscous fibre, which lowers elevated cholesterol.

BAKED GIANT LIMA BEANS IN TOMATO SAUCE

PREPARATION: 15 MINUTES, COOKING: 1 HOUR 20 MINUTES INCLUDING PRESSURE COOKER, SERVES 8

500 g (17½ oz) Lima beans
2 whole onions, peeled, cross cut
half-way down each onion
2 carrots, cut lengthwise then sliced
1 teaspoon salt
8 tablespoons extra virgin olive oil
½ cup tomato puree (passata) or
pasta sauce
1 teaspoon dried oregano
black pepper, to taste
half bunch parsley
handful of leaves from celery stalks
handful of fresh mint leaves

1. Rinse Lima beans and place with 6 cups of water into the base of a pressure cooker or ordinary pot. Bring to the boil and cook, uncovered, for 3 minutes. Drain.

2. Rinse the pressure cooker and add back the beans together with 4 cups of water, onions (half bury them with the cross-side down), carrots, salt and oil. Secure lid and bring to pressure, then turn down heat to very low and cook for 4 minutes. Remove from heat and allow the pressure to come down naturally, then remove lid. (To cook conventionally, add 6 cups of water instead, and boil for about 60 minutes until beans are soft cooked but still whole.)

3. Pre-heat oven to 180°C (350°F).

4. Remove whole onions from pressure cooker and place directly into a large baking dish (40 cm x 26 cm/16 in x 10 in). Mash onions with a fork until soft, then transfer remaining beans and contents of pressure cooker to the dish.

5. Add oregano, pepper, tomato and fresh herbs, coarsely chopped, including their stalks. Mix gently until all ingredients are evenly dispersed.

6. Bake for about 1 hour until most of the liquid has been absorbed. The dish will thicken on standing. Serve hot or cold with bread and salad.

TIP:

- Complete steps 1-2 the day before to save time.

Per serve: energy 1743 kJ (416 Cal); protein 20 g; fat 31 g; saturated fat 5 g; cholesterol 0 mg; carbohydrate 11 g; sugars 7 g; fibre 14 g; calcium 144 mg; iron 6.6 mg; sodium 314 mg

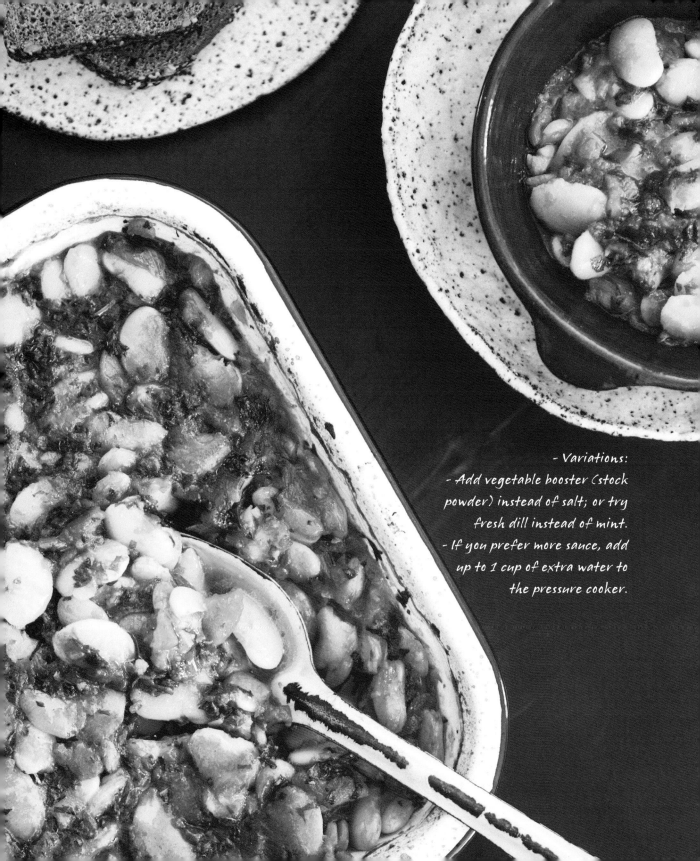

- Variations:
- Add vegetable booster (stock powder) instead of salt; or try fresh dill instead of mint.
- If you prefer more sauce, add up to 1 cup of extra water to the pressure cooker.

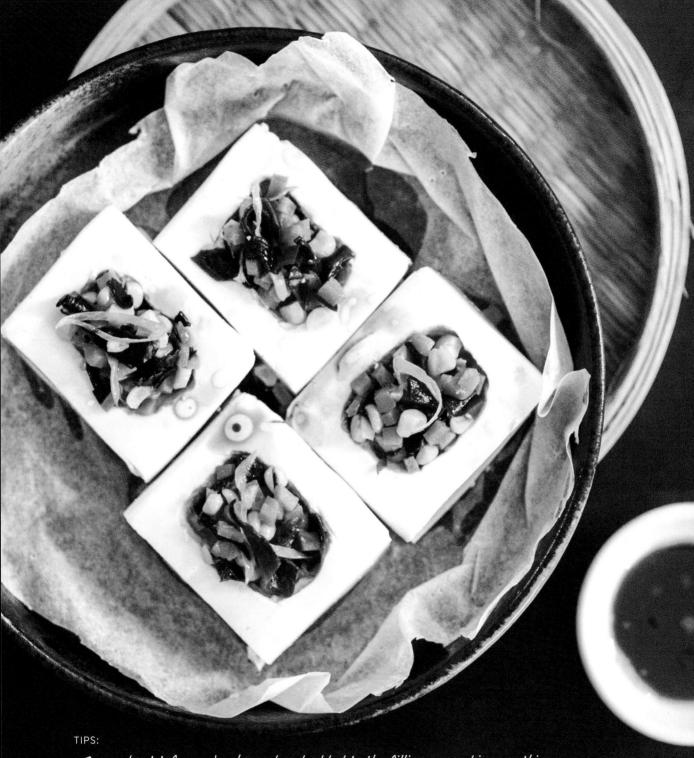

TIPS:
- Scooped out tofu can be chopped and added to the filling or used in smoothies.
- Add finely chopped red chilli to the dressing if you want more heat.

This recipe idea was shared with me by one of my Chinese dietetic staff, whose mother used to make it for her as a young girl to encourage her to eat tofu. It's delicious served as a main with a side of tenderly cooked whole-grains and steamed bok choy or you can serve it on its own as a starter. Tofu is a traditional soy food, linked in many studies with a reduced risk of breast and prostate cancers, as well as heart disease. Soy protein also lowers elevated cholesterol.

TOFU TREASURE CHESTS

PREPARATION: 15 MINUTES, COOKING: 15 MINUTES, SERVES 6

2 x 530 g (19 oz) packets firm tofu, pre-cut in 6 deep squares

Filling
1 tablespoon extra virgin olive oil
kernels removed from ¼ cob fresh corn
½ carrot, finely diced
2 shallots (scallions), finely sliced
3 dried Chinese mushrooms

Dressing
1 tablespoon extra virgin olive oil
1 tablespoon salt-reduced soy sauce

1. Cover mushrooms with boiling water and soak until soft, approximately 20 minutes. Drain and squeeze out excess moisture, then finely dice.
2. Using a melon baller or metal teaspoon, scoop out a deep hole in the middle of each tofu square to prepare a space for the filling. Position tofu squares into the base of a large steamer. Note: If bamboo, line steamer with perforated parchment (baking) paper.
3. Heat oil for the filling in a small frypan, and sauté corn, carrot, shallots and mushrooms for 5 minutes.
4. With the aid of 2 teaspoons, pile filling in the hole of each tofu square to create a "treasure chest."
5. Steam treasure chests for 7 minutes.
6. Remove from steamer, using a spatula, and place on a serving platter. Combine dressing and drizzle over just before serving. Leftovers can be stored in the fridge for several days. Recipe is unsuitable for freezing.

TIPS:
- Filling can be prepared in advance and refrigerated until required.
- Rub a little cornstarch into each tofu hole to help filling stay inside. Add a little cornstarch to the filling, as it is being sautéed, to make it more sticky.

Per serve: energy 1228 kJ (293 Cal); protein 22 g; fat 19 g; saturated fat 3 g; cholesterol 0 mg; carbohydrate 2 g; sugars 1 g; fibre 13 g; calcium 571 mg; iron 5 mg; sodium 200 mg

This tender and succulent dish was inspired from the Szechuan region in China, but it's not super spicy. It's quick to make and delicious as well! Eggplants are rich in viscous fibres and help lower blood sugar and cholesterol, if raised. The wood ear gives a lovely contrast in texture and boosts the fibre content.

SZECHUAN-STYLE EGGPLANT AND WOOD EAR

PREPARATION: 20 MINUTES, COOKING: 15 MINUTES, SERVES 5

25 g (1 oz) dried Chinese wood ears

¼ cup salt-reduced soy sauce

1 tablespoon honey

1 tablespoon balsamic vinegar

1 tablespoon cornstarch

2 fresh red birdseye chillies, finely chopped

2.5-centimetre (1-inch) knob fresh ginger, grated

2 cloves garlic, crushed

800 g (28 oz) eggplants (aubergines), about 2 medium

¼ cup extra virgin olive oil

green part of 2 shallots (scallions), thinly sliced for garnish

1. Place wood ears in a small bowl and cover with boiling water to rehydrate while preparing other ingredients. When soft, squeeze well to remove excess moisture and slice into strips.

2. To prepare marinade, combine soy sauce, honey, balsamic vinegar, cornstarch, chilli, ginger, garlic and ⅓ cup of water in a small glass jug. Mix well and put aside.

3. Using a chip slicer or knife, cut eggplants into small strips the size of French fries.

4. Heat half the oil in a large frypan or wok and add half the eggplant strips. Sauté over medium heat for about 5 minutes or until eggplant softens and turns golden. Tip: Cover with lid so eggplant will release its juices, stirring occasionally. Transfer cooked eggplant to a side plate while you repeat with the second batch of eggplant using remaining oil.

5. Return all eggplant back to pan and add wood ear slices and marinade. Cook for a few minutes, stirring constantly, until sauce thickens. Serve immediately with Asian greens over whole-grain rice, wholemeal pasta or steamed barley, and garnish with shallots. Recipe stores well in the fridge for 2 days and can be reheated.

TIP:

- *Wood ear is also known as Chinese black fungus (from the mushroom family). It is available from Asian grocery stores and some supermarkets.*

Per serve: energy 801 kJ (191 Cal); protein 5 g; fat 12 g; saturated fat 2 g; cholesterol 0 mg; carbohydrate 13 g; sugars 10 g; fibre 6 g; calcium 44 mg; iron 1 mg; sodium 454 mg

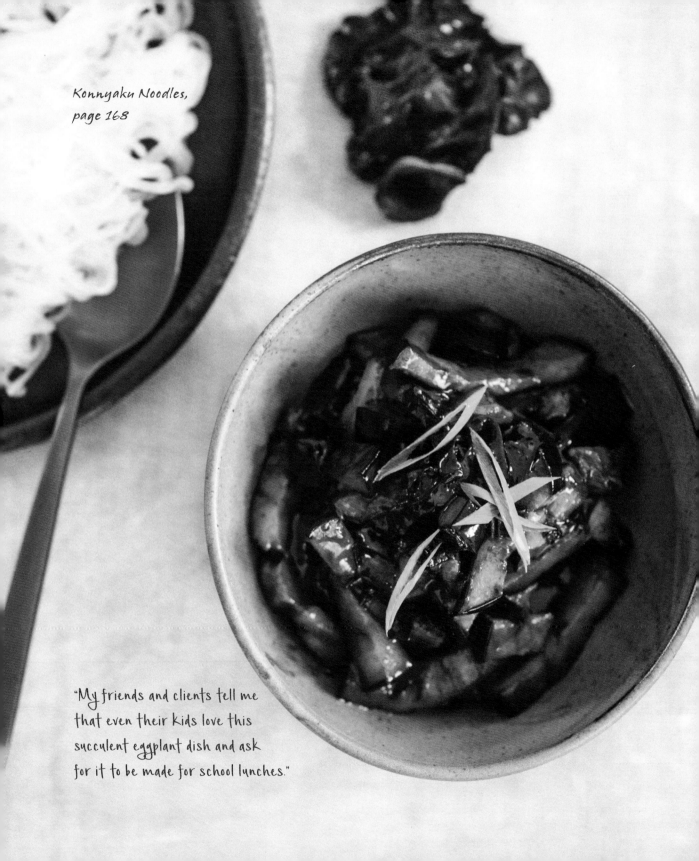

Konnyaku Noodles,
page 168

"My friends and clients tell me
that even their kids love this
succulent eggplant dish and ask
for it to be made for school lunches."

Very low in carbs and total calories, Konnyaku (as it is known in Japanese), or konjac, is made from the root of a plant in the taro family. It has a gentle, rubbery texture, a bland taste and an unforgettable fishy smell! The trick is to prepare it properly so there is no odour and the noodles can absorb more sauce. Here is the simplest way, based on how the Japanese do it, as they have been using konnyaku for centuries. Konnyaku is comprised mainly of a type of fermentable soluble fibre called glucomannan, which promotes intestinal health. Konnyaku also lowers cholesterol and improves insulin sensitivity and blood pressure. It is gluten-free. (Recipe image, page 167.)

KONNYAKU NOODLES

PREPARATION: 5 MINUTES, COOKING: 12 MINUTES, SERVES 4

500 g (17½ oz) drained konnyaku noodles
2 teaspoons extra virgin olive oil

1. Boil 6 cups of water in a medium saucepan.
2. Rinse noodles well, then place into boiling water. Bring water back to boil and cook for 3 minutes. Drain in a colander.
3. Heat a medium frypan, add noodles and dry on high heat for a few minutes, stirring constantly, until they become very bouncy and squeaky. You will hear a sizzling sound and see steam coming off. When noodles start to stick, it's a good sign they don't have much water left in them.
4. Remove from heat and stir in oil. Serve hot or refrigerate and enjoy cold as a side dish. Do not freeze konnyaku or it will become rubbery.

TIPS:

- Konjac can be purchased in supermarkets and comes in various shapes and sizes, such as spaghetti, angel hair, fettucine, lasagne sheets, noodles and rice. Traditional konnyaku is available in Asian grocery stores as blocks and balls.
- For soup noodles, simply slice a block of konnyaku into thin strips.
- Store unused, uncooked konnyaku in a bowl, submerged in water, for up to 1 week in the fridge.

Per serve: energy 135 kJ (32 Cal); protein 0 g; fat 0 g; saturated fat 0 g; cholesterol 0 mg; carbohydrate 0 g; sugars 0 g; fibre 6 g; calcium 0 mg; iron 0 mg; sodium 5 mg

This is a most delicious curry that uses coconut milk rather than dairy cream, which is more commonly used in Indian curries. Vegetables have a starring role and provide many types of antioxidants. The cabbage and eggplant will soften up and help thicken the juices. Perfect for a cool evening! (Recipe image, page 170.)

CREAMY COCONUT, POTATO AND VEGETABLE CURRY

PREPARATION: 15 MINUTES, COOKING: 55 MINUTES, SERVES 6

2 tablespoons extra virgin olive oil

2 large cloves garlic, crushed

5 tablespoons medium hot Tikka Masala paste

4 Sebago potatoes, peeled and cut into cubes

1 tablespoon medium Madras curry powder

½ teaspoon ground cumin

¼ small cabbage (250 g/9 oz), finely shredded with a knife

¼ cauliflower (250 g/9 oz), broken up into florets

2 finger eggplants (aubergines—175 g/ 6 oz), sliced lengthwise and cut into pieces

½ teaspoon salt, optional

1 x 270 g (9½ oz) can light coconut milk

7 fresh curry leaves

1. Heat oil in a large pot and sauté garlic for 30 seconds.

2. Add curry paste and cook over low heat, stirring constantly, for 3 minutes or until the oil separates.

3. Add potato chunks and cook for approximately 10 minutes on medium high, stirring frequently and scraping the bottom of the pan, until curry paste infuses into the potato and the potato starts to soften at the edges.

4. Mix in curry powder and cumin, and cook for another minute.

5. Add remaining vegetables and sauté for a few minutes until they also absorb the curry flavours.

6. Stir in salt and coconut milk followed by 2 cups of water. Cover with lid, then turn up heat and simmer for about 20 minutes or until potato is cooked through, mixing every 5 minutes to ensure vegetables don't burn.

7. Sprinkle in curry leaves and simmer for a further 10 minutes. Serve hot on top of steamed whole-grain rice. The curry flavour further improves the next day. Recipe can be stored in the fridge for several days.

TIPS:

- *Starchy potatoes are best as they soften easily around the edges.*
- *Use any leftover vegetables from your fridge, such as broccoli. Combinations of carrot, potato and frozen peas or eggplant and potato make a good curry.*
- *Add fried tofu cubes or a can of chickpeas toward the end of the cooking process to add more plant protein.*

Per serve: energy 1017 kJ (243 Cal); protein 5 g; fat 16 g; saturated fat 5 g; cholesterol 0 mg; carbohydrate 16 g; sugars 5 g; fibre 7 g; calcium 76 mg; iron 2.9 mg; sodium 834 mg

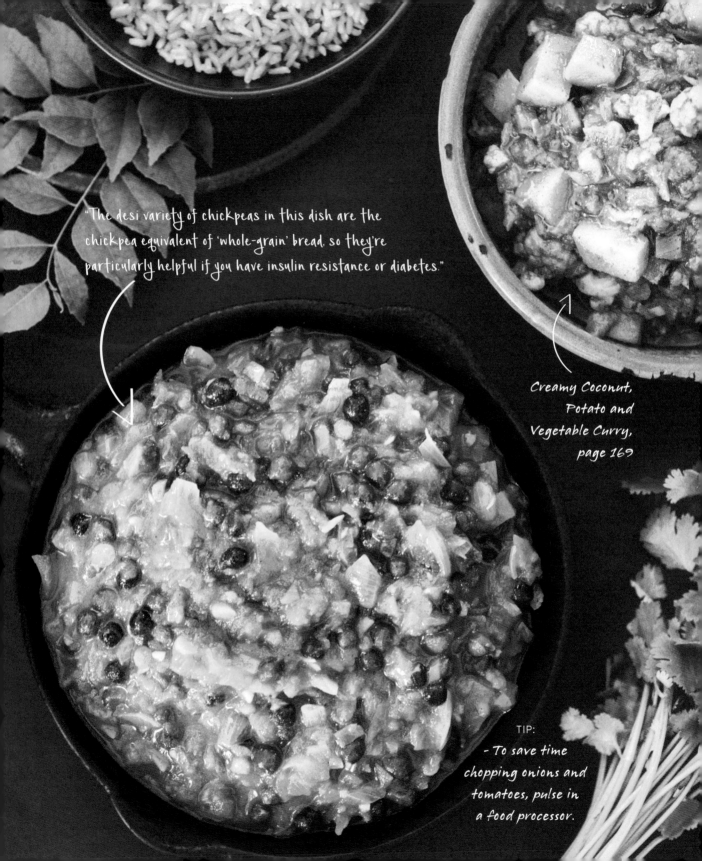

"The desi variety of chickpeas in this dish are the chickpea equivalent of 'whole-grain' bread, so they're particularly helpful if you have insulin resistance or diabetes."

Creamy Coconut, Potato and Vegetable Curry, page 169

TIP:
- To save time chopping onions and tomatoes, pulse in a food processor.

This delicious home-style Indian curry uses desi chickpeas. These are the smaller, dark brown chickpeas, which contain even higher amounts of dietary fibre and polyphenols than the more commonly available cream Kabuli variety. Desi chickpeas were traditionally considered healthier by Indian people and research has confirmed they do have a super low GI of 11! Perfect if you have diabetes or need to better control your blood sugar or insulin levels.

INDIAN BROWN CHICKPEA AND TOMATO CURRY

PREPARATION: 15 MINUTES + OVERNIGHT SOAKING, COOKING: 40 MINUTES, SERVES 5

1 cup small brown (desi variety) chickpeas (garbanzos)

3 tablespoons extra virgin olive oil

2 medium onions, finely chopped

2 cloves garlic, crushed

4 large ripe tomatoes, finely diced

1 teaspoon salt

2 teaspoons curry powder

½ cup freshly chopped coriander (cilantro) leaves + few extra for garnish

1. Soak chickpeas overnight in plenty of water. Drain, rinse and drain again, then place in a small saucepan with 2 cups of water. Cover, bring to boil and cook for 20 minutes.

2. Meanwhile, in another medium saucepan, heat oil and sauté onions until soft, adding garlic last. Stir in tomatoes, cover and cook for approximately 15 minutes until tomatoes soften and mixture forms a sauce.

3. Add half of the salt to chickpeas after 20 minutes have elapsed and continue cooking for a further 10 minutes being careful the bottom of the pan does not scorch—add a little extra water, if required. When cooked, these chickpeas will remain firm on the outside, but are tender on the inside when tested with a fork. Drain, if required, reserving the cooking water

4. Add chickpeas and remaining ingredients to tomato sauce and bring to boil. Scoop about 1 cup of mixture into a separate bowl and mash this with the back of a spoon. Return to curry to thicken, cooking for a further 2 minutes. Serve on top of steamed whole-grain rice and garnish with extra coriander. A side salad creates a complete meal. Recipe freezes well and can be refrigerated for several days.

TIPS:

- Desi chickpeas are also known as Tyson peas or kala chana. They are readily available from Indian grocery stores.

- Stir in ¼-½ cup of the reserved chickpea cooking water at the end (or some boiling water from the kettle), if you prefer a thinner curry.

Per serve: energy 1149 (274 Cal); protein 13 g; fat 18 g; saturated fat 3 g; cholesterol 0 mg; carbohydrate 11 g; sugars 8 g; fibre 10 g; calcium 95 mg; iron 4.5 mg; sodium 480 mg

This Egyptian national dish is eaten at every meal of the day with flat bread, particularly at breakfast. It is a bowl of mushy fava beans, lifted by the use of simple seasonings and the various condiments served with it. Traditionally, ful is slow-cooked overnight as fava beans take the longest time to cook compared to other beans. Condiments are offered in small bowls or sprinkled on top of the ful prior to serving. These include olive oil, finely chopped onion, diced tomatoes, fresh chilli or cayenne pepper, crushed raw garlic and an egg.

FUL MEDAMES

PREPARATION: 7 MINUTES, COOKING: 1 HOUR 15 MINUTES, SERVES 5

1 cup light-coloured dried fava beans (broad beans), soaked in water for 24 hours
½ cup red lentils, rinsed, drained
1 teaspoon salt
1½ teaspoons ground cumin
3 tablespoons lemon juice
2 tablespoons extra virgin olive oil

1. Drain and rinse soaked beans, then place in a pressure cooker, together with 4 cups of fresh water. Cover loosely and bring to boil.
2. Once boiling, stir in lentils and salt, then fit the pressure cooker lid securely. Bring to full pressure, then turn down heat to the lowest possible level and cook under pressure for 60 minutes. Note: Transfer the cooker to the smallest burner with the lowest flame so lentils don't burn on the bottom during this extended cooking time.
3. Allow for natural pressure release before opening lid. The ful will look watery but will thicken significantly on standing and refrigeration.
4. Stir in remaining ingredients and allow to sit for 1 hour, to thicken slightly, before serving. Serve ful in individual bowls with your choice of condiments. Refrigerate or freeze leftovers.

TIPS:

- Buy small (baby) fava beans as these don't need peeling after cooking. They are lighter in colour than large fava beans, which are dark brown.
- The Egyptian secret to making this recipe is to add red lentils to thicken the dish.
- If ful is too thick when serving, thin down with some boiling water.

Per serve: energy 610 kJ (146 Cal); protein 11 g; fat 8 g; saturated fat 1 g; cholesterol 0 mg; carbohydrate 3 g; sugars 3 g; fibre 10 g; calcium 50 mg; iron 3 mg; sodium 464 mg

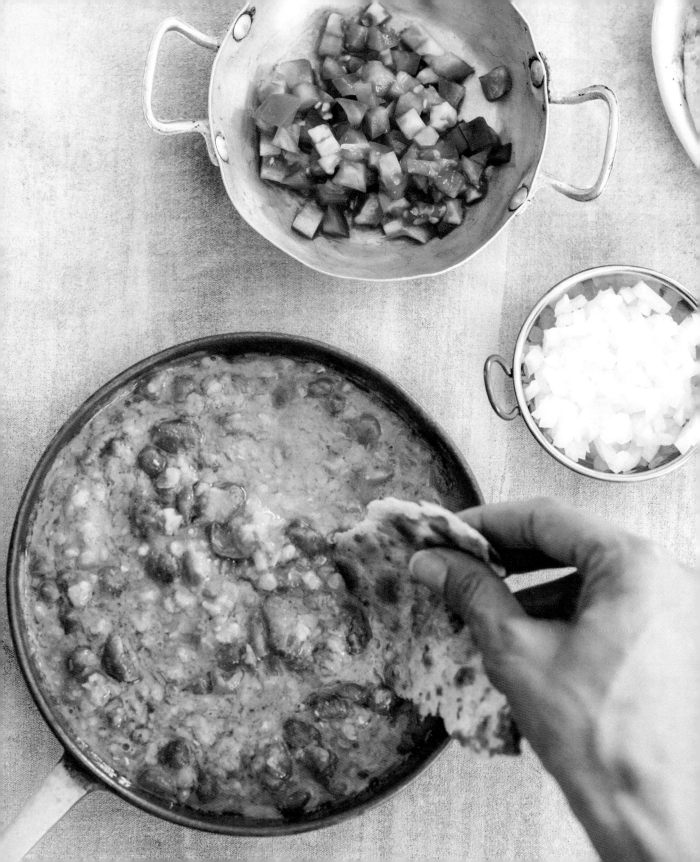

"I make this 'no fuss' dal when really time poor but craving high flavour."

Dal is an easy and delicious dish you can make ahead and serve as a main meal with whole-grain rice or as a side dish with a vegetable curry. Pakistani foods tend to be spicier. The green chilli adds a little heat but is not overly spicy. Lentils are very low GI.

PAKISTANI-STYLE DAL WITH GREEN CHILLI

PREPARATION: 10 MINUTES, COOKING: 30 MINUTES, SERVES 6

1 cup red lentils

1 cup moong dal (split and skinned mung beans)

1 teaspoon curry powder (medium or hot)

10 small curry leaves

1 green chilli, left whole

knob of fresh ginger, grated

2 cloves garlic, crushed

1 teaspoon salt

2 tablespoons extra virgin olive oil

1 onion, finely chopped

¼ bunch fresh coriander (cilantro), chopped + extra leaves for garnish

1. Place lentils and moong dal in a large saucepan, and cover with water. Soak while preparing other ingredients. Drain, rinse and drain again.

2. Add curry powder, curry leaves, chilli, ginger, garlic, salt and 5 cups of water to the rinsed lentils. Bring to boil, then turn down heat slightly and cook, half covered, for 20-25 minutes until dal is soft. Note: Never put a lid on dal when bringing it to boil as this encourages foam to form.

3. Meanwhile, make the tarka (fried onion) by heating oil in a small frypan and sautéing onion until golden brown. Stir into dal, together with chopped coriander, and garnish with extra leaves. Serve hot or cool dal and refrigerate or freeze for later use. Whole chilli can be removed after cooking.

TIPS:

- Dal thickens upon cooling and storage. To thin down, simply add a little boiling water. It will also become thinner just by re-heating.
- Turn leftover dal into rissoles/patties by adding additional binding ingredients such as rolled oats, lupin flour and "chia egg."

Per serve: energy 988 kJ (236 Cal); protein 15 g; fat 7 g; saturated fat 1 g; cholesterol 0 mg; carbohydrate 23 g; sugars 2 g; fibre 10 g; calcium 57 mg; iron 4 mg; sodium 390 mg

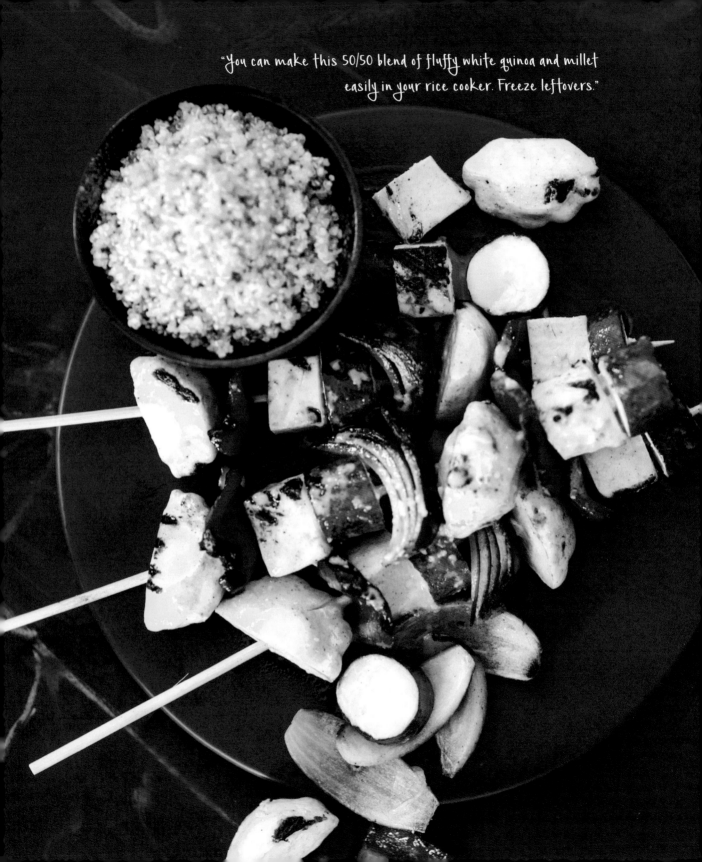

"You can make this 50/50 blend of fluffy white quinoa and millet easily in your rice cooker. Freeze leftovers."

These skewers are a kaleidoscope of colour and flavour. They are easy, fresh and nutritious! Bake them in the oven or throw onto a barbecue or grill. Vegetables and plant protein are much safer for your health than cooking meat on the barbecue or grill!

TOFU AND VEGGIE SKEWERS WITH MISO AND LIME MARINADE

PREPARATION: 20 MINUTES + 1 HOUR MARINATING, COOKING: 15 MINUTES, SERVES 4

300 g (10½ oz) firm tofu, cubed into 16 pieces
8 bamboo skewers
8 yellow baby squash, halved
1 large red capsicum (bell pepper), cubed to match size of tofu
2 zucchinis (courgettes), sliced to form 16 rings and matched to size of tofu
1 large Spanish onion, cut into 6 wedges
extra virgin olive oil spray

Marinade
1 tablespoon shiro (white) miso paste
⅓ cup extra virgin olive oil
¼ cup lime juice (about 2 limes)
1 clove garlic, crushed

1. Add marinade ingredients to a small jar and shake vigorously to combine. Check to ensure miso paste is dissolved.
2. Place tofu in a glass dish with a lid. Pour over marinade to coat all cubes, then cover and refrigerate for 1 hour, turning and shaking a few times over the sink.
3. Meanwhile, soak bamboo skewers in water for 20 minutes to prevent them from burning while cooking.
4. Remove skewers from water and thread each with tofu and vegetables in an alternating fashion, ensuring you don't overpack the skewers. For example, holding the blunt end towards you (at "the handle"), thread squash, capsicum, tofu, zucchini and onion, then repeat the sequence.
5. Pre-heat barbeque or grill and spray with extra virgin olive oil. Place skewers on heat and cook on medium-high about 5 minutes each side. Using leftover marinade, baste skewers regularly while cooking. Serve immediately on a bed of whole-grain couscous or white quinoa and drizzle with leftover marinade.

TIPS:

- Oven instructions: Bake on a lined tray at 180°C (350°F) for 45 minutes, turning once, until slightly browned. Baste well.
- A satay sauce topping is also delicious (see page 161).

Per serve: energy 1398 kJ (334 Cal); protein 14 g; fat 24 g; saturated fat 4 g; cholesterol 0 mg; carbohydrate 10 g; sugars 9 g; fibre 11 g; calcium 284 mg; iron 3.4 mg; sodium 228 mg

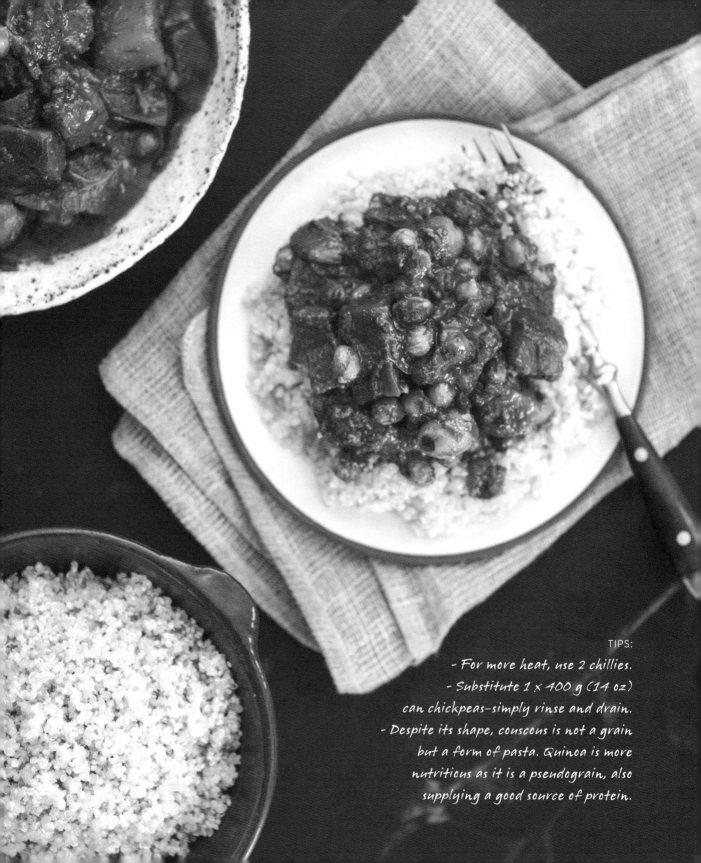

TIPS:
- For more heat, use 2 chillies.
- Substitute 1 x 400 g (14 oz)
can chickpeas—simply rinse and drain.
- Despite its shape, couscous is not a grain
but a form of pasta. Quinoa is more
nutritious as it is a pseudograin, also
supplying a good source of protein.

A hearty dish packed with loads of flavour and goodness. The chermoula paste is well worth the extra effort! It can be made the day before to speed up the cooking process. Spices are rich in antioxidant and anti-inflammatory phytonutrients.

MOROCCAN TAGINE WITH VEGETABLES AND CHICKPEAS

PREPARATION: 17 MINUTES, COOKING: 1 HOUR 5 MINUTES, SERVES 8

Chermoula Paste
1 red onion, quartered
3 cloves garlic
1 bull's eye red chilli, deseeded, chopped
1 tablespoon grated ginger
4 tablespons lemon juice
5 tablespoons extra virgin olive oil
1 tablespoon honey
1 tablespoon cumin
1 tablespoon paprika
1 tablespoon turmeric
1 loosely packed cup coriander (cilantro)

2 tablespoons extra virgin olive oil
1 red onion, cut into chunks
500 g (17½ oz) peeled butternut pumpkin
   (butternut squash), cut into chunks
4 baby eggplants (aubergines), sliced
   lengthwise then halved or cut
   into thirds
1½ cups cooked chickpeas (garbanzos)
12 dried dates
1 bottle (680 g/24 oz) passata (tomato
   puree)
1 teaspoon salt
100 g (3½ oz) green olives

1. Place all chermoula paste ingredients into a food processor and blend until a paste forms. Set aside.
2. In a large, heavy-based saucepan, heat remaining oil, and add onion, pumpkin and eggplant. Stir and cook for 2 minutes over a moderate heat.
3. Stir in chermoula paste and the remaining ingredients, except olives. Rinse out the passata jar with about ½ cup of water to extract any residual tomato and add to mixture. Bring to boil, then reduce heat and simmer, covered, for 45 minutes.
4. Add olives and continue cooking for a further 15 minutes or until vegetables are very soft. Serve hot on top of white fluffy quinoa or whole-grain couscous. Tagine can be frozen.

Per serve: energy 1441 kJ (344 Cal); protein 7 g; fat 21 g; saturated fat 3 g; cholesterol 0 mg; carbohydrate 32 g; sugars 22 g; fibre 9 g; calcium 82 mg; iron 3.1 mg; sodium 607 mg

This is a slow-cooked Greek eggplant dish that is served during the summer. Prepare it on the weekend and enjoy throughout the week with a Greek salad, some bread and olives. The dish should be moist and glossy from the oil. Eggplant is rich in viscous fibres to lower elevated cholesterol and blood sugar.

SUCCULENT EGGPLANT AND TOMATO BAKE

PREPARATION: 15 MINUTES, COOKING: 1 HOUR 5 MINUTES, SERVES 6

900 g (2 pounds) eggplants (aubergines),
   about 2 medium
1 cup extra virgin olive oil
1 large onion, halved and sliced
4 cloves garlic, sliced
600 g (21 oz) ripe Roma tomatoes,
   grated or pureed in food processor
1 teaspoon salt (+ 2 teaspoons for
   rubbing)
freshly ground pepper, to taste
½ bunch parsley, coarsely chopped

1. Cut eggplant into strips (two fingers wide), rub in 2 teaspoons of salt and allow to sit for 30 minutes. Wash and squeeze dry with a clean tea towel (dish towel) or paper towelling.
2. Pre-heat oven to 180°C (350°F).
3. Heat ½ cup of oil in a medium frypan and sauté onions on medium heat for about 10 minutes until translucent. Add garlic and continue cooking for 1 minute. Fold in tomatoes, salt, pepper and parsley, and cook for another 10 minutes until the tomatoes lose their raw appearance.
4. In another large frypan, sauté eggplant in remaining oil for about 10 minutes until just softened, being careful not to brown or overcook it.
5. Transfer eggplant into a shallow baking dish and top with the tomato-sauce mixture, dispersing it evenly. Bake for 40 minutes, then serve hot or refrigerate and enjoy cold. Recipe stores well in the fridge for several days but is unsuitable for freezing.

TIP:

- *When buying fresh parsley, wash and spin dry entire bunches, then chop and freeze for later use in cooking.*

Per serve: energy 1677 kJ (401 Cal); protein 3 g; fat 39 g; saturated fat 6 g; cholesterol 0 mg; carbohydrate 8 g; sugars 8 g; fibre 7 g; calcium 63 mg; iron 1.2 mg; sodium 404 mg

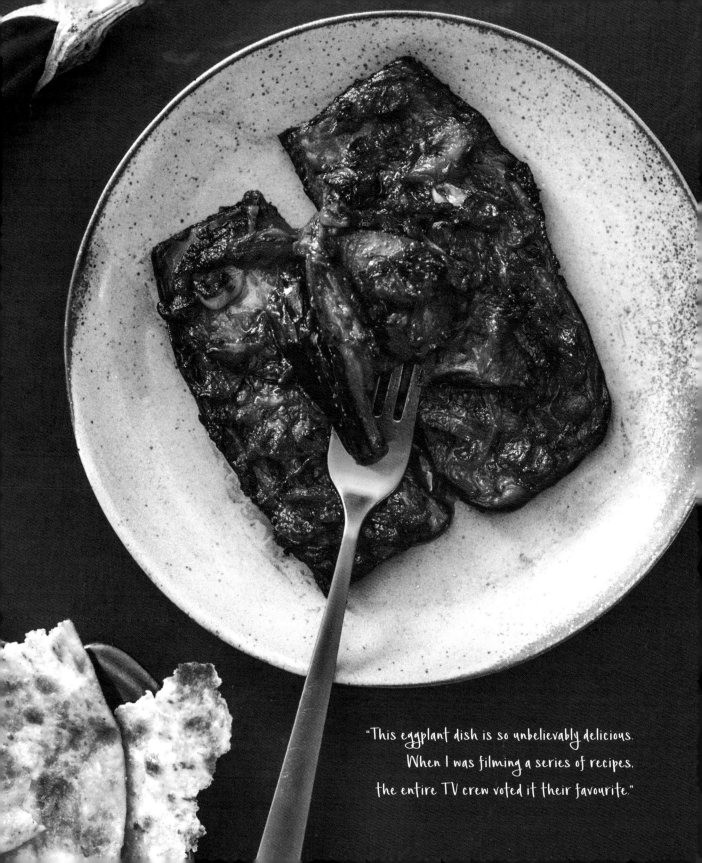

"This eggplant dish is so unbelievably delicious.
When I was filming a series of recipes,
the entire TV crew voted it their favourite."

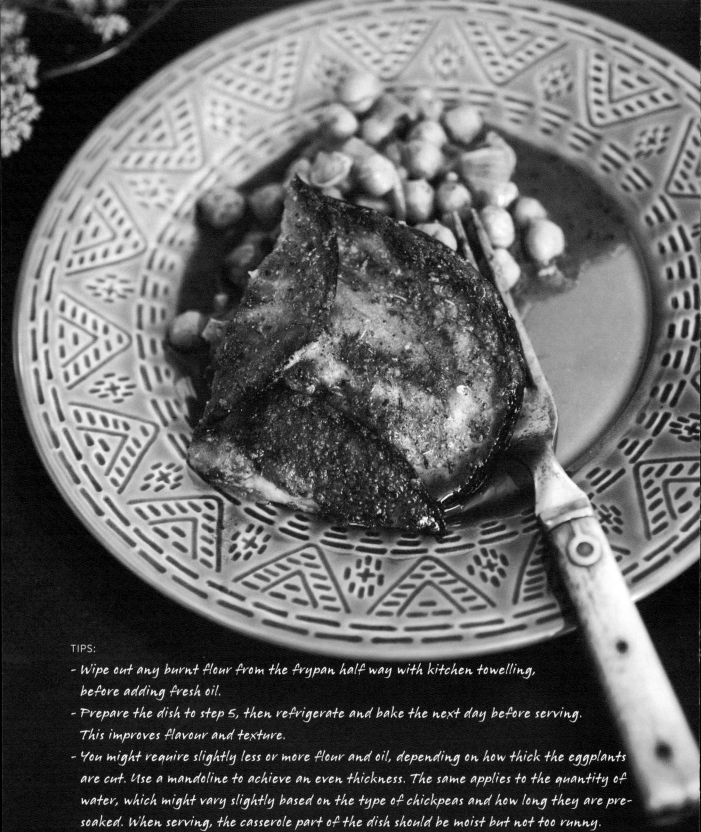

TIPS:

- Wipe out any burnt flour from the frypan half way with kitchen towelling, before adding fresh oil.
- Prepare the dish to step 5, then refrigerate and bake the next day before serving. This improves flavour and texture.
- You might require slightly less or more flour and oil, depending on how thick the eggplants are cut. Use a mandoline to achieve an even thickness. The same applies to the quantity of water, which might vary slightly based on the type of chickpeas and how long they are pre-soaked. When serving, the casserole part of the dish should be moist but not too runny.

Want to try some hearty village food from northern Greece? Try not to fight over the eggplant topping! The chickpeas are creamy and soft, and supply plant protein with low-GI carbs. Make this dish the day before and simply bake when required to crisp up. Serve with Shaved Savoy Cabbage (page 51) and you have a winner.

OVEN-BAKED CHICKPEA CASSEROLE WITH CRISPY EGGPLANT TOPPING

PREPARATION: 20 MINUTES + OVERNIGHT SOAKING, COOKING: 1 HOUR 45 MINUTES INCLUDING PRESSURE COOKER, SERVES 10

Chickpea Casserole
600 g (21 oz) chickpeas (garbanzos),
**   soaked in water overnight**
2 medium onions, coarsely chopped
4 cloves garlic, finely chopped
1 tablespoon sweet Hungarian paprika
1 teaspoon salt
2 teaspoons dried oregano
2 tablespoons extra virgin olive oil

Eggplant Topping
2 medium eggplants (aubergines,
**   800 g/28 oz), unpeeled**
⅓ cup plain white flour
1 cup extra virgin olive oil
2 teaspoons sweet Hungarian paprika
2 teaspoons dried oregano
½ teaspoon salt
freshly crushed black pepper, to taste

1. Rinse and drain chickpeas, and place in a pressure cooker with other casserole ingredients plus 2 cups of water. Mix well, cover with lid and bring to pressure. Turn down heat to very low and cook under pressure for 15 minutes, allowing for natural pressure release before removing lid. (If cooking conventionally in a saucepan, add 7 cups of water and bring to boil. Reduce heat and simmer, covered, for about 2 hours or until chickpeas are very soft, adding salt toward the end of the cooking time.)

2. Transfer cooked chickpeas with their liquid into a large, deep baking dish.

3. Meanwhile, slice eggplants lengthwise into approximately 1-centimetre (½-inch) thick cutlets (about 8 cutlets per eggplant). Pat dry with paper towelling and dust with the flour.

4. Pre-heat oven to 200ºC (390ºF).

5. Heat a small amount of oil in a large frypan and batch fry cutlets until golden, turning once and seasoning the top side with paprika, oregano and salt. Add oil gradually to the pan as the eggplant absorbs it.

6. Layer cutlets on top of the chickpea casserole in the baking dish, overlapping them slightly so they cover the entire surface. Sprinkle with any remaining seasoning and pepper.

7. Bake for 45 minutes or until the eggplant crisps up. Serve hot or at room temperature. Place leftovers immediately into meal-sized containers and freeze for lunches.

Per serve: energy 2116 kJ (506 Cal); protein 21 g; fat 39 g; saturated fat 6 g; cholesterol 0 mg; carbohydrate 14 g; sugars 7 g; fibre 15 g; calcium 140 mg; iron 6.5mg; sodium 356 mg

A delicious Sicilian pasta dish using a super-healthy vegetable–broccoli. Serve with a salad that includes another raw vegetable from the cruciferous family, such as watercress or kohlrabi. This will boost the amount of sulforaphane that can be made from the cooked broccoli. Sulforaphane has potent anti-cancer effects.

PASTA WITH BROCCOLI, SUNDRIED TOMATO AND TOASTED CRUMBS

PREPARATION: 5 MINUTES, COOKING: 30 MINUTES, SERVES 5

320 g (11 oz) broccoli, pulled apart into large florets

2 tablespoons breadcrumbs

2 teaspoons extra virgin olive oil + 5 tablespoons extra for sautéing garlic

320 g (11 oz) dry penne pasta

55 g (2 oz) large whole sun-dried tomatoes (about 6), finely chopped

4 cloves garlic, chopped not crushed

½ teaspoon salt

½ teaspoon dried chilli flakes

1. Steam broccoli for approximately 15 minutes until very soft. Chop roughly into small pieces, no longer than the length of the pasta.

2. Meanwhile, dry toast breadcrumbs in a small frypan until golden. Turn off heat and mix in 2 teaspoons of oil. Put aside.

3. Cook pasta in a large saucepan for 7 minutes or until *al dente*. Drain and place back in the saucepan.

4. Using a medium-sized frypan, heat remaining oil, and sauté tomato, garlic, salt and chilli flakes for a minute, just until they become fragrant.

5. Stir in cooked broccoli pieces, then fold this mixture through cooked pasta.

6. Divide pasta into 5 bowls and sprinkle with prepared crumbs. Serve immediately.

TIP:

- *This is an ideal way to use up leftover broccoli, including the stems, which are often thrown away.*

Per serve: energy 1953 kJ (467 Cal); protein 12 g; fat 22 g; saturated fat 4 g; cholesterol 0 mg; carbohydrate 52 g; sugars 4 g; fibre 7 g; calcium 48 mg; iron 1.9 mg; sodium 282 mg

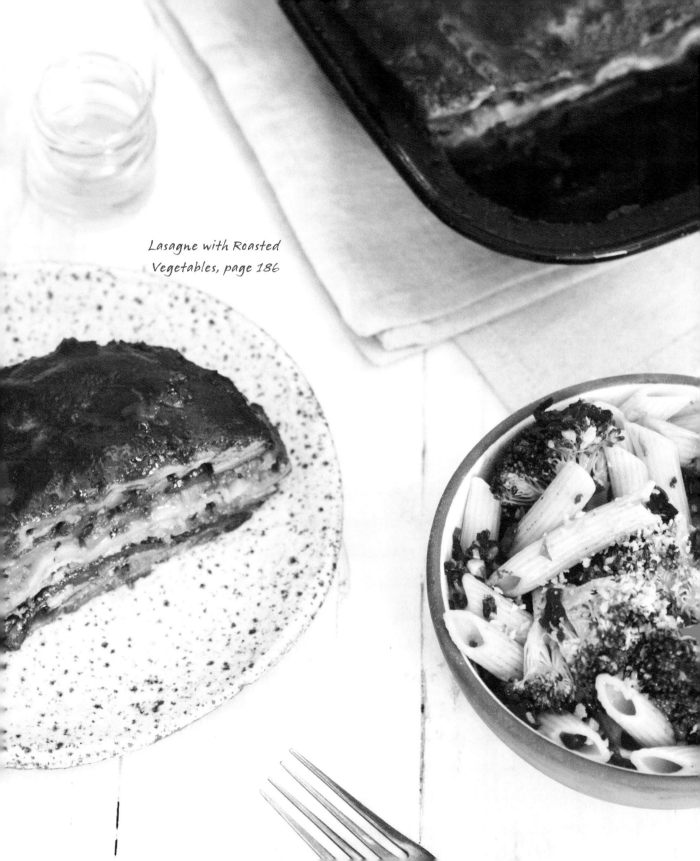

Lasagne with Roasted
Vegetables, page 186

A colourful lasagne that is both dairy-free and meat-free! As it takes a while to prepare, I always make this recipe in stages. Lasagne is also best made the day before, as it is less likely to fall apart. The good news is this recipe will feed a party—but you will require a large lasagne tray. Or halve the recipe and use a small one.

LASAGNE WITH ROASTED VEGETABLES

PREPARATION: 45 MINUTES, COOKING: 1 HOUR 45 MINUTES, SERVES 12

Vegetables

1 kg (2 lb 3 oz) cleaned butternut
   pumpkin (butternut squash), sliced
   ½-centimetre (¼-inch) thick
2 red capsicums (bell peppers), halved
   vertically and deseeded
600 g (21 oz) eggplants (aubergines),
   unpeeled and sliced lengthwise
   0.75-centimetres (⅓-inch) thick
800 g (28 oz) zucchini (courgettes),
   sliced lengthwise 0.75-centimetres/
   ⅓-inch) thick
4 tablespoons extra virgin olive oil

Tofu Ricotta

530 g (19 oz) water-packed firm tofu
½ cup tahini
⅓ cup shiro (white) miso paste
¼ cup extra virgin olive oil
5 cloves garlic
3 teaspoons dried oregano
½ teaspoon salt

Sauce and Assembly

1 tablespoon extra virgin olive oil
6 fresh lasagne sheets (wider and longer
   than dry sheets)
800 g (28 oz) Arrabbiata or tomato
   pasta sauce

Vegetables

1. Place prepared vegetables on 4 oven trays and brush with oil. Bake in a pre-heated oven for 45 minutes at 220°C (430°F). If you have a small oven, you might need to do this in 2 batches. Alternatively, use a grill.
2. When cooked, peel blackened capsicum and cut into strips.

Tofu Ricotta

3. Place all ingredients into a food processor with ⅔ cup of water and puree for a few minutes until smooth. Tofu ricotta can be made the day ahead and also used for other recipes.

Sauce and Assembly

4. Drizzle the base of a large lasagne pan (at least 36 x 25 x 7 cm/14 x 10 x 3 in) with oil and layer with 2 pasta sheets to cover. Note: Trim pasta sheets to fit.
5. Layer with half quantity of baked pumpkin, then half eggplant, capsicum and zucchini.
6. Spoon over one-third of tomato sauce.
7. Spread with half of tofu ricotta.
8. Cover with next 2 sheets of pasta and repeat steps 5-7.
9. Finish with the last 2 sheets of pasta and spoon over remaining tomato sauce.
10. Drizzle ½ cup of water around the edges, cover with foil, then prick foil heavily to allow steam to escape as this will reduce pasta buckling.
11. Bake at 180°C (350°F) for approximately 60 minutes. Allow to cool, then refrigerate for up to 3 days until required. Re-heat in oven for 40 minutes. If lasagne looks dry, add more water around the edges and across the top to hydrate while re-heating.

Per serve: energy 1670 kJ (399 Cal); protein 13 g; fat 23 g; saturated fat 3 g; cholesterol 0 mg; carbohydrate 31 g; sugars 16 g; fibre 11 g; calcium 123 mg; iron 2.9 mg; sodium 788 mg

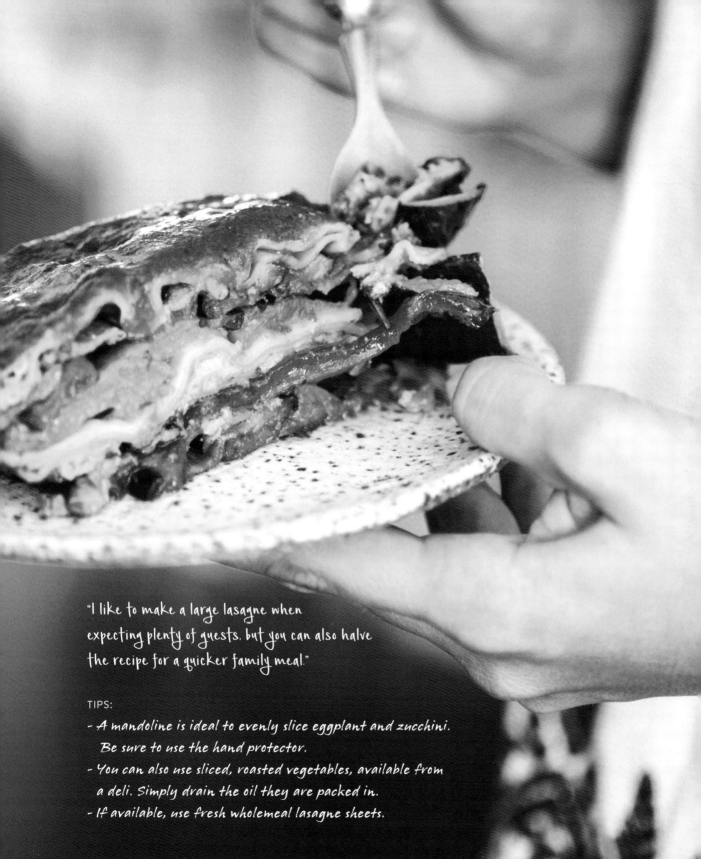

"I like to make a large lasagne when expecting plenty of guests, but you can also halve the recipe for a quicker family meal."

TIPS:
- A mandoline is ideal to evenly slice eggplant and zucchini. Be sure to use the hand protector.
- You can also use sliced, roasted vegetables, available from a deli. Simply drain the oil they are packed in.
- If available, use fresh wholemeal lasagne sheets.

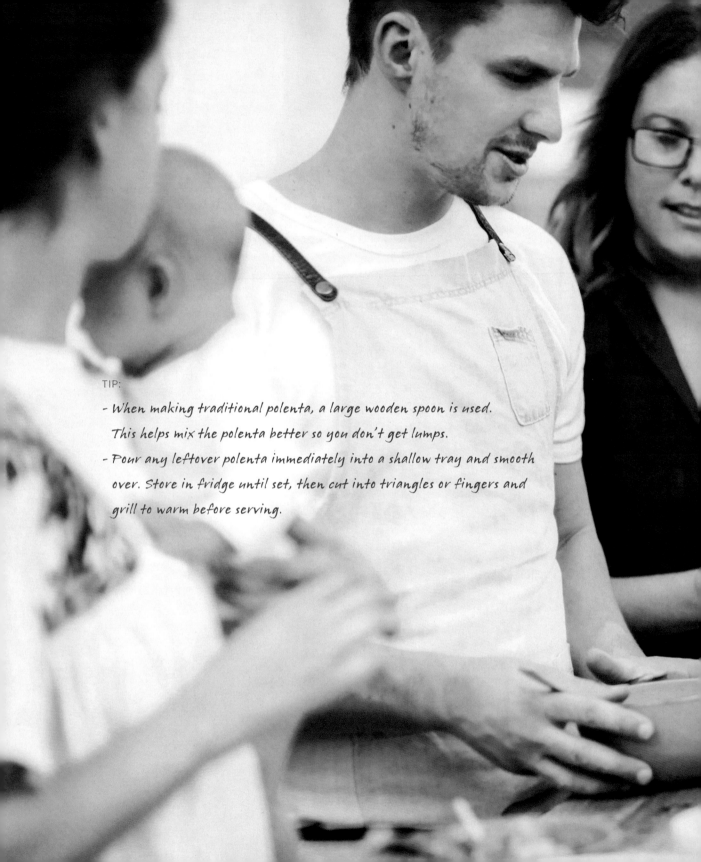

TIP:

- When making traditional polenta, a large wooden spoon is used.
  This helps mix the polenta better so you don't get lumps.
- Pour any leftover polenta immediately into a shallow tray and smooth
  over. Store in fridge until set, then cut into triangles or fingers and
  grill to warm before serving.

A delicious base for stews, dals, roasted vegetables and curries or a creamy porridge for breakfast, polenta is loaded with zeaxanthin, a phytonutrient that protects your eyes from macular degeneration. It also contains large amounts of "resistant starch," especially when cooked and cooled, to promote gut health and guard against bowel cancer. (Recipe image, page 191.)

SOFT YELLOW POLENTA

PREPARATION: 3 MINUTES, COOKING: 30 MINUTES, SERVES 4

1 teaspoon salt

2 cups polenta (yellow maize meal)

1. Place 6 cups of water and salt into a medium pot, cover and bring to boil.

2. Gradually stir in polenta, mixing vigorously with a wooden spoon so no lumps form. Be careful when you have nearly added all the polenta as the mixture will get very hot and might start to spurt.

3. Cover, turn down heat to very low, and cook for about 20 minutes, stirring every 5 minutes.

4. Serve immediately by dishing out into individual plates as the polenta will start to set quickly.

TIPS:

- *Don't use instant polenta as it is more finely ground.*
- *Variation: When fennel is in season, Italians add finely chopped fennel fronds.*
- *Cleaning: Soak the cooking pot overnight. The residual polenta will just lift off and the pot will be easy to clean.*

Per serve: energy 844 kJ (201 Cal); protein 5 g; fat 1 g; saturated fat 0 g; cholesterol 0 mg; carbohydrate 41 g; sugars 0 g; fibre 2 g; calcium 6 mg; iron 0.5 mg; sodium 573 mg

I love blending walnuts with mushrooms instead of using minced meat to make a family favourite. You can serve these hearty meatballs with their delicious sauce on soft polenta or whole-grain spaghetti. The balls are also great hot or cold as an appetiser or salad topping. This recipe is egg-free and dairy-free.

WALNUT AND MUSHROOM MEATBALLS IN TOMATO SAUCE

PREPARATION: 25 MINUTES, COOKING: 30 MINUTES FOR BALLS + 20 MINUTES FOR SAUCE, SERVES 9

Meatballs
250 g (9 oz) mushrooms
½ cup rolled oats
110 g (4 oz) walnuts
2 medium onions, quartered
4 cloves garlic
freshly ground black pepper, ,
   generous amount
1 teaspoon ground cumin
1 teaspoon dried oregano
2 tablespoons soy sauce
200 g (7 oz/about 2 cups) multigrain
   breadcrumbs

Tomato Sauce
½ cup extra virgin olive oil
2 red onions, finely chopped
680 g (24 oz) bottle passata (tomato
   puree)
1 teaspoon salt
8 fresh basil leaves, torn

1. Wipe over mushrooms with a moistened towel and chop roughly. Note: Don't wash mushrooms or they will become soggy. Transfer to a bowl and set aside.
2. Pre-heat oven to 180°C (350°F).
3. Place oats and walnuts into food processor, and process until fine.
4. Add onions and garlic, and continue blending until smooth.
5. Add mushrooms, together with spices and soy sauce, and process until smooth.
6. While the processor is running, drizzle in breadcrumbs through the chute. Continue blending until everything is well combined and mixture has a thick consistency.
7. Moisten hands and form walnut-sized balls from the mixture, then place on an oven tray lined with parchment (baking) paper and bake for 27-30 minutes until golden.
8. Meanwhile, make tomato sauce. Heat oil and sauté onions on medium heat for 7 minutes until very soft. Stir in passata, salt and 1 cup of water used to wash out the passata bottle. Continue simmering for 10 minutes until the sauce thickens. Stir in basil.
9. Serve balls on top of pasta or rice, and drizzle with tomato sauce. Alternatively, add the balls to the hot sauce and gently heat through for 1 minute, being careful not to overcook as the balls may fall apart since they are egg-free. Balls are ideal for freezing.

TIP:

- *You can also use flats or portobello mushrooms, which have a more intense flavour.*

Per serve: energy 1434 kJ (343 Cal); protein 8 g; fat 23 g; saturated fat 3 g; cholesterol 0 mg; carbohydrate 27 g; sugars 10 g; fibre 5 g; calcium 50 mg; iron 1.5 mg; sodium 728 mg

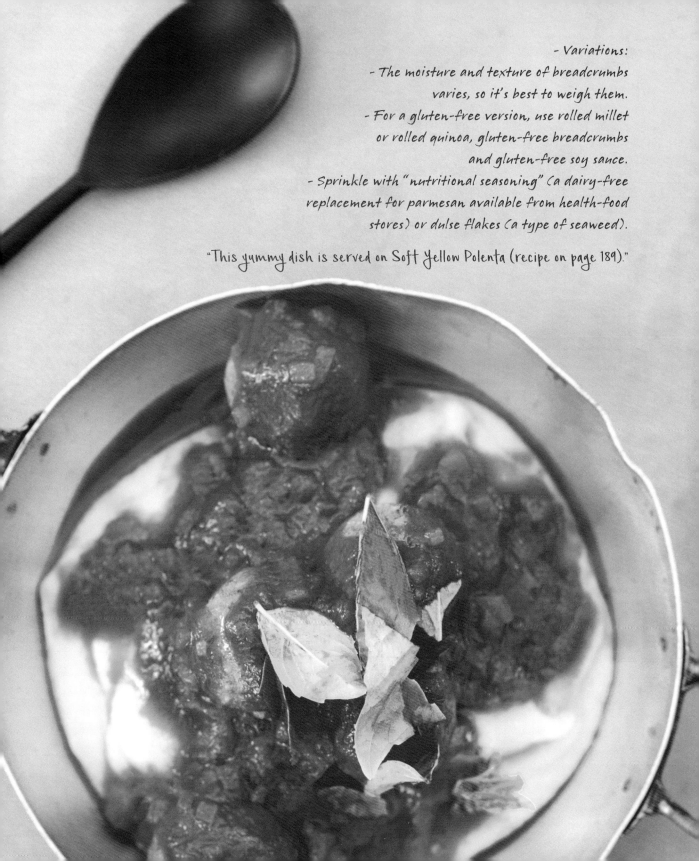

- Variations:
- The moisture and texture of breadcrumbs varies, so it's best to weigh them.
- For a gluten-free version, use rolled millet or rolled quinoa, gluten-free breadcrumbs and gluten-free soy sauce.
- Sprinkle with "nutritional seasoning" (a dairy-free replacement for parmesan available from health-food stores) or dulse flakes (a type of seaweed).

"This yummy dish is served on Soft Yellow Polenta (recipe on page 189)."

SOUPS

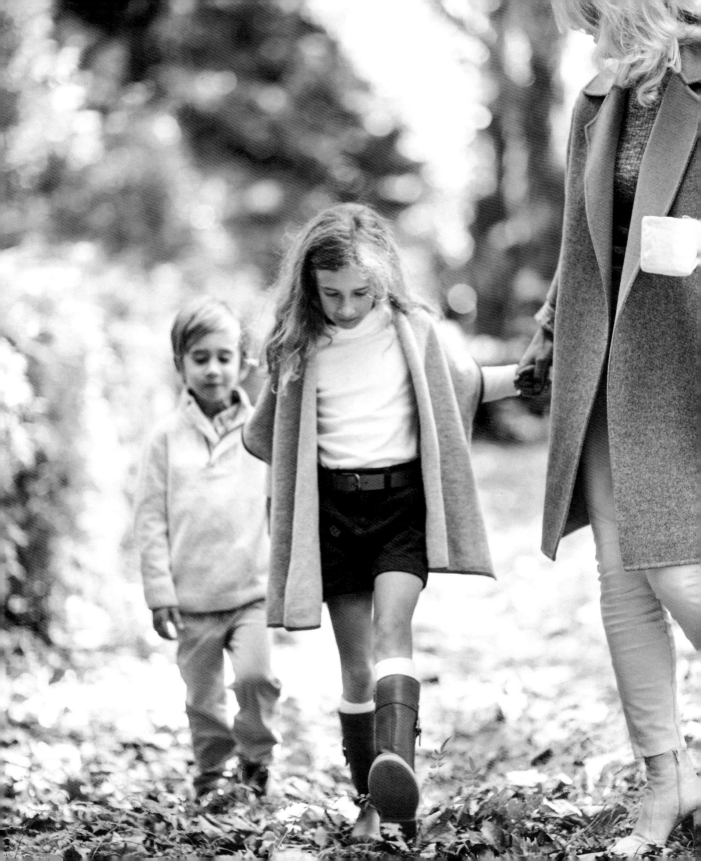

Creamy Celeriac and Cauliflower
Soup, page 197

"Stir chopped coriander through
this soup or blend it before serving."

Chilli Green Pea Soup with
Coriander, page 196

This low-GI soup provides an excellent source of antioxidants and anti-inflammatory phytonutrients –perfect for people with insulin resistance or diabetes. It's one of my favourite meals-in-a-bowl. Red lentils disintegrate with cooking, so they might be the best "gateway" legume. Just add a handful to any soup recipe and nobody knows!

SWEET POTATO, RED LENTIL AND LEMON SOUP

PREPARATION: 10 MINUTES, COOKING: 40 MINUTES, SERVES 4

200 g (7 oz) red lentils, picked over for stones and rinsed

1 x 10 g (½ oz) chicken-style vegetable stock cube, crumbled

1 large onion, peeled and roughly chopped

400 g (14 oz/1 medium) sweet potato, peeled and roughly chopped

2 cloves garlic, peeled

4 tablespoons extra virgin olive oil

1 teaspoon ground cumin

1 cup tomato pasta sauce

2 tablespoons chopped fresh dill

3 tablespoons lemon juice

1. Place washed lentils in a large saucepan with 5 cups of water and stock cube, and bring to boil. Skim the white foam that appears on the surface of the soup and simmer, half-covered, for about 15 minutes or until you prepare the other ingredients.

2. Blend onion, sweet potato and garlic in a food processor until vegetables are finely chopped.

3. Heat oil in a large frypan and add chopped vegetables, cumin and tomato pasta sauce in turn, sautéing for 10 minutes.

4. Add sautéed vegetables to pot of boiling lentils and simmer for a further 15 minutes, stirring occasionally, until flavours amalgamate.

5. Mix in dill and lemon juice and serve hot with some grainy or rye bread. Soup freezes well and the flavour continues to improve. To garnish, top each portion with a round slice of lemon.

TIP:

- Use up any over-ripe tomatoes you might have sitting on the bench, by chopping them and adding to this soup.

Per serve: energy 1855 kJ (443 Cal); protein 16 g; fat 21 g; saturated fat 3 g; cholesterol 0 mg; carbohydrate 44 g; sugars 15 g; fibre 11 g; calcium 97 mg; iron 5.3 mg; sodium 624 mg

A sophisticated yet simple-to-make soup, guaranteed to impress. Research suggests coriander has anti-tumour properties in the colon and enhances insulin secretion from the pancreas, with the seeds having the highest concentration of phytonutrients. In this soup, the leaves add a vibrant note, which blends with the sweetness of the peas and light spiciness of the chilli. (Recipe image, page 194.)

CHILLI GREEN PEA SOUP WITH CORIANDER

PREPARATION: 6 MINUTES, COOKING: 18 MINUTES, SERVES 4

1 tablespoon extra virgin olive oil

1 medium onion, finely chopped

1 small red chilli, deseeded, finely chopped

500 g (17½ oz) frozen green peas

1 x 10 g (⅓ oz) chicken-style vegetable stock cube

½ small bunch coriander (cilantro), finely chopped

1. Heat oil in a medium soup pot, and sauté onion and chilli until very soft.

2. Add frozen peas, crumble in stock cube and add 4 cups of boiling water.

3. Bring contents to boil again, then turn down heat and simmer for 5 minutes.

4. Add chopped coriander leaves and purée soup, using an immersion (stick) blender. Alternatively, allow soup to cool, then transfer to a blender and whiz until smooth. Adjust the flavour with extra pepper, if required. Soup stores well in the fridge for 2 days.

TIP:

- *The flavour of this soup is even better the next day and it can be served cold, similar to gazpacho.*

Per serve: energy 589 kJ (141 Cal); protein 8 g; fat 6 g; saturated fat 1 g; cholesterol 0 mg; carbohydrate 10 g; sugars 4 g; fibre 10 g; calcium 45 mg; iron 2.6 mg; sodium 321 mg

Celeriac is a knobby root vegetable derived from wild celery, which has been used in Europe since ancient times. It is lower in calories than potato, is a good source of vitamin K and contains phytonutrients with possible anti-cancer effects. The strong fragrance of celeriac is reminiscent of a blend of celery and parsley. When cooked, celeriac has an earthy, nutty taste and is simply delicious! (Recipe image, page 194.)

CREAMY CELERIAC AND CAULIFLOWER SOUP

PREPARATION: 15 MINUTES, COOKING: 50 MINUTES, SERVES 6

2 tablespoons extra virgin olive oil

1 medium onion, finely chopped

½ teaspoon cumin

800 g (1 lb 12 oz) peeled celeriac root, roughly chopped into small pieces, leaves washed

400 g (14 oz) cauliflower pieces

1 large potato, peeled and cubed

freshly ground pepper, to taste

2 x 10 g (⅓ oz) chicken-style vegetable stock cubes, made up to 6 cups of stock with boiling water

sprigs fresh parsley, for garnish

1. Heat oil in a soup pot and sauté onion for about 5 minutes until soft. Stir in cumin and cook for 15 seconds.

2. Add celeriac and its leaves, cauliflower, potato, pepper and stock, and bring to boil. Turn down heat and simmer, covered, for 30 minutes until vegetables are soft.

3. Remove from stove, discard leaves and puree soup until smooth using an immersion (stick) blender. Garnish with parsley and serve. Alternatively, cool and refrigerate, then puree soup the next day before re-heating.

TIP:

- Drizzle some truffle oil on top or swirl in some pesto for an amazing flavour boost.

Per serve: energy 658 kJ (157 Cal); protein 5 g; fat 7 g; saturated fat 1 g; cholesterol 0 mg; carbohydrate 13 g; sugars 6 g; fibre 10 g; calcium 81 mg; iron 1.1 mg; sodium 491 mg

This Japanese soup will introduce you to a healthy sea vegetable and two soy products—tofu and miso. Miso is made from fermented soybeans and has a satisfying savoury flavour, while silken tofu is unfermented and melts in the mouth. This soup is a wonderful starter and quick to make. Soy products and sea vegetables are an important part of the traditional Asian diet and their regular use is associated with longevity and a reduced risk of cancer.

MISO SOUP WITH WAKAME AND SILKEN TOFU

PREPARATION: 7 MINUTES, COOKING: 15 MINUTES, SERVES 4

1 tablespoon dried wakame seaweed

4 fresh shiitake mushrooms, washed, stems removed and sliced

150 g (5 oz) silken tofu, cubed into 36 small pieces

2½ tablespoons shiro (white) miso paste

1. Soak wakame in 1 cup of water for 5 minutes, then squeeze dry.

2. Boil 6 cups of water in a medium saucepan. Add wakame and mushrooms to boiling water, and cook for 3 minutes.

3. Turn down heat to medium and add tofu cubes to heat through.

4. Place miso paste into a small bowl and ladle in small amounts of the cooking broth. Dissolve the miso until it forms a thin paste. Gradually stir the paste back into soup and heat through for just 1 minute. Important: Do not boil.

5. Remove soup from heat and serve immediately or cover with lid and re-heat gently when required, but never to boiling point. Soup is unsuitable for freezing.

TIPS:

- Buy wakame and miso in Asian grocery stores. Wakame will expand to about 3 times its volume once rehydrated.

- For a more robust stock, soak dried shiitake mushrooms and a strip of kombu seaweed in the 6 cups of water overnight, then strain prior to using. Slice the mushrooms and kombu, and use in the soup instead of fresh mushrooms.

Per serve: energy 235 kJ (56 Cal); protein 5 g; fat 2 g; saturated fat 0 g; cholesterol 0 mg; carbohydrate 5 g; sugars 3 g; fibre 2 g; calcium 18 mg; iron 1.4 mg; sodium 287 mg

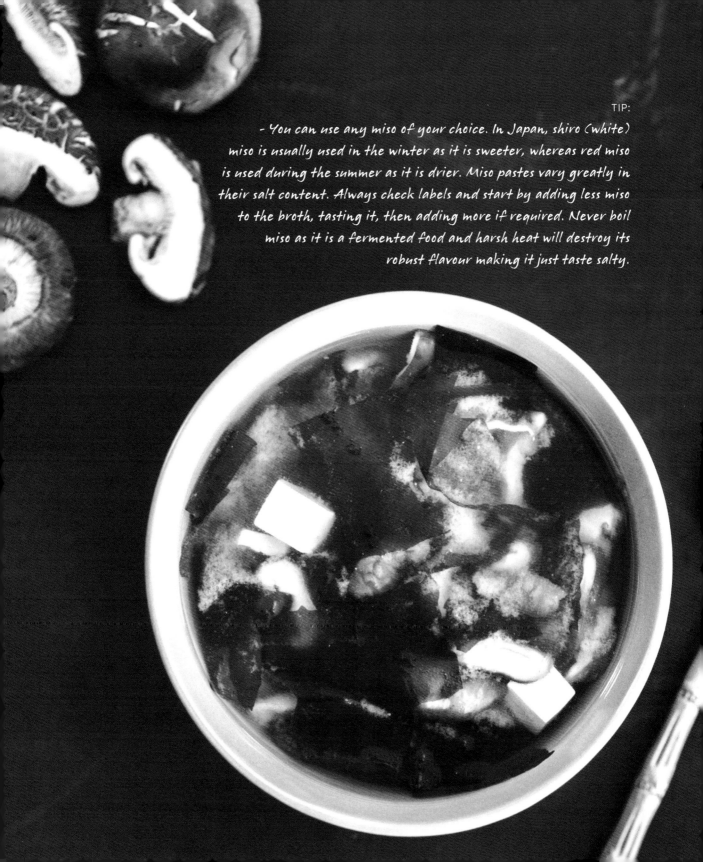

TIP:

– You can use any miso of your choice. In Japan, shiro (white) miso is usually used in the winter as it is sweeter, whereas red miso is used during the summer as it is drier. Miso pastes vary greatly in their salt content. Always check labels and start by adding less miso to the broth, tasting it, then adding more if required. Never boil miso as it is a fermented food and harsh heat will destroy its robust flavour making it just taste salty.

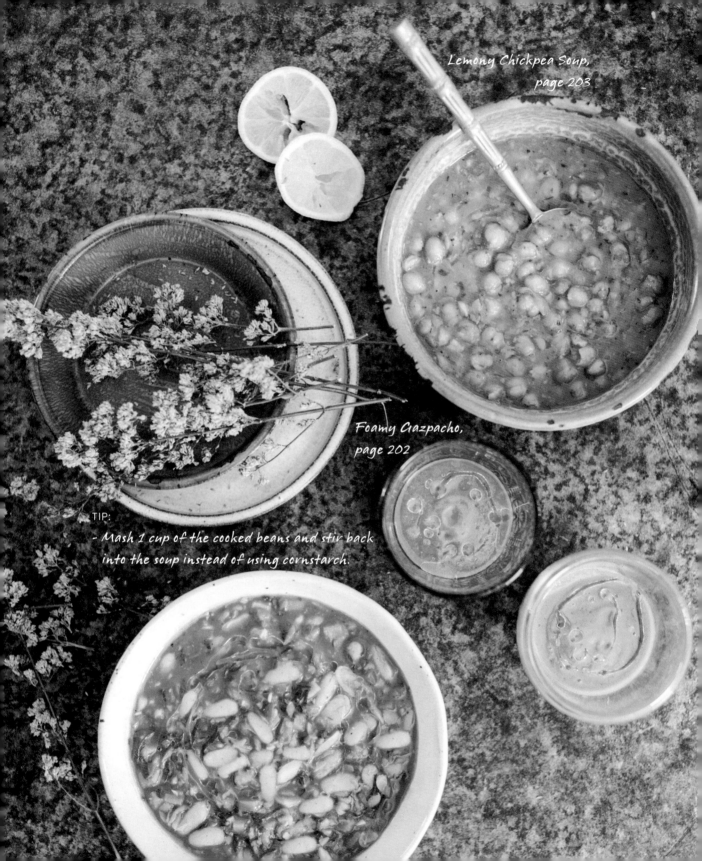

Lemony Chickpea Soup,
page 203

Foamy Gazpacho,
page 202

TIP:
- Mash 1 cup of the cooked beans and stir back
  into the soup instead of using cornstarch.

This traditional Croatian soup is particularly satisfying in winter, but I cook it all year round. Leftovers taste even better the next day, and it's a great recipe to cook in bulk and freeze in meal-sized portions. Bean soup is traditionally served as a main meal with fresh cabbage salad. Try my Shaved Savoy Cabbage with Lemon Dressing (page 51).

CANNELLINI BEAN AND CARROT SOUP WITH PARSLEY

PREPARATION: 10 MINUTES + OVERNIGHT SOAKING, COOKING: 50 MINUTES INCLUDING PRESSURE COOKER, SERVES 5

1½ cups dry cannellini beans, soaked
    overnight in plenty of water
5 tablespoons extra virgin olive oil
1 large onion, finely chopped
2 cloves garlic, crushed
2 medium carrots, peeled and chopped
    into small pieces
1 large soft tomato, coarsely chopped
1½ teaspoons salt
cracked black pepper to taste
2 tablespoons ground sweet paprika
2 tablespoons cornstarch
3 tablespoons parsley, finely chopped

1. Heat oil in pressure cooker and sauté onion until golden for approximately 5 minutes. Stir in garlic and cook for another minute.
2. Rinse and drain soaked beans, and add to the pressure cooker with carrots, tomato, salt, pepper and 6 cups of water. Mix well.
3. Cover the pressure cooker and turn up heat. Once pressurised, turn down heat to very low and cook for 20 minutes, then remove from stove and allow for natural pressure release before opening lid. (If cooking in a conventional pot, cover with lid until soup comes to boil, then turn down heat and simmer until beans are very soft, stirring occasionally. This method will require about 2 hours cooking time. You will also need to add an extra ½ cup of water.)
4. Blend ground paprika with cornstarch, and gradually stir in ½ cup of water until a smooth, thin paste forms. Make sure there are no lumps. Mix paste into bean soup and bring back to boil. Boil soup for about 5 minutes until it thickens slightly.
5. Stir in parsley and serve hot with crusty whole-grain bread. Add a squeeze of lemon juice, if desired.

TIPS:

- Variation: Try using navy or borlotti beans as an alternative.
- Use passata or tomato pasta sauce to replace fresh tomato.

Per serve: energy 1945 kJ (465 Cal); protein 21 g; fat 31 g; saturated fat 5 g; cholesterol 0 mg; carbohydrate 19 g; sugars 11 g; fibre 18 g; calcium 166 mg; iron 7.8 mg; sodium 729 mg

Gazpacho is from southern Spain and is always served chilled during the summer when tomatoes are in season. Super refreshing, this totally raw soup is loaded with lycopene, a powerful antioxidant best known for its role in protecting against prostate cancer. Start this recipe an hour before needed to allow for chilling time. (Recipe image, page 200.)

FOAMY GAZPACHO

PREPARATION: 10 MINUTES + 1 HOUR CHILLING, COOKING: 0 MINUTES, SERVES 6

1 kg (2 lb 3 oz) soft red tomatoes (peel skin only if very tough)

1 small onion

½ green capsicum (bell pepper)

½ Lebanese cucumber, peeled

2 cloves garlic

½ teaspoon salt

¼ teaspoon ground cumin

1 tablespoon extra virgin olive oil + 3 teaspoons extra for garnish

2 teaspoons apple cider vinegar

1. Roughly chop vegetables and, together with salt and cumin, place into a powerful blender with at least 6-cup capacity. Blend for a few minutes until smooth, using the tamper if required.

2. Drizzle in olive oil and vinegar, and continue blending until emulsified.

3. Refrigerate until chilled.

4. Pour into glasses or soup bowls and drizzle with extra oil as garnish. Gazpacho will store well for up to 3 days in the fridge but is unsuitable for freezing.

TIPS:

- Authentic gazpacho is pinky-orange in colour, not red as commonly depicted. If you prefer it more red, add tomato juice.
- For a thicker consistency, sprinkle some water over stale bread to soften, then add to the blender with the remaining ingredients.
- Traditional Spanish condiments include croutons, chopped hard-boiled egg, finely diced red/green capsicum, sliced shallot and small sweet white grapes.

Per serve: energy 351 kJ (84 Cal); protein 2 g; fat 6 g; saturated fat 1 g; cholesterol 0 mg; carbohydrate 5 g; sugars 5 g; fibre 3 g; calcium 24 mg; iron 0.6 mg, sodium 209 mg

A Greek-style white chickpea soup with a creamy texture from the tenderly cooked chickpeas. The emulsion of extra virgin olive oil and lemon juice creates a most delicious flavour! In Greece, this soup is usually served with bread, olives and feta. It also goes well with a crunchy raw salad of celery, radish and mint. Chickpeas are low GI and promote intestinal health. (Recipe image, page 200.)

LEMONY CHICKPEA SOUP

PREPARATION: 5 MINUTES + OVERNIGHT SOAKING, COOKING: 1 HOUR 10 MINUTES INCLUDING PRESSURE COOKER, SERVES 6

500 g (17½ oz) chickpeas (garbanzos), soaked overnight in water with 2 tablespoons salt

2 medium onions, peeled, with stem part left intact

2 cloves garlic, peeled, left whole

¼ cup extra virgin olive oil

1½ teaspoons salt

1 teaspoon dried oregano or freshly chopped parsley, to taste

1 tablespoon cornstarch

¼ cup lemon juice (about 1 juiced lemon)

1. Drain soaked chickpeas and rinse well. Transfer to the base of a pressure cooker and add water to cover by 2.5 centimetres (1 inch), then boil for 5 minutes.

2. Drain chickpeas again and discard the cooking water. Wash out the pressure-cooker base, then return the chickpeas, together with 6 cups of boiling water.

3. Add garlic and half bury the onions into the chickpeas, close the pressure-cooker lid and bring to pressure, then turn down heat to very low and cook under pressure for 35 minutes until very soft. Allow for natural pressure release. (Alternatively, boil conventionally for at least 1½ hours, adding an extra 7 cups of water.)

4. Remove pressure-cooker lid, and discard onion and garlic using a large slotted spoon to squeeze their juices back into the soup.

5. Add oil, salt and oregano, and bring back to boil.

6. Meanwhile, blend cornstarch with lemon juice to form a thin paste, then stir into the soup and cook for a further 5 minutes, uncovered, until it becomes creamy. Serve hot or cool and refrigerate or freeze as meal-sized portions.

TIPS.

- By soaking the chickpeas in salt water, you will soften their skins and the beans will come out creamier.

- Soup tastes best after standing for half an hour—and it's even better the next day!

- For extra flavour, add 1 hot red chilli.

Per serve: energy 1752 kJ (418 Cal); protein 27 g; fat 26 g; saturated fat 4 g; cholesterol 0 mg; carbohydrate 14 g; sugars 7 g; fibre 18 g; calcium 166 mg; iron 8.3 mg; sodium 583 mg

The striking orange colour of this soup comes from the antioxidants alpha and beta carotene. But carrots also contain lutein and zeaxanthin, which are deposited in the macula of your eyes where they act as a type of "sunscreen" to protect against UV damage and macular degeneration.

SMOOTH CARROT AND ORANGE SOUP

PREPARATION: 20 MINUTES, COOKING: 30 MINUTES, SERVES 8

2 tablespoons extra virgin olive oil

1 medium onion, chopped

2 cloves garlic, crushed

3 teaspoons fresh grated ginger

2 teaspoons ground cumin

1 teaspoon ground coriander

shake of cayenne pepper

1 kg (2 lb 3 oz) carrots, peeled and roughly sliced into 1-centimetre (½-inch) rings

1 medium sweet potato, peeled and roughly sliced into 1-centimetre (½-inch) rings

5 cups stock (can be from stock cubes)

juice of 1 orange

½ bunch coriander (cilantro), chopped

1. Heat oil, and sauté onion and garlic until soft.

2. Add ginger, spices and cayenne, and cook for a further 30 seconds.

3. Add carrot, sweet potato and stock, cover and bring to boil.

4. Reduce heat and simmer, half covered, for about 15 minutes until vegetables are cooked.

5. Puree until smooth and stir through orange juice. Add a little more boiling water for a thinner consistency.

6. Serve hot, garnished with coriander.

Per serve: energy 622 kJ (149 Cal); protein 3 g; fat 5 g; saturated fat 1 g; cholesterol 0 mg; carbohydrate 19 g; sugars 13 g; fibre 7 g; calcium 73 mg; iron 1.4 mg; sodium 226

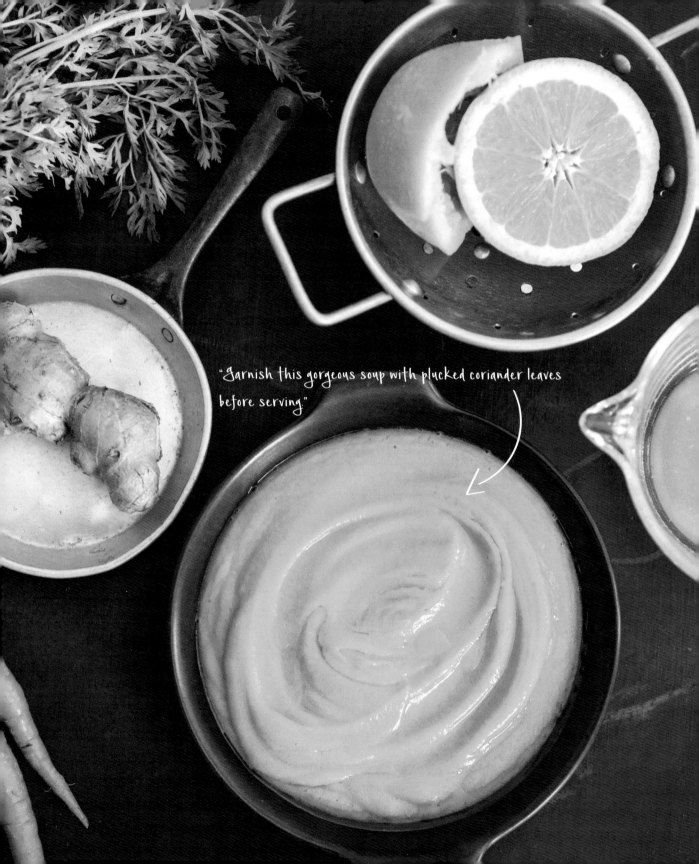

"garnish this gorgeous soup with plucked coriander leaves before serving."

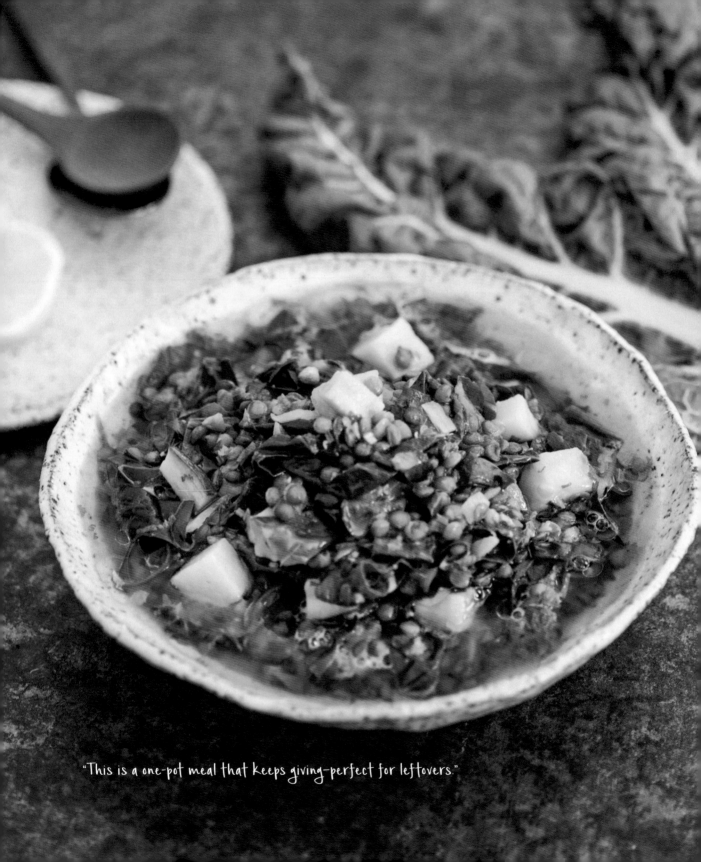

"This is a one-pot meal that keeps giving—perfect for leftovers."

This delicious Lebanese-style brown lentil soup with the goodness of greens can be served as a main course. Eating one serve of dark leafy green vegetables each day can cut your risk of developing type 2 diabetes and macular degeneration. This soup is great for making ahead of time as the flavour continues to improve. Freeze leftovers in meal-sized glass containers for an easy lunch.

TANGY LENTIL SOUP WITH SILVERBEET AND ZUCCHINI

PREPARATION: 20 MINUTES, COOKING: 45 MINUTES, SERVES 8

2 tablespoons extra virgin olive oil

1 large onion, chopped

500 g (17½ oz) brown lentils, picked over for stones and washed

1 teaspoon salt

2 medium potatoes, peeled and cut into 1-centimetre (½-inch) cubes

2 medium zucchinis (courgettes), cut into 1-centimetre (½-inch) cubes

1 bunch silverbeet (chard), trimmed, washed and shredded into 1-centimetre (½-inch) strips making up 600 g (about 21 oz)

2 cloves garlic, crushed

freshly ground black pepper, optional

1 bunch fresh coriander (cilantro), chopped

juice of 2 lemons

1. Warm oil in a large soup pot (at least 8 litres/2 gallons) capacity) and sauté onions until soft.

2. Add lentils, salt and 8 cups of water, cover with lid and bring to boil. Turn down heat and simmer for 15 minutes.

3. Add potato cubes and continue cooking for 10 minutes.

4. Add zucchini, silverbeet, garlic, pepper and 4 cups of extra boiling water, and cook for a further 5 minutes until the greens just start to soften.

5. Stir in coriander and lemon juice, and ladle hot into soup bowls. Serve with wholemeal Lebanese bread, if desired.

Per serve: energy 1201 kJ (287 Cal); protein 19 g; fat 6 g; saturated fat 1 g; cholesterol 0 mg; carbohydrate 34 g; sugars 5 g; fibre 13 g; calcium 130 mg; iron 7.7 mg, sodium 457 mg

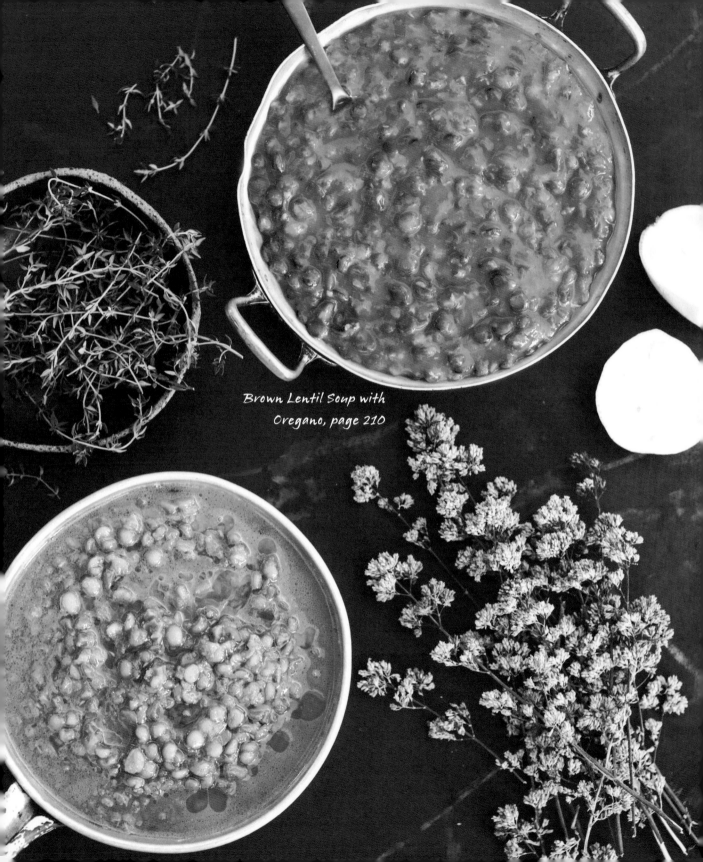

Brown Lentil Soup with
Oregano, page 210

A sweet-tasting soup with the subtle perfume of fresh thyme. Enjoy it with lightly toasted bread rubbed with a clove of fresh garlic. Soup will thicken on standing and tastes even better the next day!

YELLOW SPLIT PEA SOUP WITH LEEK AND THYME

PREPARATION: 15 MINUTES, COOKING: 1 HOUR, SERVES 5

2 cups yellow split peas, picked over for stones and rinsed

2 tablespoons extra virgin olive oil

1 onion, finely chopped

1 leek, finely sliced

1 carrot, finely diced

2 sticks celery, stringed and finely diced

3 large sprigs fresh thyme + extra thyme leaves, to serve

1 x 10 g (⅓ oz) chicken-style vegetable stock cube, crumbled

pinch salt, optional

freshly cracked black pepper

1. Place split peas in a large pot with 6 cups of water. Bring contents to boil, then turn down heat and simmer for 15 minutes until half cooked.

2. Meanwhile, in a large frypan, heat oil and sauté onion until soft. Add leek, carrots and celery, and continue cooking for a further 5 minutes until all vegetables are tender.

3. Transfer sautéed vegetables to the soup pot, and add sprigs of thyme, stock cube, salt and 3 cups of boiling water. Cover and bring to boil again. Reduce heat and simmer for a further 20-30 minutes until peas are very soft. Note: Stir every so often to ensure soup doesn't stick to the bottom of the pot.

4. Rest soup for 10 minutes and remove thyme stems before serving. Ladle into bowls, and garnish with pepper and a scattering of fresh thyme leaves. Freeze leftovers.

TIPS:

- Unlike most hard beans, split peas don't require soaking. But you can soak them in water overnight to speed up the cooking process.

- The tiny thyme leaves will loosen and easily come off their stems during cooking. If you prefer to strip them beforehand, run them through the tines of a fork. If you don't have fresh thyme, use 1 teaspoon of dried thyme.

Per serve: energy 1422 kJ (340 Cal); protein 19 g; fat 9 g; saturated fat 2 g; cholesterol 0 mg; carbohydrate 41 g; sugars 7 g; fibre 12 g; calcium 92 mg; iron 4.2 mg; sodium 321 mg

This is possibly the quickest and easiest brown-lentil soup you can make! It's also delicious, inexpensive and good for your whole body—from blood vessels to bowels. I love making it year round and storing leftovers in the fridge or freezer for an instant lunch. (Recipe image, page 208.)

BROWN LENTIL SOUP WITH OREGANO

PREPARATION: 8 MINUTES, COOKING: 25 MINUTES, SERVES 5

2 cups brown lentils, picked over for stones and rinsed

1 onion, coarsely chopped

2 cloves garlic, sliced thinly

1 teaspoon dried oregano

1 teaspoon salt

freshly ground black pepper, generous amount

4 tablespoons extra virgin olive oil

5 teaspoons lemon juice

1. Place lentils, onion, garlic, oregano, salt, pepper and oil in a pressure cooker. Mix in 6 cups of water and cover with lid.

2. Turn up heat until the pressure builds up, then turn down to very low and cook soup for 10 minutes under pressure. (Alternatively, simmer for 25-30 minutes in a conventional saucepan, until lentils are very soft and creamy.)

3. Remove from stove and allow for natural pressure release so you can open the lid easily.

4. Ladle into bowls, stir 1 teaspoon of lemon juice into each serve, then drizzle with more extra virgin olive oil, if desired. Crusty bread is typically eaten with this soup to make it a main meal. Wilted greens, such as spinach, or raw cabbage salads are a perfect match.

TIPS:

- *Variation: Add diced carrot, celery or halved baby potatoes and a little more water.*
- *You can also swap marjoram for oregano–it's from the same family.*

Per serve: energy 1520 kJ (363 Cal); protein 19 g; fat 16 g; saturated fat 2 g; cholesterol 0 mg; carbohydrate 31 g; sugars 3 g; fibre 12 g; calcium 71 mg; iron 6.2 mg; sodium 467 mg

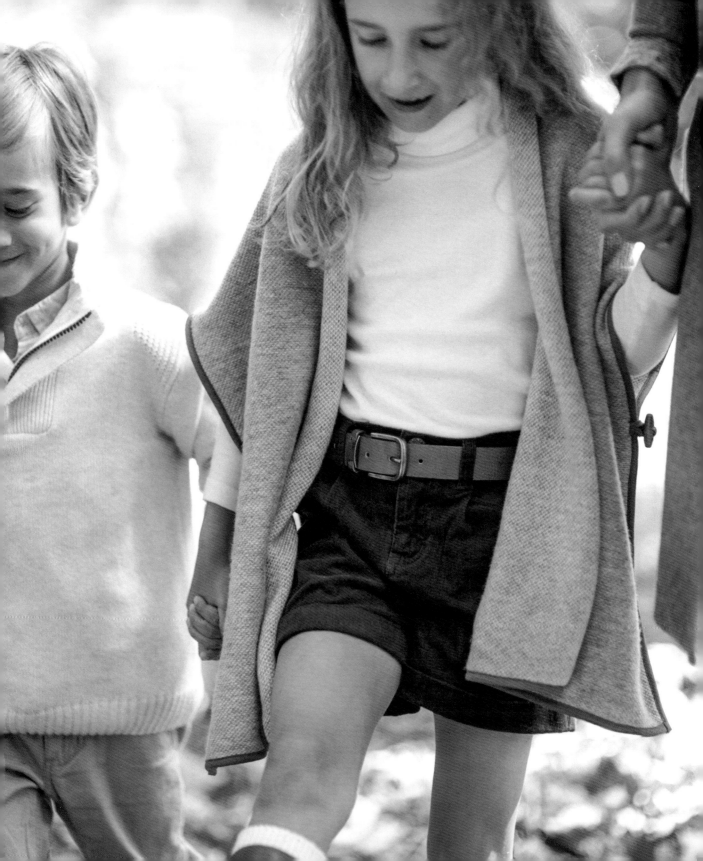

DIPS, SPREADS & PASTES

CREAMY HUMMUS

recipe on page 216

ALMOND AND SAGE PESTO

recipe on page 215

SUNFLOWER SEED SOUR CREAM

recipe on page 218

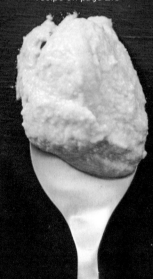

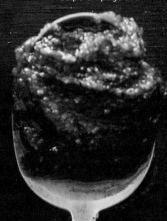

recipe on page 222

GREEK-STYLE YOGURT DIP WITH CUCUMBER AND MINT

Get dipping!

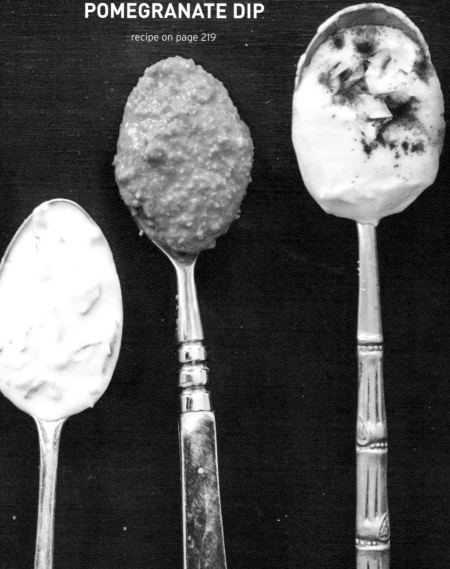
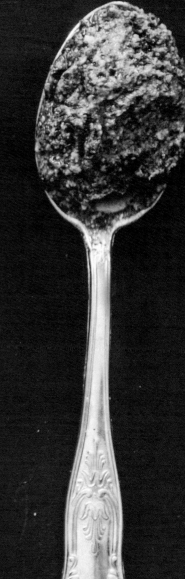

ROASTED RED CAPSICUM, WALNUT AND POMEGRANATE DIP

recipe on page 219

SANTORINI FAVA DIP

recipe on page 214

PESTO WITH BASIL AND PINE NUTS

recipe on page 223

This dip comes from the island of Santorini, Greece. It is traditionally served as an appetiser or on a meze platter. Fava has a sweet flavour, peppered by the raw onion and extra virgin olive oil, which are a vital part of how it is served. (Recipe image, page 213.)

SANTORINI FAVA DIP

PREPARATION: 10 MINUTES, COOKING: 1 HOUR 30 MINUTES, SERVES 12

1 cup yellow split peas, picked over for stones and rinsed
2 cloves garlic, crushed
1 onion, finely chopped
½ teaspoon salt
6 tablespoons extra virgin olive oil
1 tablespoon sweet paprika
¼ onion, finely chopped, for serving

1. Place peas, garlic, the 1 onion and salt in a medium saucepan with 2½ cups of water and bring to boil. Turn down heat and simmer, covered, for 1 hour, stirring occasionally. The peas should become very soft.
2. Place mixture in a blender, add 3 tablespoons of oil and puree until creamy.
3. Transfer to a serving platter. Just before serving, run the back of a spoon over the top to form a well, then drizzle with remaining olive oil. Sprinkle with paprika and raw onion, and serve with wholemeal Lebanese bread or whole-grain crackers.

TIPS:

- If you triple the split peas–use 3 cups–and cook on a very low heat with 7½ cups water for 1½ hours, they will turn completely mushy and you will not need to puree mixture.

- A few olives or capers are also traditionally served as a garnish.

- Lemon juice can be stirred through after blending or balsamic vinegar can be drizzled on top, if desired.

- Leftover dip can be stored in the fridge for several days and re-warmed. It thickens on cooling and softens with heating.

Per serve: energy 572 kJ (137 Cal); protein 4 g; fat 10 g; saturated fat 2 g; cholesterol 0 mg; carbohydrate 8 g; sugars 1 g; fibre 2 g; calcium 12 mg; iron 0.8 mg; sodium 99 mg

Sage is a high-antioxidant herb that brings amazing flavours to your plate. When I was in Sicily, I discovered this simple paste idea that goes well with whole-grain pasta. Keep pasta portion modest—80 g (about 3 oz) dry pasta per person—and cook only until al dente to reduce the effect the carbohydrate will have on blood sugar levels. Serve with a fresh salad. (Recipe image, page 212.)

ALMOND AND SAGE PESTO

PREPARATION: 7 MINUTES, COOKING: 0 MINUTES, SERVES 8 FOR PASTA

1 cup almonds

20 g (1 oz) soft sage leaves, plucked
   from stalks

1 clove garlic

1 teaspoon finely ground salt

1 cup extra virgin olive oil

1. Pulverise almonds in a medium food processor bowl, then add sage leaves, garlic and salt. Process to form a paste.

2. While the motor is running, drizzle in olive oil through the chute and process until all ingredients are well combined. Serve pesto tossed through hot pasta. Or transfer to a glass jar for storage. Pesto will store in the fridge for at least 1 week and freezes well.

TIPS:

- Use about 1 tablespoon of pesto per 1 cup of cooked pasta. Loosen with some cooking water, reserved from draining the pasta, until a desired creamy consistency is reached.
- Sprinkle with freshly grated pecorino or nutritional yeast seasoning for a dairy-free alternative.
- To achieve a thicker pesto for use on crispbread, reduce the amount of oil.

Per serve: energy 1470 kJ (351 Cal); protein 3 g; fat 37 g; saturated fat 5 g; cholesterol 0 mg; carbohydrate 1 g; sugars 1 g; fibre 2 g; calcium 80 mg; iron 1.3 mg; sodium 287 mg

Try this delicious recipe for an authentic creamy hummus, taught to me by my Lebanese friend Claudia. It takes a little more effort than if using canned chickpeas, but tastes so much better! Store hummus in the fridge for a week in an airtight container and use as a dip or spread in place of butter. (Recipe image, page 212.)

CREAMY HUMMUS

PREPARATION: 15 MINUTES + OVERNIGHT SOAKING, COOKING: 45 MINUTES, SERVES 14

250 g (9 oz) dried chickpeas (garbanzos), soaked overnight in water
¼ cup lemon juice (about 1 juiced lemon)
⅓ cup hulled tahini
1 clove garlic, crushed
1 teaspoon salt

1. Drain soaked chickpeas and rinse twice. Place in a large pot with half of the salt and 5 cups of water. Cover and bring to boil, then remove lid and skim any foam that appears on the surface. Cook, uncovered, for 30-40 minutes or until chickpeas are soft. Test with the back of a spoon to ensure they can be mashed easily.

2. Remove chickpeas from the stove and drain, reserving 1 cup of the cooking liquid.

3. In a food processor, place chickpeas, lemon juice, tahini, garlic and remaining salt, and puree for several minutes until very smooth and creamy. Scrape down the sides of the bowl with a spatula, then turn on the processor again and gradually drizzle in half, or more, of the reserved cooking water until you reach the desired consistency. Hummus will thicken upon refrigeration but is unsuitable for freezing.

Per serve: energy 469 kJ (112 Cal); protein 7 g; fat 8 g; saturated fat 1 g; cholesterol 0 mg; carbohydrate 3 g; sugars 1 g; fibre 5 g; calcium 55 mg; iron 2.1 mg; sodium 170 mg

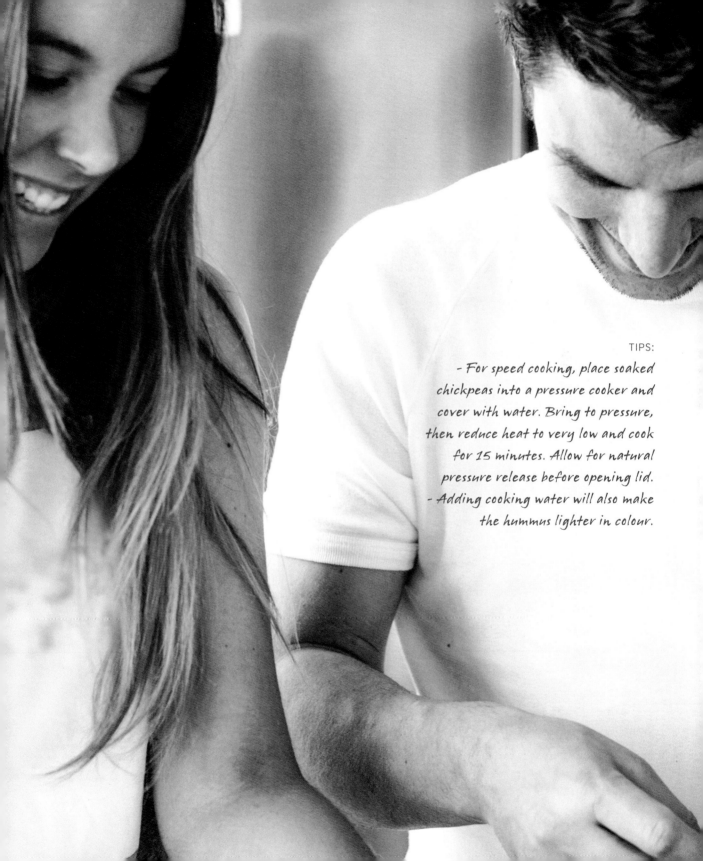

TIPS:
- For speed cooking, place soaked chickpeas into a pressure cooker and cover with water. Bring to pressure, then reduce heat to very low and cook for 15 minutes. Allow for natural pressure release before opening lid.
- Adding cooking water will also make the hummus lighter in colour.

An easy dairy-free "sour cream." Seeds are useful alternatives for people who cannot tolerate nuts. They're also one-third of the price of most nuts! Sunflower seeds are rich in vitamin E and plant sterols, and they provide an impressive array of vitamins and minerals. (Recipe image, page 212.)

SUNFLOWER SEED SOUR CREAM

PREPARATION: 7 MINUTES, COOKING: 0 MINUTES, SERVES 8

1 cup sunflower seeds
¼ cup lemon juice (about 1 juiced lemon)
½ teaspoon onion powder
¼ teaspoon garlic powder
¾ teaspoon salt

1. Place all ingredients into a powerful blender with 1¼ cups of water. Puree for several minutes until the mixture becomes white, smooth and creamy.

2. Transfer to a storage jar and refrigerate. The cream will thicken on cooling. Use as required over 1 week. Unsuitable for freezing.

TIPS:

- Use this everywhere you would use sour cream.
- Once chilled and thickened, this sour cream is also perfect to use as a spread for sandwiches.
- Turn up the flavour by stirring in some grated horseradish or wasabi.
- To use as a thin dressing, simply add more water and adjust seasonings.

Per serve: energy 439 kJ (105 Cal); protein 4 g; fat 9 g; saturated fat 1 g; cholesterol 0 mg; carbohydrate 1 g; sugars 1 g; fibre 2 g; calcium 22 mg; iron 0.9 mg; sodium 215 mg

Traditionally known as "muhamarra," this Middle Eastern dip is extremely versatile and delicious. Serve with Lebanese bread triangles or use as a paste for pasta. The walnuts will drop the GI of any carbohydrates that you serve this with. The roasted capsicums add antioxidants and the pomegranate molasses give a special sweet-and-sour tang! (Recipe image, page 213.)

ROASTED RED CAPSICUM, WALNUT AND POMEGRANATE DIP

PREPARATION: 10 MINUTES + 1 HOUR SOAKING, COOKING: 0 MINUTES, SERVES 20

2 cups walnuts, soaked in water
   for 1 hour
1 x 450 g (16 oz) jar fire-roasted peeled
   whole peppers, drained
1½ tablespoons pomegranate molasses
3 cloves garlic, crushed
2 teaspoons ground cumin
½ teaspoon salt
½ cup breadcrumbs
pinch chilli powder
½ cup extra virgin olive oil

1. Drain walnuts, place in a food processor and blend.
2. Add remaining ingredients, except for olive oil, and puree until smooth.
3. Slowly drizzle in oil through the chute with the motor running until you have a creamy texture.
4. Store in an airtight container in the fridge for up to 1 week.
To serve as a dip, spread onto a plate, indent channels with the back of a spoon and drizzle with a little extra olive oil. Garnish with mint, olives or pomegranate seeds, if desired.

TIPS:

–If using roasted peppers from a larger jar, you will need at least 330 g (11½ oz) of drained peppers.

- You can also roast fresh capsicums yourself using a gas burner or oven until the skin blackens. Allow to cool before peeling and removing the seeds and stalk. Do not wash.

- Soaking nuts increases the calcium available to the body.

Per serve: energy 669 kJ (160 Cal); protein 3 g; fat 15 g; saturated fat 1 g; cholesterol 0 mg; carbohydrate 4 g; sugars 2 g; fibre 1 g; calcium 16 mg; iron 0.5 mg; sodium 80 mg

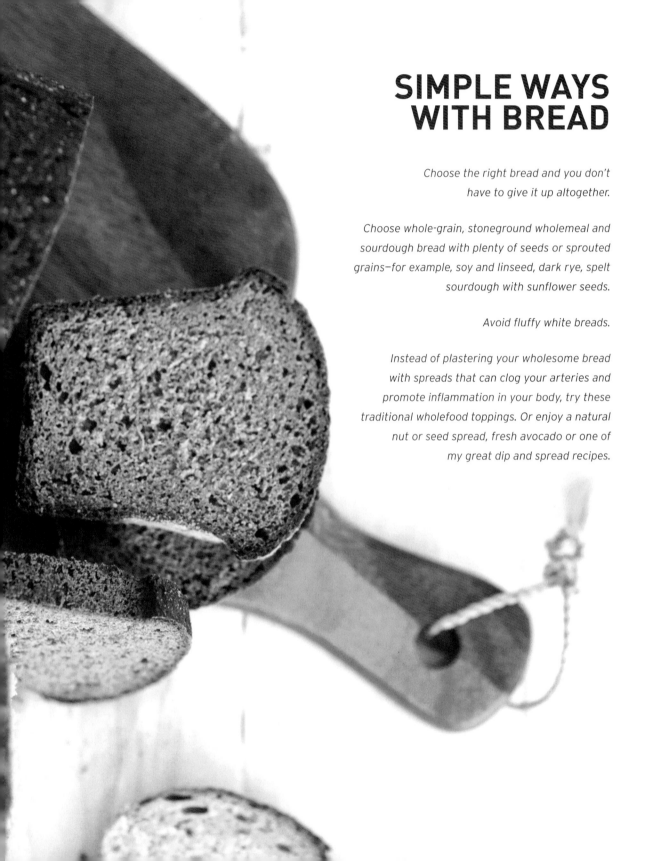

SIMPLE WAYS
WITH BREAD

*Choose the right bread and you don't
have to give it up altogether.*

*Choose whole-grain, stoneground wholemeal and
sourdough bread with plenty of seeds or sprouted
grains—for example, soy and linseed, dark rye, spelt
sourdough with sunflower seeds.*

Avoid fluffy white breads.

*Instead of plastering your wholesome bread
with spreads that can clog your arteries and
promote inflammation in your body, try these
traditional wholefood toppings. Or enjoy a natural
nut or seed spread, fresh avocado or one of
my great dip and spread recipes.*

• Garlic rub

*Lightly toast your bread and rub the surface with a clove of fresh garlic.
You will notice the clove disappearing as the garlic juice is pressed into the bread.
Europeans have known this secret for a long time.*

• Olive oil and oregano

*Drizzle your bread with a good quality extra virgin olive oil
and sprinkle with dried oregano. This is so Greek!*

• Zataar

*Turn zataar (a good spoonful) into a paste with extra virgin olive oil. Then spread
onto fresh Lebanese bread. Cut into triangles, like a pizza pro. A Middle Eastern
makeover!*

• Juicy tomato

*Go Spanish. Grate an overripe tomato and season with a little salt.
Spoon over your bread and drizzle with some extra virgin olive oil.*

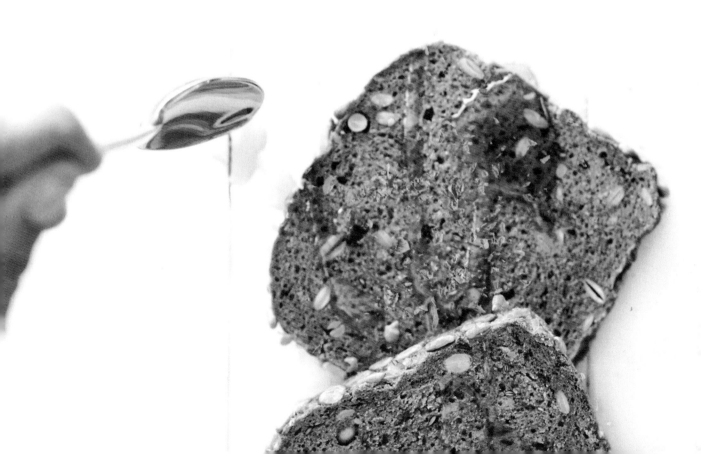

Here is the authentic way to make tzatziki, the world-famous Greek yogurt sauce and dip.
(Recipe image, page 213.)

GREEK-STYLE YOGURT DIP WITH CUCUMBER AND MINT

PREPARATION: 10 MINUTES, COOKING: 0 MINUTES, SERVES 8

2 Lebanese cucumbers, unpeeled

2 cups low-fat Greek-style plain yogurt

7 large mint leaves, rolled into a cigar shape and finely sliced

juice of ¼ juicy lemon

1 clove garlic, crushed

¼ teaspoon salt, optional

1. Grate cucumber and place in a strainer over sink. Press down with a spoon to remove as much juice as possible.

2. Transfer grated cucumber into a bowl, and fold in yogurt and remaining ingredients. Place in a serving bowl and enjoy immediately or refrigerate for several days. The flavour continues to improve. Recipe is unsuitable for freezing.

TIPS:

- Variation: Substitute fresh dill for the mint or experiment with using herbs in combination.
- Swap dairy yogurt for Homemade Soy Yogurt (page 294), which you have strained for at least 4 hours (or overnight) using a a fine-meshed nylon nut bag to thicken.

Per serve: energy 239 kJ (57 Cal); protein 4 g; fat 1 g; saturated fat 1 g; cholesterol 11 mg; carbohydrate 6 g; sugars 6 g; fibre 1 g; calcium 158 mg; iron 0.2 mg; sodium 66 mg

This classic paste is simple and incredibly tasty—it's one of my favourites! While it contains fat, this is entirely from the extra virgin olive oil and nuts. Such fat is healthy as it comes packaged with phytonutrients that provide antioxidant and anti-inflammatory benefits, as nature intended. Enjoy pesto stirred through cooked pasta, swirled into soups or spread on whole-grain bread. (Recipe image, page 213.)

PESTO WITH BASIL AND PINE NUTS

PREPARATION: 10 MINUTES, COOKING: 0 MINUTES, SERVES 6

1 very large bunch basil
¼ cup pine nuts
2 cloves garlic, crushed
cracked black pepper, to taste
¼ teaspoon salt
⅓ cup extra virgin olive

1. Pluck basil leaves from stalks. Wash, then spin dry.
2. Grind pine nuts in a food processor for 30 seconds. Add remaining ingredients, including basil leaves, and puree for 3 minutes or until a smooth paste forms.
3. Transfer paste from the processor into a small airtight container. This will reduce exposure to air and help maintain the bright-green colour. Pesto can be made in advance and frozen or stored in the fridge for up to 1 week. Serve with farfalle or penne pasta and sprinkle with parmesan or nutritional yeast (a dairy-free alternative), if desired.

TIPS:

- To loosen the pesto when mixing through pasta, stir in a few tablespoons of reserved cooking water from the pasta.
- To lighten the calories or reduce the carbohydrate load, serve with kelp noodles, konnyaku noodles or zucchini linguine instead of regular pasta. Many vegetables can be turned into noodles by using a spiraliser, mandoline or julienne peeler. Try carrot, beetroot, kohlrabi, jicama or daikon radish. You can enjoy them raw or soften in a pan with a drop of olive oil, chilli flakes and garlic powder.

Per serve: energy 721 kJ (172 Cal); protein 2 g; fat 18 g; saturated fat 2 g; cholesterol 0 mg; carbohydrate 1 g; sugars 0 g; fibre 2 g; calcium 59 mg; iron 0.8 mg; sodium 99 mg

This delicious cream cheese is made with the goodness of almonds, which provide only healthy fats and plant protein. Although it's easy to make, you will need to start this recipe about 48 hours before you want to eat it. Nuts lower your cholesterol and dampen the blood sugar raising effect of carbohydrate foods that you serve them with.

ALMOND CREAM CHEESE TOPPED WITH HERBS

PREPARATION: 15 MINUTES + 6 HOURS SOAKING + 12 HOURS SETTING, COOKING: 0 MINUTES, SERVES 8

1 cup blanched almonds, soaked in water for at least 6 hours

3 tablespoons extra virgin olive oil + 1 tablespoon extra for garnish

¼ cup lemon juice (about 1 juiced lemon)

1 teaspoon salt

1 clove garlic, peeled

1 tablespoon fresh rosemary

1 teaspoon dried oregano

1. Drain soaked almonds and rinse well, then place in a high-powered blender.

2. Add oil, lemon juice, salt, garlic and ½ cup of water. Puree for a few minutes until really smooth and creamy white, resembling thick whipped cream. You might need to stop and re-start the blender a few times to scrape down the sides.

3. Remove cream from blender and divide into 2 portions. Spoon each portion onto 3 layers of cheesecloth, which you have placed over a small strainer and sit each over a bowl. Pull up the sides of the cloth and twist into a ball to remove any excess water. Transfer to the fridge to firm for at least 12 hours.

4. Unwrap the cloths to remove the 2 cheese mounds and invert each onto a serving plate. Press down to slightly flatten to about 2-centimetre (¾-inch) thickness and smooth edges. Sprinkle with herbs and drizzle with extra olive oil just before serving. Serve with whole-grain bread or crispbread. Recipe freezes well.

TIPS:

- *A fine-meshed nylon nut bag can also be used. Purchase online or from health-food stores.*

- *Blanch your own almonds: After soaking overnight, simply cover with boiling water for 20 minutes, squeeze almonds with 2 fingers to slip off their skin. This will require an extra 8 minutes of preparation time.*

Per serve: energy 856 kJ (205 Cal); protein 4 g; fat 20 g; saturated fat 2 g; cholesterol 0 mg; carbohydrate 1 g; sugars 1 g; fibre 2 g; calcium 49 mg; iron 0.8 mg; sodium 289 mg

"I serve this cream cheese at dinner parties with crispbread and it's so smooth and creamy that my guests cannot believe it's dairy-free!"

TIP:

- To dry cheese and turn it into a crumbly "feta," place portions onto a tray lined with parchment (baking) paper and bake for about 20 minutes at 140°C (280°F). Cool then freeze until required.

SWEET ENDINGS

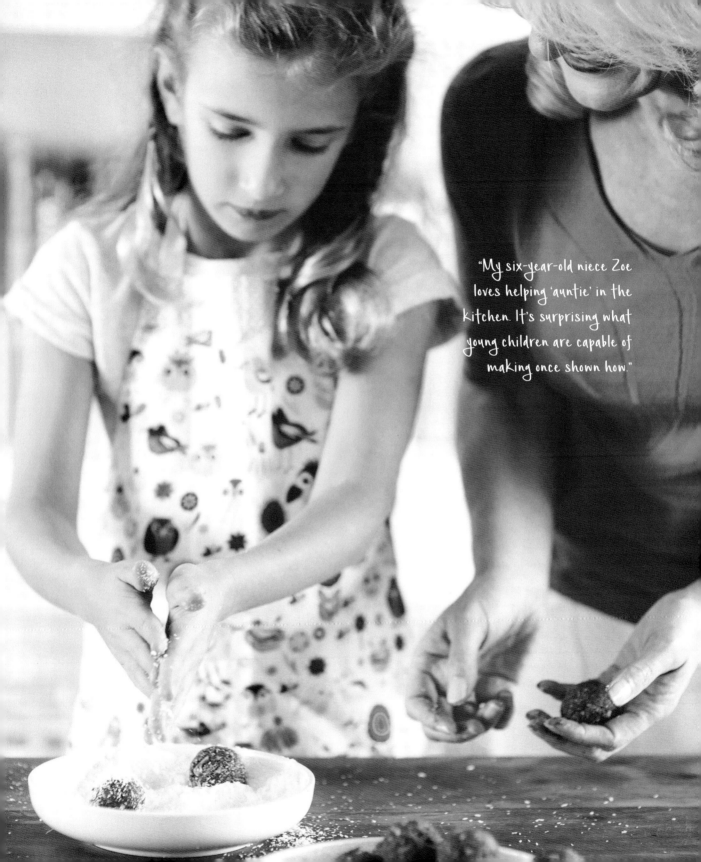

"My six-year-old niece Zoe loves helping 'auntie' in the kitchen. It's surprising what young children are capable of making once shown how."

Here's what you should give them when the kids call for ice-cream! You can also use other frozen fruit, such as mango, or add in some berries. This recipe needs to be started the day before. It is the perfect way to use up over-ripe bananas.

REAL BANANA ICE-CREAM

PREPARATION: 15 MINUTES + FREEZING, COOKING: 0 MINUTES, SERVES 4

4 over-ripe bananas, peeled
¼ teaspoon cinnamon, nutmeg or wattleseed
¼ teaspoon alcohol-free pure vanilla extract

1. Slice or break up bananas into small chunks of even size, place in a glass container then freeze until solid, preferably overnight.
2. Remove bananas from freezer and defrost for 5-10 minutes. Place into a food processor with remaining ingredients and puree until a smooth ice-cream-like texture is formed.
3. Scoop immediately into small bowls or re-freeze for later use.

Per serve: energy 360 kJ (86 Cal); protein 1 g; fat 0 g; saturated fat 0 g; cholesterol 0 mg; carbohydrate 19 g; sugars 16 g; fibre 2 g; calcium 6 mg; iron 0.3 mg; sodium 0 mg

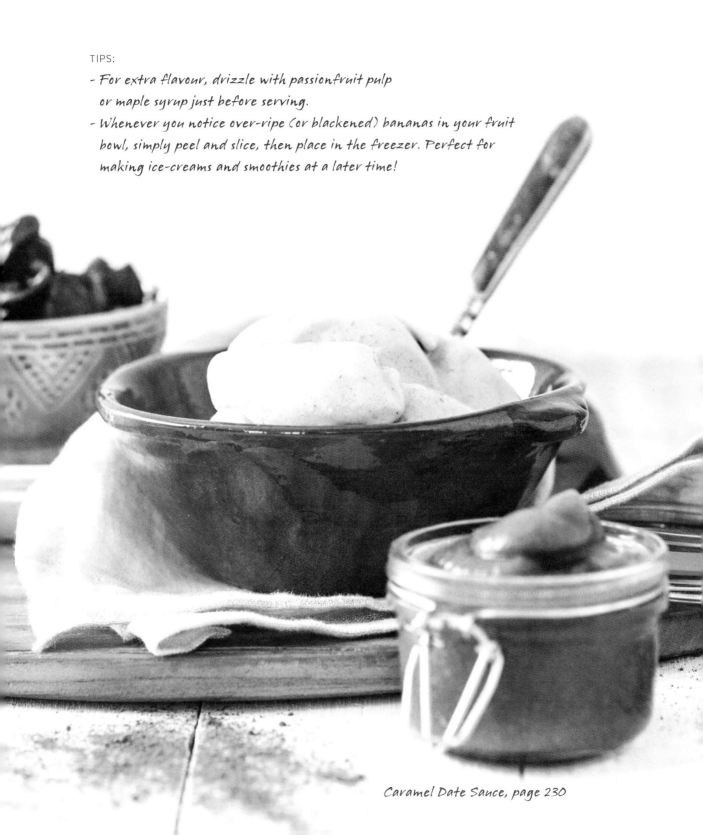

TIPS:

- For extra flavour, drizzle with passionfruit pulp
  or maple syrup just before serving.
- Whenever you notice over-ripe (or blackened) bananas in your fruit
  bowl, simply peel and slice, then place in the freezer. Perfect for
  making ice-creams and smoothies at a later time!

Caramel Date Sauce, page 230

Instead of sugar, use this wonderful caramel sweetener on cereal, to top desserts or with ice-cream. The best news? It comes with plenty of antioxidants and soluble fibre to lower an elevated cholesterol. (Recipe image, page 229.)

CARAMEL DATE SAUCE

PREPARATION: 4 MINUTES, COOKING: 0 MINUTES, SERVES 20

300 g (about 2 cups) pitted, dried dates
2 teaspoons lemon juice

1. Place dates in a bowl and cover with 2 cups of boiling water. Allow 5 minutes to soften.
2. Transfer dates together with their soaking water to a high-powered blender or food processor, add lemon juice and puree until really smooth.
3. Pour sauce into a glass jar with a screw-top lid and store in the fridge for up to 2 weeks.

TIPS:

- The lemon juice adds a tang and helps preserve the puree.
- Variation: Use orange juice instead of the boiling water and soak dates for 4 hours prior to pureeing.
- If you hear a crunch during processing from overlooked date stones, sieve the sauce before use.

Per serve: energy 182 kJ (44 Cal); protein 0.3 g; fat 0 g; saturated fat 0 g; cholesterol 0 mg; carbohydrate 10 g; sugars 10 g; fibre 1.5 g; calcium 7 mg; iron 0.4 mg; sodium 2 mg

This luscious sauce, which requires no cooking, is a great match for baked cheesecake and can also be used to top other desserts or porridge. Berries are loaded with anthocyanins and other powerful antioxidants and have a very low GI, so I try to include them at breakfast every day. (Recipe image, page 233.)

MIXED BERRY SAUCE

PREPARATION: 3 MINUTES, COOKING: 0 MINUTES, SERVES 6

2 cups frozen mixed berries
juice of 1 orange
2 teaspoons raw agave syrup

1. Blend all ingredients in a food processor for about 30 seconds and transfer to a small jug. Sit for 20–30 minutes, if required, until the ice melts and the sauce thins, then serve. Sauce stores well in the fridge for several days but is unsuitable for re-freezing.

TIPS:
- Fresh berries can be used in place of frozen.
- If you prefer the sauce to look more pink, use at least half raspberries.

Per serve: energy 138 kJ (33 Cal); protein 1 g; fat 0 g; saturated fat 0 g; cholesterol 0 mg; carbohydrate 6 g; sugars 6 g; fibre 2 g; calcium 10 mg; iron 0.2 mg; sodium 2 mg

You won't believe that this incredibly easy-to-make mousse is also good for you! It contains soy protein and psyllium husks to help lower cholesterol and better regulate blood sugar and bowel function.

STRAWBERRY AND BANANA MOUSSE

PREPARATION: 10 MINUTES + 5 HOURS CHILLING, COOKING: 0 MINUTES, SERVES 4

1 punnet strawberries, hulled and washed
1 large banana
1½ cups lite soy milk
1 tablespoon honey
3 tablespoons psyllium husks
4 extra strawberries for garnish, halved

1. Place all ingredients, except for garnish, in a blender and whiz until smooth. Note: Leave a few fruit lumps for extra texture, if preferred.
2. Pour into tall glasses and chill for 5 hours or overnight until set. Top each glass with extra strawberries and serve. Enjoy within 2 days as the mousse does not contain preservatives and the top will discolour. Unsuitable for freezing.

Per serve: energy 529 kJ (126 Cal); protein 6 g; fat 2 g; saturated fat 0 g, cholesterol 0 mg; carbohydrate 19 g; sugars 14 g; fibre 5 g; calcium 134 mg; iron 1.3 mg; sodium 65 mg

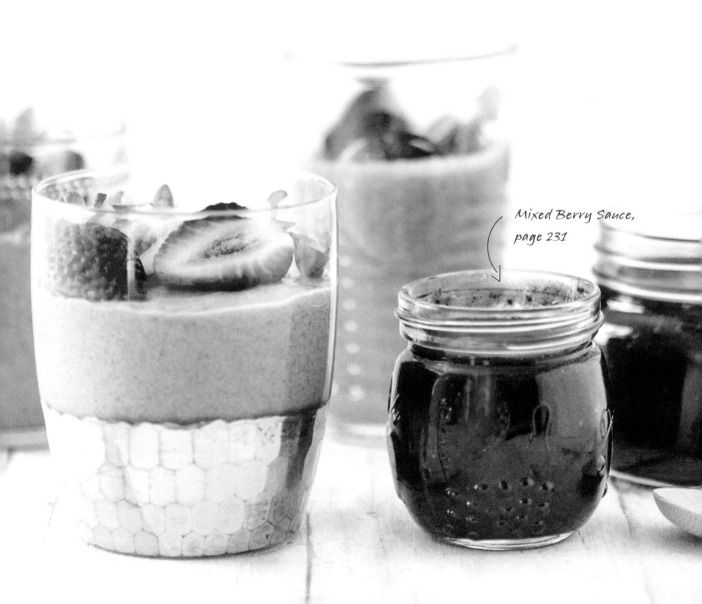

"Swap the strawberries with other berries to vary colour and flavour of the mousse."

Mixed Berry Sauce,
page 231

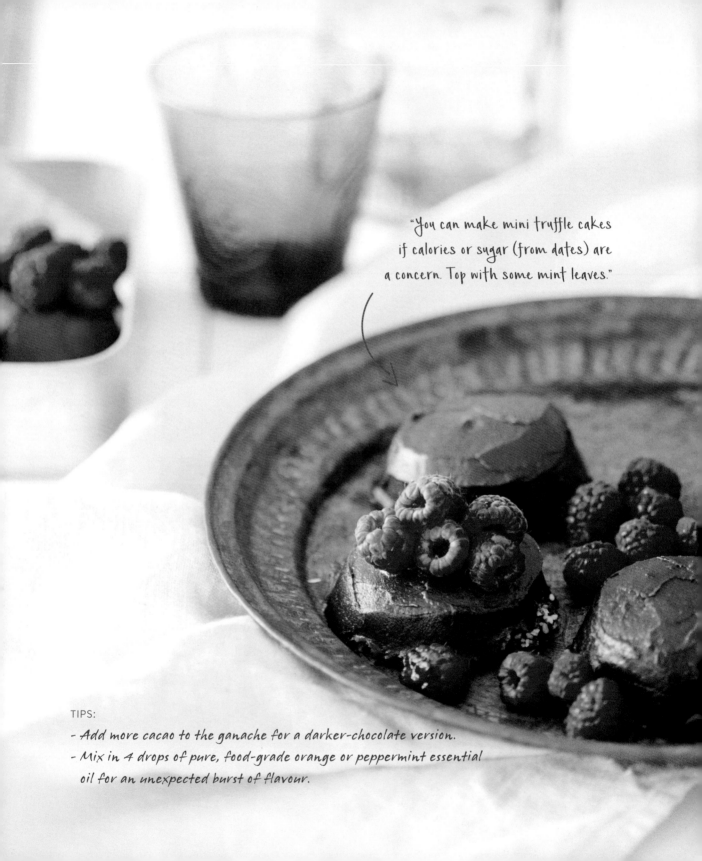

"You can make mini truffle cakes if calories or sugar (from dates) are a concern. Top with some mint leaves."

TIPS:
- Add more cacao to the ganache for a darker-chocolate version.
- Mix in 4 drops of pure, food-grade orange or peppermint essential oil for an unexpected burst of flavour.

Want something healthy but indulgent? This super delicious raw-food recipe uses only wholefoods. The nuts and avocado drop the GI, and the dates and raspberries add sweetness and a high dose of antioxidants. To save time, create the truffles in advance and freeze, then whip up the ganache just before serving.

CHOCOLATE TRUFFLE CAKES WITH RASPBERRIES

PREPARATION: 30 MINUTES + 30 MINUTES SETTING, COOKING: 0 MINUTES, SERVES 6

Truffles
¾ cup almonds
¾ cup pecans
210 g (7½ oz) pitted medjool dates (about 14 dates or 1½ cups, depending on size)
2 tablespoons raw cacao powder

Ganache
1 small avocado (180 g/6½ oz)
120 g (4 oz) pitted medjool dates (about 7 dates)
2 tablespoons raw cacao powder

Topping
180 g (6½ oz) fresh or frozen raspberries
6 large fresh mint leaves

1. Line 6 cups of a regular muffin tray with squares of plastic film so it hangs over the sides and can be folded inward to cover and lift out each truffle.

2. Place nuts in food processor and pulse until ground, but not too fine so they don't become oily. Add dates and cacao, and blend for 1 minute until well combined and the texture of moist sand.

3. Distribute mixture equally between the lined muffin cups (about ½ cup each) and press down firmly with the back of a metal spoon to form an even surface. Cover with the overhanging film and place in the fridge for about 30 minutes to set. Tip: Once set, truffles can be removed from muffin tray and frozen for future use.

4. Meanwhile, place ganache ingredients in food processor and blend until very smooth.

5. Before serving, invert truffles onto a board. Using a palette knife, cover top and build up the sides of each truffle with the ganache to create a rounded shape.

6. Transfer truffles to individual serving plates and pile each with 6 raspberries, allowing any juice to drizzle over the sides. Garnish with a mint leaf. Serve immediately.

TIPS:
- Use a mini-muffin tray to make 12 bite-sized serves.
- Decorate with extra red fruits, such as fresh cherries or red currants, when in season.

Per serve: energy 1879 kJ (449 Cal); protein 9 g; fat 25 g; saturated fat 3 g; cholesterol 0 mg; carbohydrate 43 g; sugars 40 g; fibre 11 g; calcium 124 mg; iron 2.6 mg; sodium 4 mg

An amazing dairy-free and wheat-free "cheesecake" using healthy ingredients including tofu and almond meal to create the texture of a traditional cheesecake. Unlike traditional cheesecake, it leaves a "light" feeling after eating!

SMOOTH VANILLA BEAN TOFU CHEESECAKE

PREPARATION: 30 MINUTES + 4 HOURS CHILLING, COOKING: 1 HOUR 15 MINUTES, SERVES 16

Crust
3 cups almond meal
½ cup brown rice flour
1½ cups rolled oats
1 teaspoon salt
⅓ cup extra virgin olive oil
5 tablespoons natural maple syrup

Filling
600 g (21 oz) vacuum-packed silken firm tofu, drained
450 g (16 oz) extra-firm plain tofu, drained
1 cup natural maple syrup
½ cup arrowroot
2 tablespoons extra virgin olive oil
1 tablespoon finely grated lemon zest
⅓ cup lemon juice
1 vanilla bean, cut lengthwise, middle scraped out with a sharp knife
pinch salt
½ teaspoon baking powder

1. Mix all the dry crust ingredients in a medium bowl. In a separate small jug, stir the liquid ingredients for the crust with 2 tablespoons of water until well combined. Using a fork, gradually mix oil mixture into the dry crust ingredients until a moist dough forms.
2. Pre-heat oven to 180°C (350°F).
3. Transfer dough to a greased 25-centimetre (10-inch) springform tin and press down firmly with clean hands or the back of a spoon to form an even base and sides about 5 centimetres (2 inches) high. Place in oven and blind bake for 15 minutes.
4. Meanwhile, blend filling ingredients in a food processor for several minutes until smooth and creamy.
5. Once crust has cooked, remove from oven and pour in the filling mixture.
6. Bake cheesecake for a further 1 hour until it is set around the edges and almost set in the middle. The top will start to brown. Transfer to a wire rack. Don't remove the edge ring; just loosen it by running around the sides with a large knife. Cool completely and remove the ring, then refrigerate cheesecake for at least 4 hours.
7. Just prior to serving, remove from the fridge and cut into 16 slices. Drizzle each portion with a fruity sauce such as Mixed Berry Sauce (page 231) or top with a few berries and mint garnish. Chill leftover cheesecake immediately to prevent it from going soft. It will keep in the fridge, covered, for several days.

Per serve: energy 1361 kJ (325 Cal); protein 10 g; fat 18 g; saturated fat 2 g; cholesterol 0 mg; carbohydrate 28 g; sugars 19 g; fibre 5 g; calcium 160 mg; iron 2.8 mg; sodium 228 mg

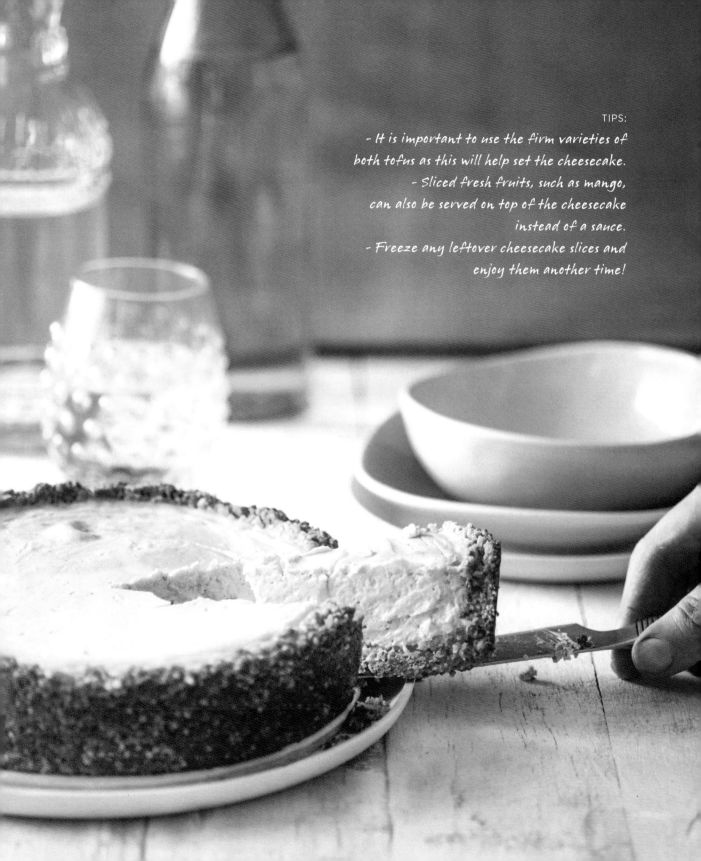

TIPS:
- It is important to use the firm varieties of both tofus as this will help set the cheesecake.
- Sliced fresh fruits, such as mango, can also be served on top of the cheesecake instead of a sauce.
- Freeze any leftover cheesecake slices and enjoy them another time!

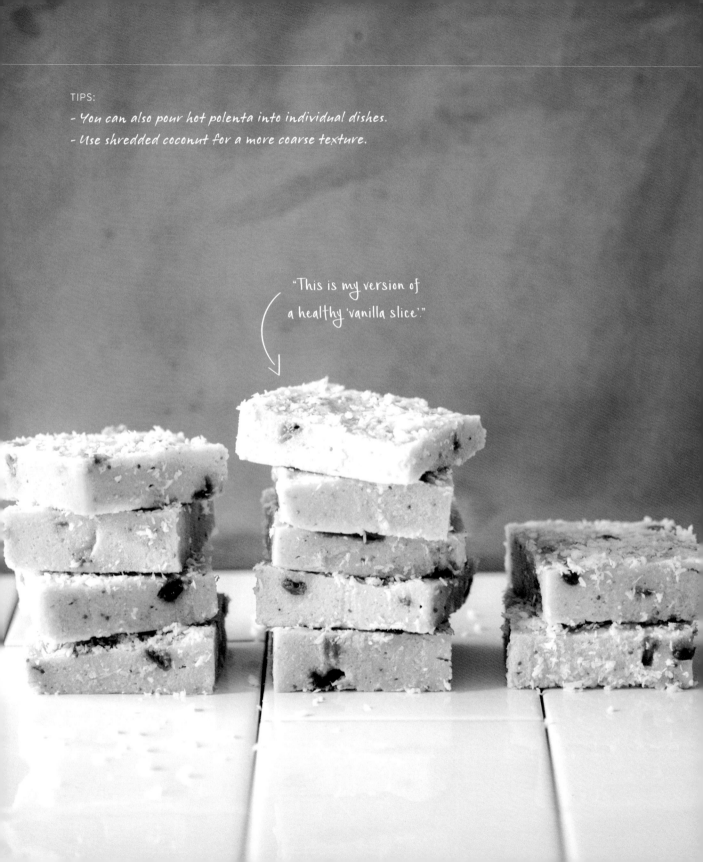

TIPS:
- You can also pour hot polenta into individual dishes.
- Use shredded coconut for a more coarse texture.

"This is my version of a healthy 'vanilla slice'."

This nutritious and delicious dessert—called "Poudine mais" in French—was a popular sweet in Mauritius in the 1960s and frequently sold by street vendors. The bright yellow colour is due to zeaxanthin, an antioxidant pigment, which is important to protect your eyes from macular degeneration. Polenta is also high in resistant starch, a type of dietary fibre recognised for its protective effects against bowel cancer.

FIG AND VANILLA POLENTA PUDDING

PREPARATION: 3 MINUTES + 40 MINUTES SETTING TIME, COOKING: 18 MINUTES, SERVES 12

1 cup polenta (yellow maize meal)
4 cups lite soy milk
¼ cup honey
3 large dried white figs, finely chopped
1 teaspoon alcohol-free pure vanilla extract
¼ cup desiccated coconut

1. Place milk with ½ cup of water in a medium saucepan and heat until almost boiling. Note: Be watchful as milk can easily boil over.

2. Gradually mix in polenta, stirring constantly until the milk has just been absorbed. This should take about 1 minute.

3. Add in honey, chopped figs and vanilla extract, and continue stirring constantly over a low heat for about 7 minutes. Note: If your heat source is too high and the polenta becomes too thick, add a little more boiling water to thin it down.

4. Sprinkle half the coconut onto the bottom of a rectangular baking dish (approximately 30 cm x 23 cm/12 in x 9 in). Pour in hot polenta and immediately smooth out the top. Sprinkle with remaining coconut.

5. Allow to cool slightly, then refrigerate for at least 30 minutes until set.

6. Cut into 12 squares and serve cold. Garnish with extra sliced fresh figs or a scattering of berries, if desired.

Per serve: energy 596 kJ (142 Cal); protein 4 g; fat 3 g; saturated fat 1 g; cholesterol 0 mg; carbohydrate 24 g; sugars 10 g; fibre 2 g; calcium 115 mg; iron 0.2 mg; sodium 55 mg

A very easy "no-cook" desert to wow family and guests! Chia seeds are rich in soluble fibre and omega-3, making them a perfect addition to everyone's diet. Start this recipe a day before required and simply assemble when ready to serve.

BLOOD ORANGE, POMEGRANATE AND CHIA SEED PUDDING

PREPARATION: 15 MINUTES + OVERNIGHT CHILLING, COOKING: 0 MINUTES, SERVES 6

½ cup black chia seeds

2 tablespoons natural maple syrup

2 cups sweetened almond milk

1 teaspoon orange blossom water

3 blood oranges, peeled, segmented and cut into small pieces

6 teaspoons pomegranate seeds

1. Place chia into a medium glass bowl and stir in maple syrup until mixture resembles wet cement.

2. Mix in milk and orange blossom water, and let sit for 5 minutes until chia starts to swell.

3. Stir contents again so there are no clumps. Cover and refrigerate overnight or until thickened. Makes 2½ cups of pudding, which stores in the fridge for several days.

4. Before serving, stir chia pudding slightly to soften before spooning equal amounts into 6 dessert glasses or small bowls. Top with orange pieces and pomegranate seeds, and drizzle with any remaining juice from the oranges.

TIPS:

- To remove seeds from a pomegranate, trim both ends, then cut 4 slits into the fruit vertically as if cutting it into quarters. Place in a bowl and cover with water. Put your hands under the water and slowly pull apart the pomegranate, working the seeds out of their casing until they drop to the bottom of the bowl. The white pith will float to the top. Drain and rinse with extra water until seeds are clean.

- Swap blood oranges for other brightly coloured and tangy fruit, such as berries with their juice, or use diced fuyu fruit, mango or papaya with passionfruit pulp.

Per serve: energy 626 kJ (150 Cal); protein 4 g; fat 7 g; saturated fat 0.6 g; cholesterol 0 mg; carbohydrate 15 g; sugars 14 g; fibre 6 g; calcium 123 mg; iron 1.2 mg; sodium 67 mg

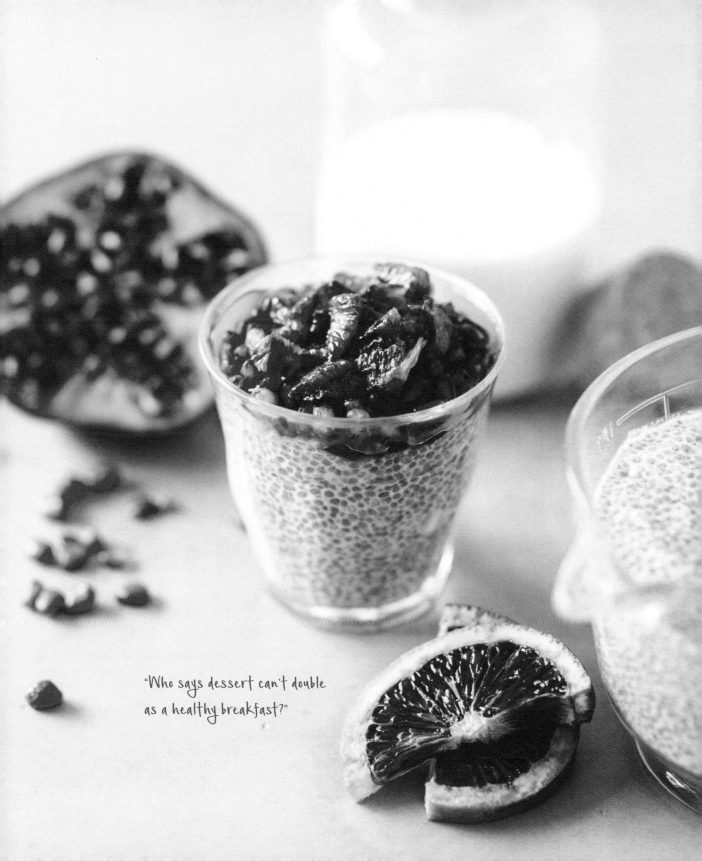

"Who says dessert can't double as a healthy breakfast?"

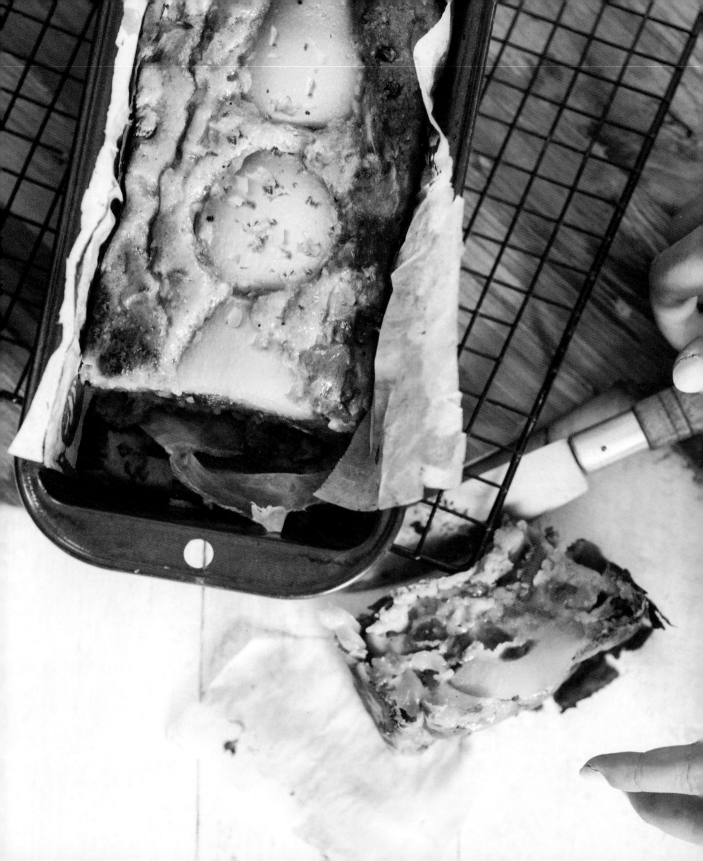

Need a wonderfully moist loaf recipe without butter or margarine? Enjoy this for dessert, breakfast or afternoon tea. Walnuts have cholesterol-lowering properties and the dried muscatel grapes are full of polyphenol antioxidants to protect your cholesterol from being oxidised into a harmful form.

SPICED PEAR, WALNUT AND MUSCATEL LOAF

PREPARATION: 15 MINUTES, COOKING: 55 MINUTES, SERVES 10

90 g (¾ cup) rye flour
150 g (1 cup) wholemeal self-raising flour
1 teaspoon baking powder
½ cup seeded muscatel raisins
½ cup walnut pieces, plus an extra
   2 tablespoons for decoration
1 x 825 g (29 oz) can pear halves
   in natural juice
2 tablespoons honey
¼ teaspoon baking spice

1. Pre-heat oven to 180°C (350°F). Line a standard loaf tin (21 x 11 x 7 cm/8 x 4½ x 3 in) with parchment (baking) paper, so it goes up the sides to the top.

2. Place flours, baking powder, muscatels and walnuts into a large bowl. Stir with a wooden spoon to break up any raisins that are stuck together.

3. Drain pears, reserving the juice. Set aside 3 shapely pear halves and roughly chop the remainder into 1-centimetre (½-inch) pieces.

4. Add chopped pears to the flour and nut mixture, along with 1 cup of reserved pear juice. Fold ingredients gently to combine. The mixture should be moist and sticky.

5. Spoon mixture into prepared loaf tin. Spread evenly. Arrange the 3 reserved pear halves along the top, cut sides face down.

6. In a small bowl, mix together the honey and spice, and spoon this over each pear. Sprinkle with extra walnuts.

7. Bake for approximately 55 minutes. Allow loaf to cool for at least 30 minutes in tin. Using the paper sides, lift gently from tin and slice with a serrated knife. Serve warm or enjoy at room temperature. Store sliced loaf in fridge in an airtight container.

TIP:
- Serve with a dollop of Cashew Nut Cream (page 244).

Per serve: energy 831 kJ (200 Cal); protein 4 g; fat 5 g; saturated fat 0 g; cholesterol 0 mg; carbohydrate 34 g; sugars 19 g; fibre 6 g; calcium 36 mg; iron 1.4 mg; sodium 174 mg

Mild-tasting nuts like cashews, almonds and peanuts can be used to whip up a deliciously light and fluffy cream to serve alongside any dessert. Unlike dairy cream, which is high in saturated fat and will clog your arteries, this cream lowers high cholesterol and tones down the effect of carbohydrates on blood sugar levels. Enjoy it, knowing it's doing your body good!

CASHEW NUT CREAM

PREPARATION: 5 MINUTES, COOKING: 0 MINUTES, SERVES 6

1 cup raw cashews
4 canned pear halves, drained
½ teaspoon alcohol-free pure vanilla extract

1. Place all ingredients in a food processor. Puree for several minutes until smooth and ivory in colour, scraping down sides of the bowl half way with a spatula.
2. Transfer cream to a glass jar and refrigerate, ready for use when required. Recipe is unsuitable for freezing. Makes 1½ cups.

TIPS:

- Variation: Substitute ½ cup of apple juice for pears.
- If using peanuts, rub off their skins first, or blanch almonds to remove their skin for a whiter colour.

Per serve: energy 674 kJ (161 Cal); protein 4 g; fat 12 g; saturated fat 2 g; cholesterol 0 mg; carbohydrate 8 g; sugars 5 g; fibre 3 g; calcium 10 mg; iron 1 mg; sodium 5 mg

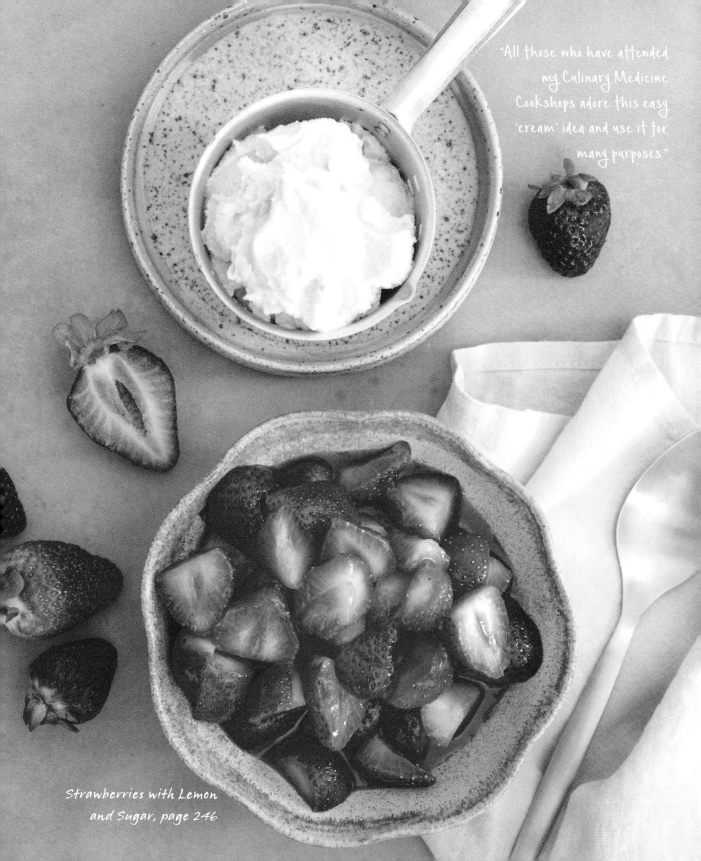

"All those who have attended my Culinary Medicine Cookshops adore this easy 'cream' idea and use it for many purposes."

Strawberries with Lemon and Sugar, page 246

"Fragole al limone" is a classic and classy Italian dessert served in restaurants and homes. It's easy to make and perfect for when strawberries are in season. While this recipe includes a small amount of sugar, Italians don't add any extra ice-cream or cream and neither should you! (Recipe image, page 245.)

STRAWBERRIES WITH LEMON AND SUGAR

PREPARATION: 6 MINUTES, COOKING: 0 MINUTES, SERVES 4

2 x 250 g (9 oz) punnets strawberries
4 teaspoons castor sugar
¼ cup lemon juice (about 1 juiced lemon)

1. Wash and hull strawberries, then cut into halves or quarters, depending on their size, and place in a bowl.
2. Sprinkle with sugar and lemon juice. Toss well to combine and place in the fridge, covered, for at least 2 hours to macerate. Strawberries will soften as they are "cooked" by the acid from the lemon.
3. Taste before serving to ensure the mixture is not too tart. Adjust with a little extra sugar, if required, depending on the natural sweetness of the berries and the tartness of the lemon. Serve chilled. Recipe is unsuitable for freezing.

TIPS:

- For extra presentation, shred a handful of mint leaves and sprinkle on top before serving.
- In Italy, they also use balsamic vinegar as the acid instead of lemon.

Per serve: energy 197 kJ (47 Cal); protein 2 g; fat 0 g; saturated fat 0 g; cholesterol 0 mg; carbohydrate 8 g; sugars 8 g; fibre 2 g; calcium 18 mg; iron 0.8 mg; sodium 8 mg

A perfect-sized treat for the kids, set with "Asian jelly" made from seaweed, so also suitable for vegetarians and vegans. (Recipe image, page 248.)

JAPANESE-STYLE GRAPE JELLY

PREPARATION: 5 MINUTES + 30 MINUTES CHILLING, COOKING: 5 MINUTES, SERVES 4

**12 purple grapes, washed, dried with
paper towelling**
2 cups grape juice at room temperature
2 teaspoons agar agar
1 tablespoon lemon juice

1. Place grape juice in a small saucepan together with agar agar. Bring to boil, then turn down and cook, stirring constantly, for 1-2 minutes until the agar agar dissolves. Remove from heat and stir in lemon juice. Allow to cool slightly, so there is no visible steam.
2. Swirl water into each small serving glass or dish, then pour out. (This will prevent jelly from sticking, so washing up is easier.) Add 3 grapes to each glass.
3. Drizzle grape juice mixture evenly over the grapes—approximately 3 large serving spoons per glass—then place in the fridge for 30 minutes to set. Serve chilled.

TIPS:

- You can buy agar agar from Asian grocery stores or health-food stores. It comes in powder form or noodle-like strands.
- While you can peel the grape skin to make the grapes softer, I don't advise this as it will remove most of their valuable polyphenols.
- Agar agar will not set in the presence of some foods, such as kiwi fruit, pineapple, rhubarb or papaya.

Per serve: energy 385 kJ (92 Cal); protein 1 g; fat 0 g; saturated fat 0 g; cholesterol 0 mg; carbohydrate 23 g; sugars 23 g; fibre 1 g; calcium 21 mg; iron 0.6 mg; sodium 20 mg

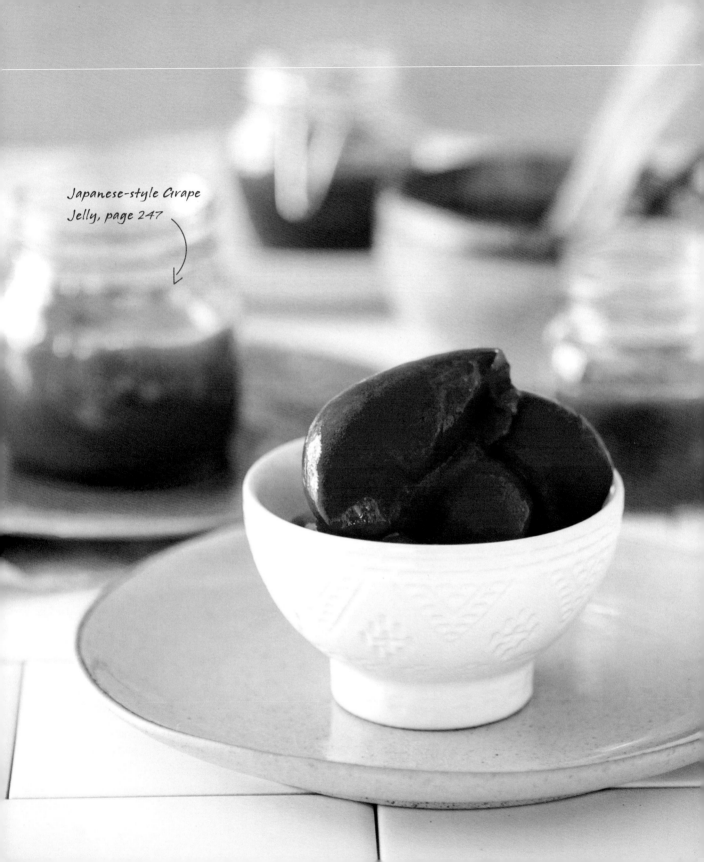

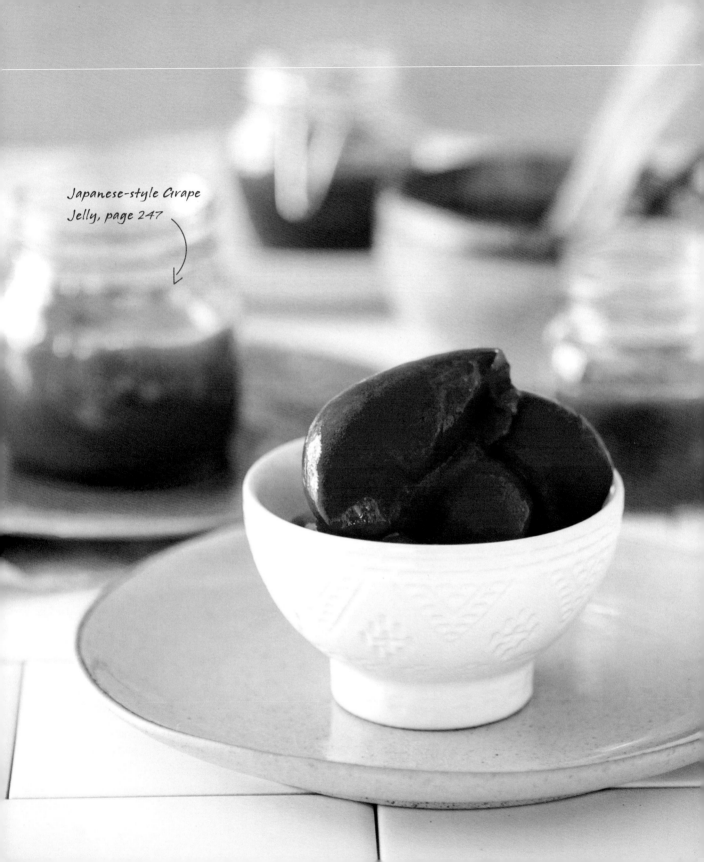Japanese-style Grape
Jelly, page 247

This easy tangy recipe has all the goodness of whole fruit without the additives that usually hide in ice-cream. Perfect for an elegant ending to a dinner party. Berries are some of the highest antioxidant foods you can find. Like strawberries, raspberries are low GI and contain ellagic acid, but they have 50 per cent more of this phytonutrient and double the fibre.

REAL RASPBERRY SORBET

PREPARATION: 5 MINUTES, COOKING: 0 MINUTES, SERVES 6

2 large (approximately 120 g/4 oz each) very ripe bananas, peeled, chopped and frozen
2 cups frozen raspberries
2 tablespoons natural maple syrup
2 tablespoons lemon juice

1. Remove bananas from freezer and place in a food processor. Let sit for 5–7 minutes to soften slightly, then pulse until broken down.
2. Add remaining ingredients and blend until a thick, creamy pink mixture is formed, pausing once or twice to scrape down sides.
3. Serve immediately in cups or cones, or transfer to a glass bowl with a lid and freeze for later.

TIPS:

– This recipe is great for using up bananas that are starting to go brown. Simply peel, chop and pop into the freezer for later use.
– The pink colour will intensify with freezing and turn raspberry red.
– You can also use other berries of your choice.
– Freeze leftover sorbet in an ice-cube tray to make your own smoothie cubes. Then just pop them into a blender with dairy or soy milk or yogurt!

Per serve: energy 405 kJ (97 Cal); protein 2 g; fat 0 g; saturated fat 0 g; cholesterol 0 mg; carbohydrate 19 g; sugars 17 g; fibre 6 g; calcium 29 mg; iron 0.7 mg; sodium 2 mg

If you're not a lover of traditional fruitcakes, this is for you! It isn't sickly sweet and it's full of the more delicious fruits. Celebrate the season and stay healthy at the same time! Think tangy apricots, and the seeded texture and sweetness of figs. You'll want to also make it in a loaf pan and sneak slivers all year round!

HEALTHY CHRISTMAS CAKE

PREPARATION: 20 MINUTES, COOKING: 50 MINUTES, SERVES 12

3 free-range eggs

3 tablespoons extra virgin olive oil

zest of 1 whole orange

½ cup orange juice (from about 1 juiced
   orange)

1 teaspoon ground cassia

¼ teaspoon ground nutmeg

1 teaspoon alcohol-free pure vanilla extract

600 g dried apricots, figs and raisins
   (use equal amounts of each), chopped

1 cup almond meal

1 cup plain wholemeal flour

½ cup walnuts, lightly broken up or chopped

20 blanched almonds

1 tablespoon apricot jam

1. Grease a round 18-centimetre (7-inch) baking tin or rectangular 13 x 23-centimetre (5 x 9-inch) loaf pan with a small amount of olive oil, then line with parchment (baking) paper, leaving some overhang so you can easily lift the cake from the tin when baked. The paper will stick to the tin as it has been greased. Pre-heat oven to 180°C (350°F).

2. In a large mixing bowl, whisk eggs, oil, zest and juice, and stir in spices and vanilla extract.

3. Coarsely chop dried fruits and add to mixture, together with almond meal, flour and walnuts. Fold until well combined so there are no clumps of fruit.

4. Transfer mixture into the baking tin, packing it down so there are no air pockets. Level the surface with the back of a spoon. Make a gentle hollow in the middle to prevent the cake from peaking. Press almonds on top into a pattern and bake for 50–55 minutes until cooked. Cover with foil for the last 10 minutes to prevent raisins from burning. Test by inserting a skewer in the middle, which should come out fairly dry.

5. Remove cake from oven but leave in tin for about 30 minutes, then transfer to a rack, peel off the parchment paper and cool completely before slicing. Warm jam and brush over the top for a glaze. Store in an airtight container in the pantry for up to 2 weeks or freeze. Note: Refrigerating the cake will dry it out and should only be done under humid conditions.

TIP:

- Australian dried apricots have a tangier flavour than Turkish dried apricots. Greek dried white figs are moist and delicious!

Per serve: energy 1432 kJ (342 Cal); protein 8 g; fat 16 g; saturated fat 2 g; cholesterol 46 mg; carbohydrate 40 g; sugars 31 g; fibre 7 g; calcium 94 mg; iron 2.2 mg; sodium 38 mg

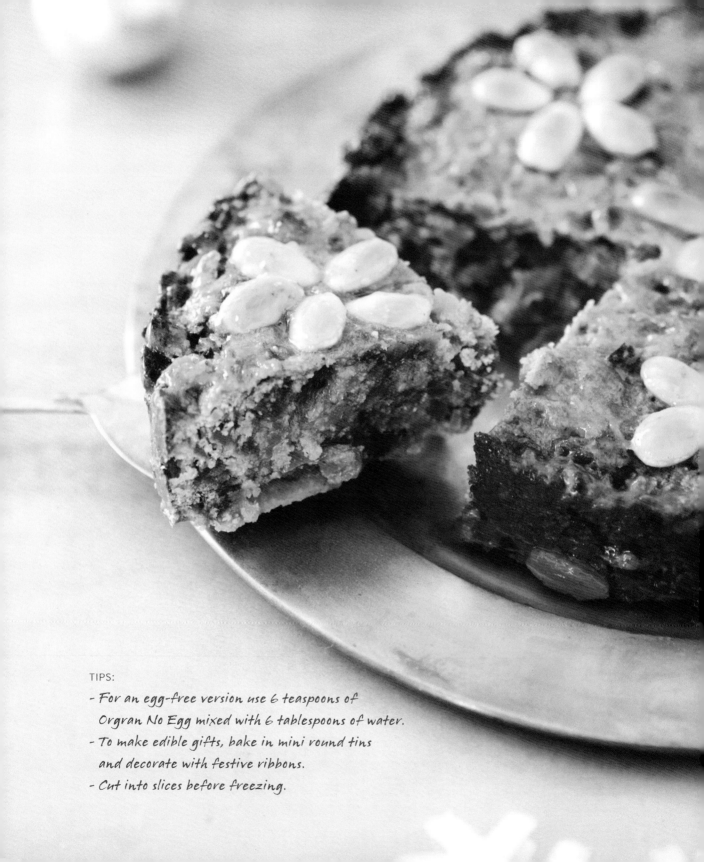

TIPS:
- For an egg-free version use 6 teaspoons of
  Orgran No Egg mixed with 6 tablespoons of water.
- To make edible gifts, bake in mini round tins
  and decorate with festive ribbons.
- Cut into slices before freezing.

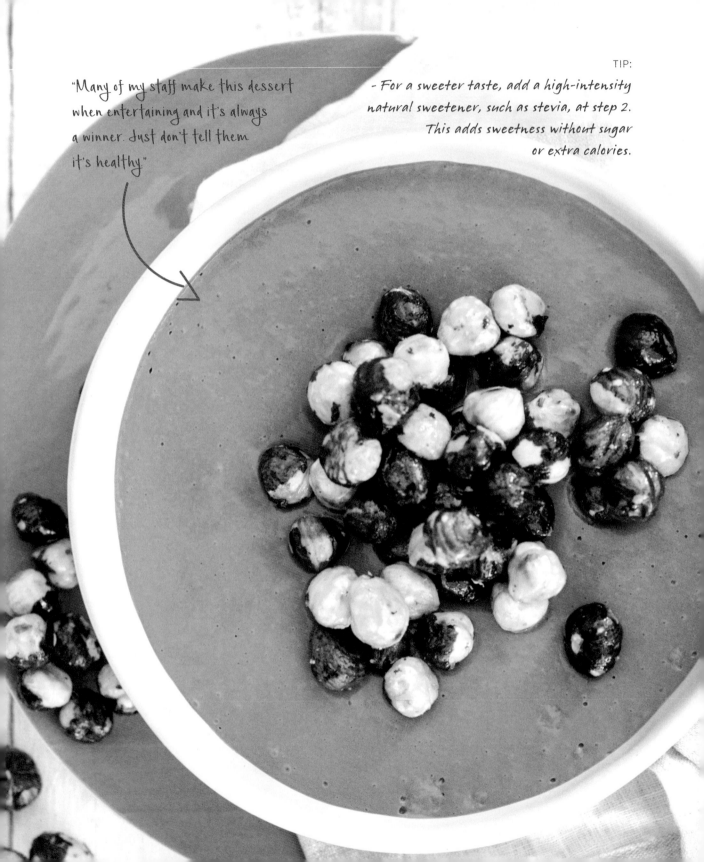

"Many of my staff make this dessert when entertaining and it's always a winner. Just don't tell them it's healthy."

TIP:
- For a sweeter taste, add a high-intensity natural sweetener, such as stevia, at step 2. This adds sweetness without sugar or extra calories.

This sweet treat is a great dessert for guests, offering all the satisfaction without the guilt! Depending on the processing method, dark chocolate can be rich in flavonoids, which impart a bitter flavour but help relax blood vessels and lower blood pressure. The hazelnut topping adds a lovely sweet contrast. Tofu delivers extra food-as-medicine power by lowering high cholesterol.

BITTERSWEET CHOCOLATE MOUSSE WITH HAZELNUT MAPLE CRUNCH

PREPARATION: 15 MINUTES + 1 HOUR CHILLING, COOKING: 5 MINUTES, SERVES 6

100 g (3½ oz) dark (85% cocoa) chocolate, chopped
¼ cup soy milk
300 g (10½ oz) silken tofu (medium firm)
2 tablespoons natural maple syrup

Topping
100 g (3½ oz) hazelnuts, whole
2 tablespoons natural maple syrup

1. Place chocolate and soy milk in a small saucepan, and heat until just melted and combined, being careful not to cook the chocolate.
2. Wipe excess moisture from tofu with paper towelling and place together with 2 tablespoons of the maple syrup in a food processor. Blend until just smooth, then add chocolate mixture and continue blending until a very smooth paste forms.
3. Transfer mixture to 6 individual serving cups or glasses and place in the fridge for at least 1 hour to set.
4. While the mousse is setting, toast hazelnuts in a frypan, until they are aromatic and begin to brown. Remove from heat and add remaining maple syrup. Stir to combine until mixture comes together. Pile up over each chocolate mousse and return them to the fridge until firm. Serve chilled.

TIPS:

- Look for dark chocolate where cocoa mass, not sugar, is the first ingredient. Avoid "Dutched chocolate" as this type of chocolate is stripped of flavonoids due to the alkaline processing. The type of processing is not always declared on the label so you might need to contact the manufacturer.

- Variation: Replace a third of the hazelnuts with slivered almonds.

Per serve: energy 1140 kJ (272 Cal); protein 7 g; fat 16 g; saturated fat 3 g; cholesterol 0 mg; carbohydrate 24 g; sugars 21 g; fibre 3 g; calcium 61 mg; iron 2.4 mg; sodium 28 mg

This delicious gluten-free, low-sodium dessert is inspired from Thailand, where fragrant flavours abound. It's easy to create and a much healthier option compared to usual puddings. Tapioca pearls are made from starch derived from the root of the cassava plant. The essential oils from the spices provide a subtle contrast to the creamy texture of the pudding. The tangy mango and passionfruit topping adds a refreshing note.

TAPIOCA PUDDING WITH MANGO, COCONUT CREAM AND KAFFIR LIME

PREPARATION: 10 MINUTES + 3 HOURS SOAKING, COOKING: 15 MINUTES, SERVES 9

1 cup small tapioca pearls, soaked
   in cold water for 3-4 hours or overnight,
   drained
1 stalk lemongrass, finely sliced
4 fresh kaffir lime leaves, rolled and
   finely sliced
5-centimetre (2-inch) knob ginger, peeled
   and finely sliced or grated
2 cups lite soy milk
5 tablespoons natural maple syrup

Topping
1 large mango, peeled, cheeks cut into
   small cubes
pulp from 4 passionfruit
9 tablespoons coconut cream
9 kaffir lime leaves, rolled and very finely
   shredded

1. Place lemongrass, kaffir lime and ginger into a small saucepan with 1 cup of water, cover and bring to boil. Turn off heat and steep for at least 20 minutes. Pour through a strainer into a larger saucepan (about 8-cup capacity), pressing down on the solids with a spoon to release all the flavoured liquid. Discard the solids.
2. Add milk and maple syrup, and bring almost to boil. Stir in drained tapioca pearls and bring to boil, then turn down heat and simmer for about 5 minutes, stirring constantly, until the pearls are translucent.
3. Divide tapioca into 9 glasses or small Asian dessert bowls, and allow to cool slightly, then refrigerate until required.
4. Prior to serving, top each pudding with cubed mango and passionfruit pulp, and drizzle with some coconut cream. Garnish with the kaffir lime.

TIPS:

- Do not use boiling water to soak tapioca or it will turn to mush.
   If in a hurry, quick soak it for 20 minutes in warm water.
- Use a saucepan with a thick bottom when cooking tapioca to prevent sticking.

Per serve: energy 809 kJ (193 Cal); protein 3 g; fat 5 g; saturated fat 4 g; cholesterol 0 mg; carbohydrate 33 g; sugars 14 g; fibre 2 g; calcium 88 mg; iron 0.8 mg; sodium 50 mg

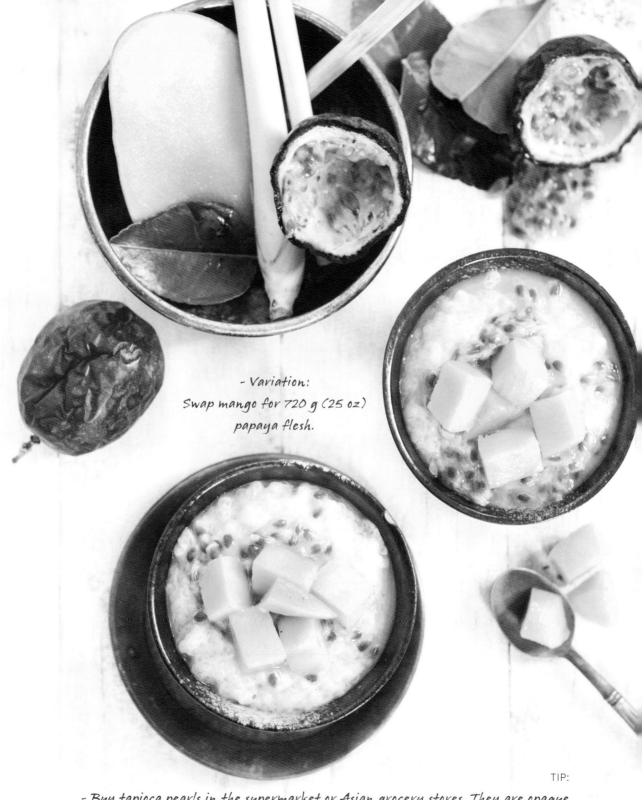

- Variation:
Swap mango for 720 g (25 oz)
papaya flesh.

TIP:
- Buy tapioca pearls in the supermarket or Asian grocery stores. They are opaque
white in colour when dry but become translucent after cooking.

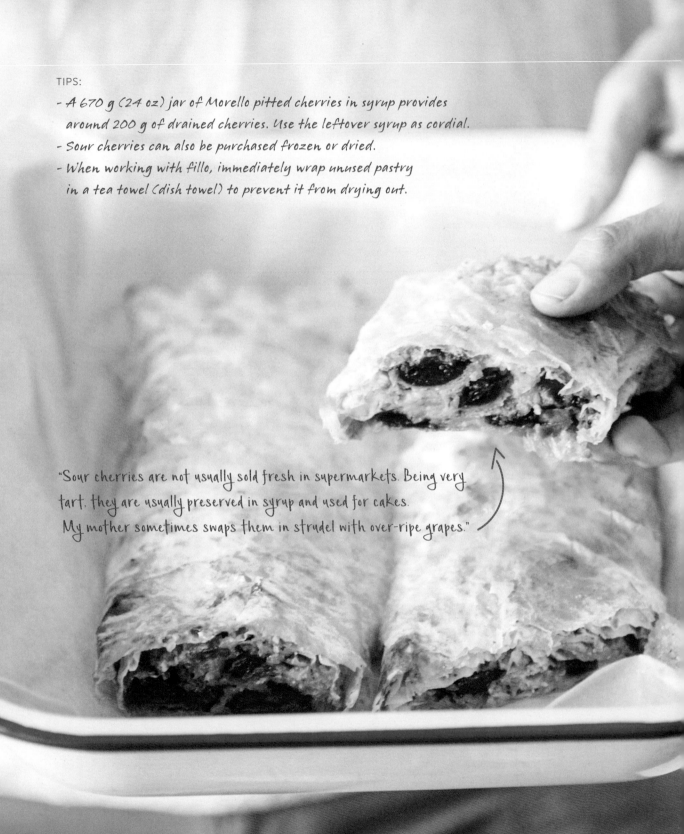

TIPS:
- A 670 g (24 oz) jar of Morello pitted cherries in syrup provides around 200 g of drained cherries. Use the leftover syrup as cordial.
- Sour cherries can also be purchased frozen or dried.
- When working with fillo, immediately wrap unused pastry in a tea towel (dish towel) to prevent it from drying out.

"Sour cherries are not usually sold fresh in supermarkets. Being very tart, they are usually preserved in syrup and used for cakes. My mother sometimes swaps them in strudel with over-ripe grapes."

A delicious sweet-sour filling, wrapped in light flaky pastry, to enjoy as dessert. Morello is a dark, sour cherry used for making cakes in Europe and the Middle East. Sour cherries and their juice have been shown to provide unique anti-inflammatory effects. Walnuts supply omega-3s to further tone down inflammation. Remove fillo from the fridge 2 hours before use to ensure it is pliable, rather than brittle and prone to cracking.

APPLE, SOUR CHERRY AND WALNUT STRUDEL

PREPARATION: 30 MINUTES, COOKING: 35 MINUTES, SERVES 12

4 large green apples (about 800 g/28 oz)
¼ cup brown sugar
9 sheets fillo pastry
½ cup extra virgin olive oil
½ cup breadcrumbs
200 g (7 oz) drained, pitted sour cherries
⅓ cup walnuts, chopped

Lemon Syrup
1 tablespoon lemon juice
2 teaspoons extra virgin olive oil
2 teaspoons brown sugar

1. Pre-heat oven to 200°C (390°F). Brush a large baking tray with some of the oil.

2. Grate apples with their skin on. Sprinkle with sugar.

3. Place 3 sheets of pastry, vertically, beside each other on a clean bench. Brush well with oil, being sure to cover edges. Sprinkle one-third of breadcrumbs on the pastry sheets, then place another layer of pastry on top of each sheet. Repeat with the oil brushing, bread-crumbs and the third layer of pastry, so you have 3 reinforced fillo sheets ready for filling.

4. Divide grated apple mixture, cherries and walnuts evenly over the 3 fillo pastries using a spoon. Spread out contents so there are no large clumps. Roll each pastry, in turn, toward yourself, wrapping it up so you end with the seam on the bottom.

5. Transfer strudels onto oiled tray. Brush with leftover oil and extra water to soften. Bake for 30 minutes until golden, basting with more water half way through baking.

6. Meanwhile, prepare syrup by placing ingredients into a small saucepan and boiling for 1 minute.

7. Remove baked strudel from oven and brush with syrup until it soaks in.

8. Place back in the oven for a further 5 minutes, then remove and cool before cutting.

9. Trim both ends of each strudel at 45 degrees, then cut each into 4 diamond-shaped pieces. Serve at room temperature or store in a cool cupboard for up to 2 days and re-heat in oven before serving.

Per serve: energy 942 kJ (225 Cal); protein 3 g; fat 13 g; saturated fat 2 g; cholesterol 0 mg; carbohydrate 24 g; sugars 14 g; fibre 3 g; calcium 18 mg; iron 0.7 mg; sodium 114 mg

People fight over these delicious waffles, yet they contain no flour, eggs or butter. With eight whole grains and four kinds of nuts and seeds, these waffles are very nutritious, high in fibre and a good source of iron. Strawberries raise the antioxidant capacity of your blood and their ellagic acid boosts your body's natural detox enzymes. Adding strawberries to a meal has been shown to reduce the insulin response in overweight people!

CRISPY MULTIGRAIN WAFFLES WITH WARM STRAWBERRY AND RHUBARB SAUCE

PREPARATION: 15 MINUTES, COOKING: 45 MINUTES, SERVES 8

Waffles

olive oil spray

¼ cup LSA (linseed, sunflower seed and almond mixture)

¼ cup rolled amaranth

½ cup buckwheat or buckwheat pieces

½ cup rolled millet

½ cup rolled grain mix (barley, triticale, rye, wheat)

½ cup rolled oats

1 tablespoon soy flour

2 tablespoons brown sugar

¼ cup raw cashew pieces

pinch of salt

Sauce

2 x 250 g (9 oz) punnets strawberries, washed, hulled and halved

400 g (14 oz) rhubarb stalks, washed and cut into 3-centimetre (1-inch) pieces

¼ cup brown sugar

1. Place all waffle ingredients into a blender, together with 3 cups of water, and process for a few minutes until batter is milky and smooth.

2. Heat waffle iron on high. When hot, coat with olive oil spray.

3. Pour in ½ cup of the batter and cook several minutes until crispy and golden brown. This may take 3–5 minutes, depending on your waffle maker. Do not overfill, as the mixture will spill over the edges.

4. Mix a further ½ cup of water into the batter, as it will have thickened while standing. The consistency should be similar to pancake batter.

5. Repeat step 3 until all the batter is used up. (Tip: If you have a non-stick waffle iron, you might not need to add more spray after the first waffle.)

6. Meanwhile, place all the sauce ingredients, together with ½ cup of water, in a saucepan, then cover and gradually bring to boil. Reduce heat immediately to low and simmer for about 10 minutes until fruit has just softened and released its juices, being careful not to overcook it.

7. Serve waffles with sauce or freeze for later with freezer-go-between paper.

Per serve: energy 1148 kJ (274 Cal); protein 9 g; fat 8 g; saturated fat 1 g; cholesterol 0 mg; carbohydrate 38 g; sugars 11 g; fibre 7 g; calcium 66 mg; iron 2.8 mg; sodium 35 mg

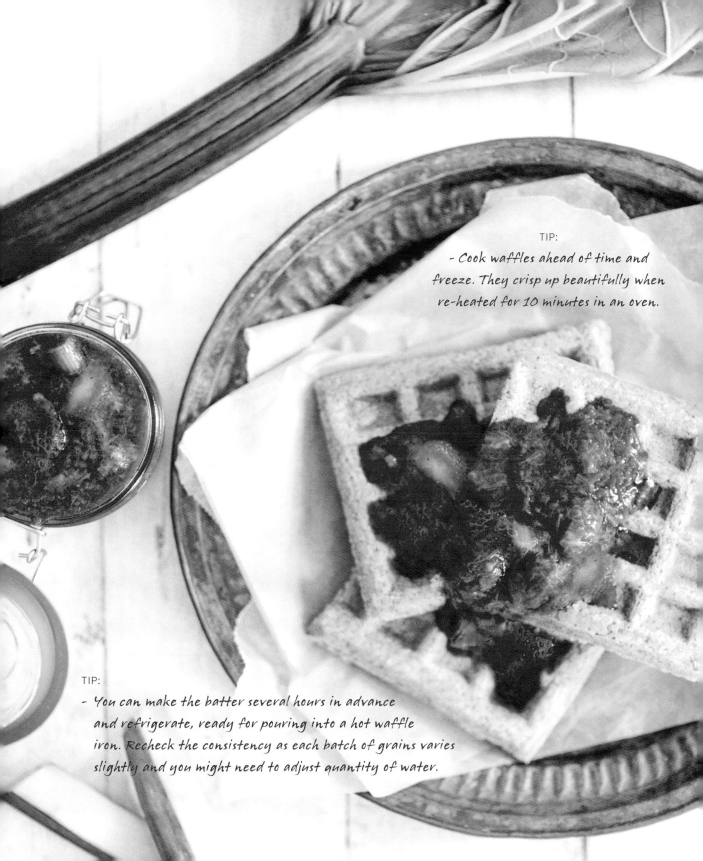

TIP:
- Cook waffles ahead of time and freeze. They crisp up beautifully when re-heated for 10 minutes in an oven.

TIP:
- You can make the batter several hours in advance and refrigerate, ready for pouring into a hot waffle iron. Recheck the consistency as each batch of grains varies slightly and you might need to adjust quantity of water.

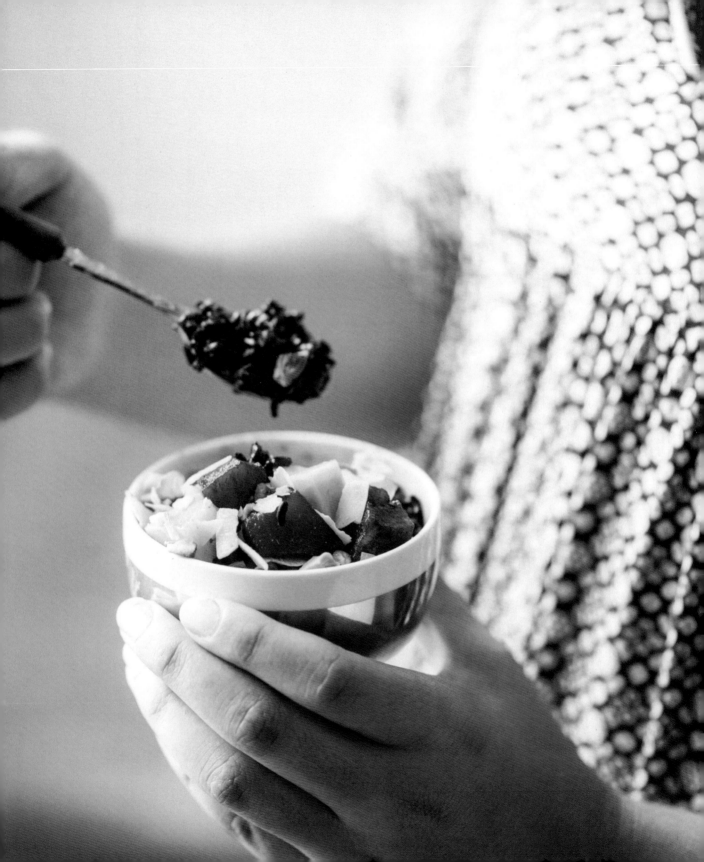

This Asian-style pudding tastes decadent with the coconut cream. Despite the longer cooking time, it's well worth the effort. Black glutinous rice does not contain any gluten—its name describes the sticky texture when cooked. The purplish colour is due to phytonutrients.

BLACK RICE PUDDING WITH PISTACHIO AND COCONUT

PREPARATION: 10 MINUTES, COOKING: 40 MINUTES, SERVES 4

½ **cup black glutinous rice, rinsed**

¼ **cup flaked dried coconut**

¼ **cup pistachio kernels, roughly chopped**

¼ **teaspoon ground cassia**

¼ **teaspoon ground cardamom**

pinch of ground cloves

1 tablespoon honey

165 ml (5½ fl oz) lite coconut cream

1 cup diced fresh fruits, such as mango, peach or plum

1. Place rinsed rice in a small saucepan with 2 cups of water and bring to boil. Fast simmer with the lid on for about 30 minutes, stirring occasionally, until rice is soft.

2. Meanwhile, lightly toast coconut and pistachio nuts in a small dry pan until golden and fragrant. Place in a bowl to cool while making pudding. (Note: Coconut will continue to brown if you leave it in the hot pan.)

3. When rice is cooked, add spices, honey and about three-quarters of coconut cream. Stir well for about 5 minutes over low heat until rice has absorbed most of the liquid. The rice should be sticky and soft.

4. Divide mixture into 4 small bowls or glasses. Drizzle with remainder of coconut cream, sprinkle with toasted flaked coconut and pistachios, and top with the fresh fruit and serve. Recipe is unsuitable for freezing.

Per serve: energy 644 kJ (154 Cal); protein 5 g; fat 9 g; saturated fat 4 g; cholesterol 0 mg; carbohydrate 31 g; sugars 12 g; fibre 2 g; calcium 20 mg; iron 1.7 mg; sodium 9 mg

An easy dessert with a good dose of sour cherries. Sour cherries are loaded with phytonutrients that fight inflammation to ease arthritis, prevent gout attacks and aid in muscle recovery. One study suggests half a cup of frozen sour cherries is the equivalent of approximately two aspirin! You will need to start this recipe the night before.

SOUR CHERRY SAGO

PREPARATION: 5 MINUTES + OVERNIGHT SOAKING + 3 HOUR CHILLING, COOKING: 20 MINUTES, SERVES 4

⅓ cup small sago pearls (or seed tapioca)
2 tablespoons natural maple syrup
½ cassia or cinnamon stick
1½ cups drained pitted sour cherries
    in syrup

1. Place sago in a bowl and cover with cold water. Leave to soften overnight, then drain and rinse excess starch before use.
2. Place 1½ cups of water in a small saucepan and bring to boil. Add sago, maple syrup and cassia, and simmer for approximately 15 minutes, stirring constantly, until the pearls turn transparent.
3. Remove cassia and add cherries, then simmer for a further 5 minutes, stirring occasionally. The mixture should turn a lovely pink, and be sticky and gelatinous.
4. Remove from heat and divide into 4 individual serving bowls. Refrigerate for at least 3 hours to set before serving.

TIPS:

- Sago and tapioca pearls are available from Asian grocery stores and most supermarkets. Although sago comes from the sago palm and tapioca from the cassava plant, they are used interchangeably.
- To wash the sticky saucepan after cooking, simply fill with water and soak for 5 hours or overnight. The residual sago will be easily removed.
- Serve with a dollop of vanilla-bean yogurt and grated dark chocolate for garnish, if desired.

Per serve: energy 547 kJ (131 Cal); protein 1 g; fat 0 g; saturated fat 0 g; cholesterol 0 mg; carbohydrate 32 g; sugars 18 g; fibre 1 g; calcium 18 mg; iron 1 mg; sodium 4 mg

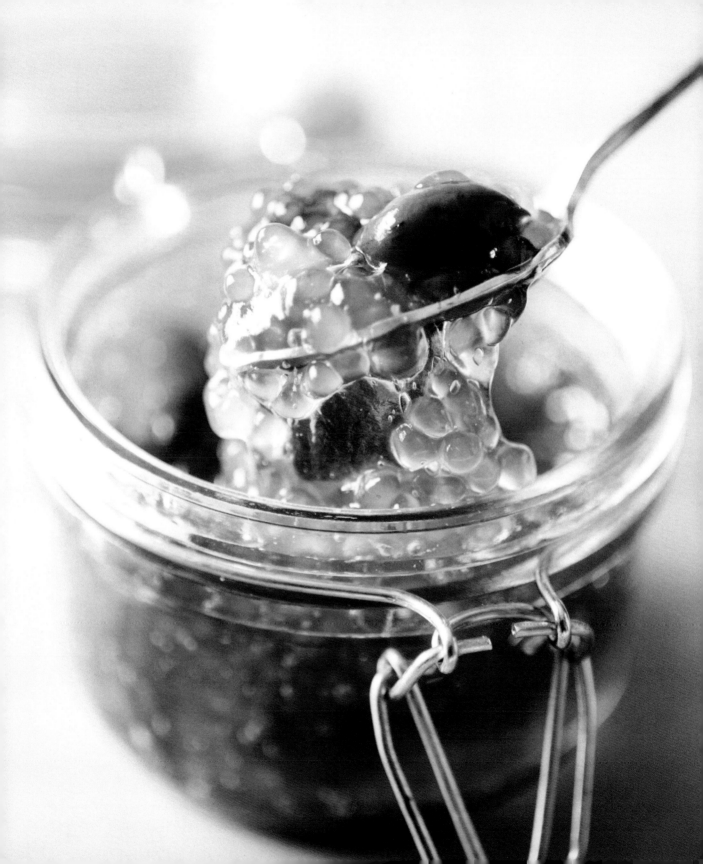

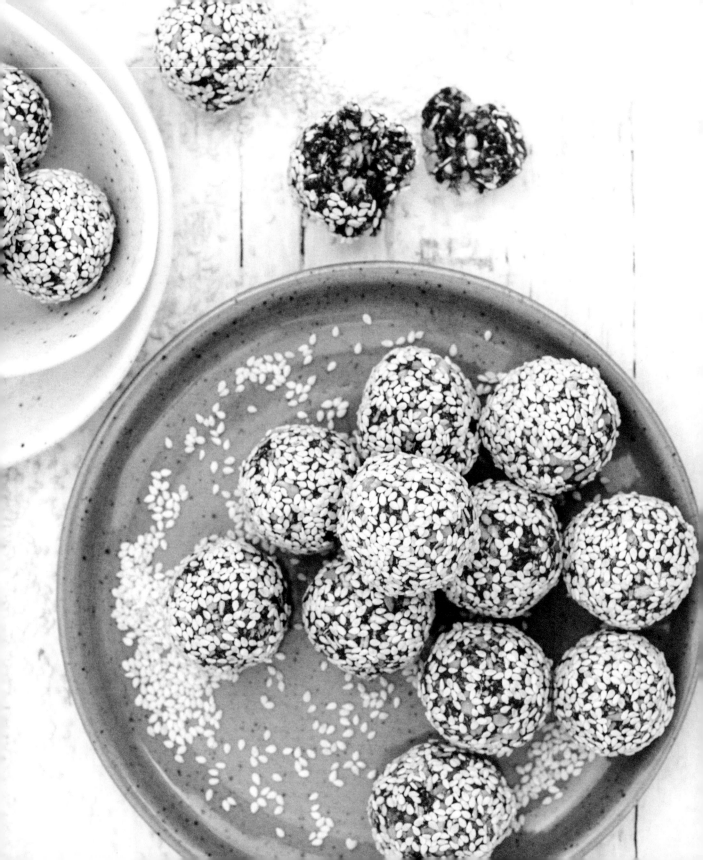

These energy balls are designed to give you an instant buzz pre- or post-workout, or simply a quick treat on the go. They're based on the goodness of nuts, seeds and fresh dates, which make an excellent sweetener while adding texture.

HIGH ENERGY BALLS

PREPARATION: 20 MINUTES, COOKING: 0 MINUTES, SERVES 10

½ cup walnuts

200 g (7 oz) pitted fresh medjool dates

½ cup almond meal

1 cup traditional rolled oats

½ cup sunflower seeds

¼ cup raw cacao powder

3 tablespoons natural maple syrup

¼ cup white sesame seeds

1. Using a food processor, lightly pulse walnuts into coarse pieces and put aside.

2. Place remaining ingredients in the food processor, except for sesame seeds, and blend until the mixture comes together.

3. Transfer mixture to a bowl and fold in walnuts.

4. Using moistened hands, grab walnut-sized amounts of the mixture and shape into balls.

5. Place sesame seeds into a small bowl and roll the balls in seeds to coat their surface. Serve immediately or store in the fridge or freezer and enjoy later. Freezing makes the balls more chewy.

TIPS:

- Add a couple of drops of pure, food-grade essential oil (mint or orange) for flavour variation!

- For additional protein, add 3 tablespoons of a plant protein powder, such as pea protein powder.

- Variation: Roll balls in raw cacao powder for a more bitter flavour or substitute ground pistachios for sesame seeds. Simply press more firmly into the balls.

Per serve: energy 1002 kJ (239 Cal); protein 6 g; fat 12 g; saturated fat 0 g; cholesterol 0 mg; carbohydrate 25 g; sugars 19 g; fibre 5 g; calcium 52 mg; iron 1.6 mg; sodium 3 mg

SNACKS, NIBBLES & SWEET MORSELS

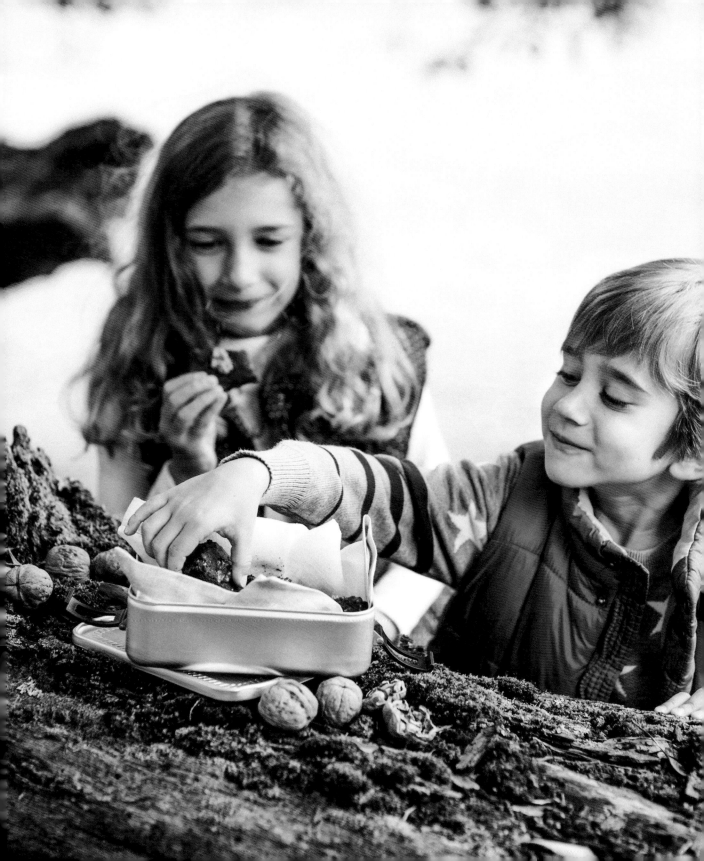

A decadent, yet super-healthy, sweet for that chocolate hit. Perfect to take to picnics and parties, and not as sickly sweet as some brownies. Black beans are low GI and high in polyphenols, as are nuts and seeds. The spices add further antioxidants and tone down inflammation!

CHOCOLATE BROWNIES WITH WALNUTS

PREPARATION: 15 MINUTES, COOKING: 30 MINUTES, SERVES 24

1 cup walnuts + 24 walnut pieces for garnish
3 cups cooked black beans
1 cup extra virgin olive oil
300 g (10½ oz) pitted fresh medjool dates
½ cup white sesame seeds
½ cup raw cacao powder
2 tablespoons ground cinnamon
1 teaspoon ground cardamom
3 tablespoons natural maple syrup
2 teaspoons alcohol-free pure vanilla extract
½ cup sunflower seeds

1. Pre-heat oven to 180ºC (350ºF).
2. Lightly pulse 1 cup of walnuts in a food processor.
3. Add black beans and oil, and blend until combined. Add dates, sesame seeds, cacao powder, spices, maple syrup and vanilla extract, and continue to process until smooth.
4. Transfer mixture into a large bowl and fold in sunflower seeds with a wooden spoon.
5. Spread into a lined baking pan (30 x 23 cm/12 x 9 in) and flatten with a spatula. Cut into 24 squares and press an additional walnut piece in the centre of each square. Tip: Lining the pan with parchment (baking) paper will enable you to easily lift out the brownies when they are cooled.
6. Bake for 30 minutes. Leave to cool in the pan before removing brownies. Enjoy brownies freshly baked or store in the fridge for up to 1 week. They can also be frozen.

TIPS:

- Remove brownies from oven after 30 minutes even if they appear not fully cooked, otherwise they might burn on the bottom.
- Variation: For a spicy version, swap cardamom with ¼ teaspoon ground cayenne pepper.

Per serve: energy 1079 kJ (258 Cal); protein 6 g; fat 18 g; saturated fat 2 g; cholesterol 0 mg; carbohydrate 16 g; sugars 11 g; fibre 6 g; calcium 38 mg; iron 1.9 mg; sodium 4 mg

SIMPLE NATURAL SNACKS

I don't recommend regular snacking for most adults as it often means empty calories and can promote weight gain. My preference is to drink water between meals, allowing 4-5 hours rest to the stomach between eating. However, small stomachs or poor appetites can benefit from regular snacks, and encouraging nutritious snacks between meals is a trusted strategy used in hospitals to promote weight gain.

In the event that your requirements are higher—or you enjoy a healthy nibble between meals—here are a few suggestions for nature's wholefood snacks (in addition to the delicious recipe ideas that follow):

- Fruit in season
- Corn on the cob
- Homemade vegetable soup
- Handful of unsalted, unroasted nuts or seeds
- Roasted chickpeas or fava beans

- Vegetable sticks
- Small sweet potato (steamed or baked)
- Vegetable juice
- Handful of dried fruits

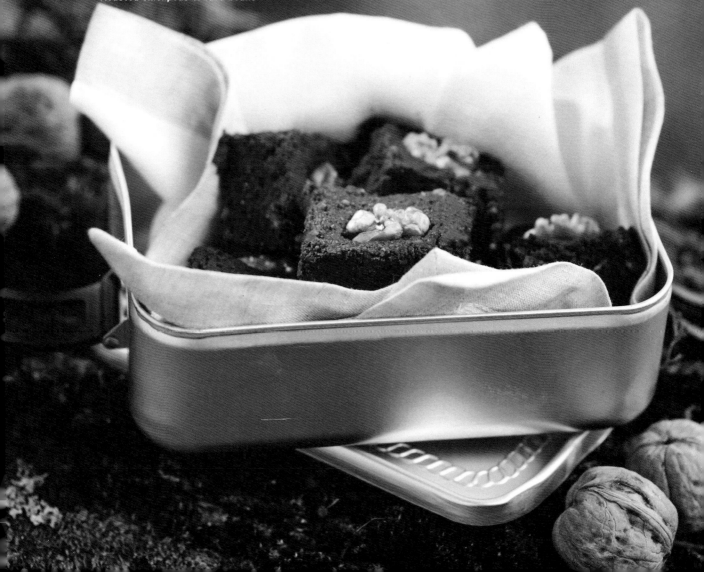

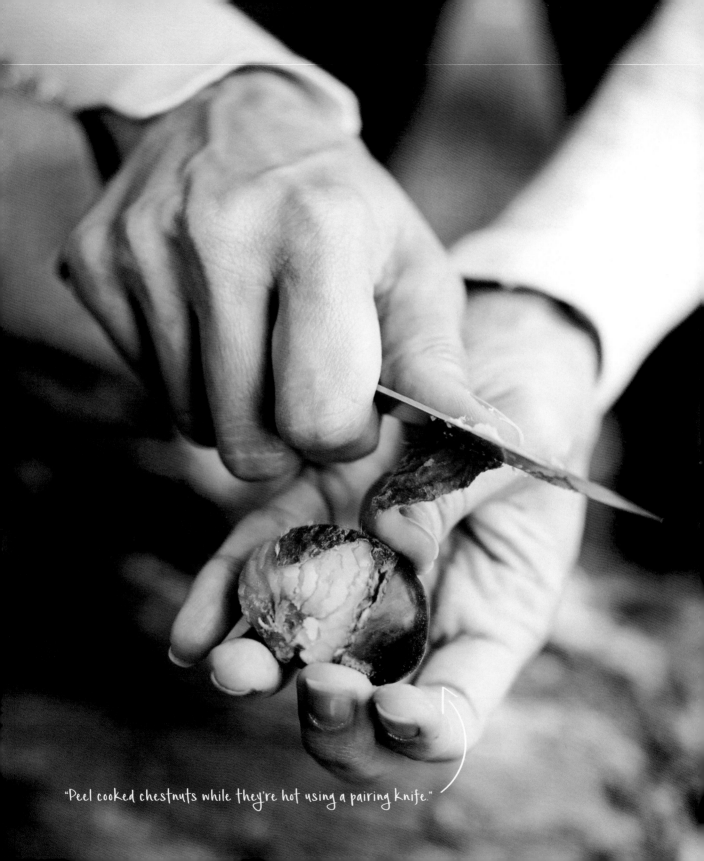

"Peel cooked chestnuts while they're hot using a pairing knife."

For both Europeans and Asians, chestnuts are a favourite snack. Used in the time of Alexander the Great and the Romans, they are still popular and sold roasted by street vendors, when in season. Chestnuts have a delicate, sweet nutty flavour and, unlike other nuts, are very low in fat. They're also loaded with fibre, making them ideal for the whole family. Try this easy recipe, which is just as delicious as roasted chestnuts but doesn't require an oven.

BOILED CHESTNUTS

PREPARATION: 1 MINUTE, COOKING: 40 MINUTES, SERVES 10

1 kg (2 lb 3 oz) fresh chestnuts

1. Place chestnuts in a large saucepan and cover with plenty of cold water.
2. Boil with the lid on for approximately 35 minutes, until the flesh is cooked through and soft like mashed potato. Be careful that the saucepan does not run dry. Add extra boiling water if you notice the water has almost evaporated.
3. Remove from stove and allow chestnuts to remain in the hot water for a further 10 minutes, then drain and serve in a bowl. Eat chestnuts by peeling their skin with a sharp knife or slitting each chestnut in half and sucking out the sweet flesh.

TIPS:

- To test whether chestnuts are cooked, pull one out of the boiling water, cut it in half with a sharp knife and suck out filling, being careful not to burn your tongue. If still firm or crunchy, continue cooking for a little longer. A good-quality, fresh chestnut should be creamy and smooth when cooked.
- To reheat leftover chestnuts, boil for 1-2 minutes. Do not reheat in a microwave as chestnuts might explode.

Per serve: energy 724 kJ (173 Cal); protein 3 g; fat 1 g; saturated fat 0 g; cholesterol 0 mg; carbohydrate 34 g; sugars 4 g; fibre 8 g; calcium 13 mg; iron 0.8 mg; sodium 1 mg

Delicious, easy to make and perfect to replace ordinary biscuits or cookies, which usually hide saturated and trans fats that raise cholesterol. You will enjoy these with a hot drink.

PECAN AND GINGER DROPS

PREPARATION: 25 MINUTES, COOKING: 15 MINUTES, SERVES 12

2 cups pecans

2.5-centimetre (1-inch) knob of fresh ginger, finely grated

200 g (7oz) pitted medjool dates (approximately 10 large dates with pits removed)

4 extra pecans, broken into 6 pieces each, for garnishing

1. Place pecans in a food processor and pulse until coarsely chopped.

2. Add dates and grated ginger, and continue processing until combined and a doughy mixture starts to form.

3. Pre-heat oven to 180°C (350°F).

4. Divide mixture into 4 and form 6 walnut-sized balls from each quarter. Tip: Moisten hands with water so the mixture is less sticky.

5. Place balls onto an ungreased baking tray and gently press down 1 piece of pecan in the middle of each drop. If the balls appears to be splitting around the sides, gently smooth back together before placing in oven. Note: Balls will not spread when baking so they can be placed close together.

6. Bake for 12–15 minutes until golden brown using the upper rack in the oven so the bottoms do not burn. Drops store well in an airtight container for several days.

Per serve: energy 686 kJ (164 Cal); protein 2 g; fat 12 g; saturated fat 1 g; cholesterol 0 mg; carbohydrate 12 g; sugars 12 g; fibre 3 g; calcium 19 mg; iron 0.6 mg; sodium 1 mg

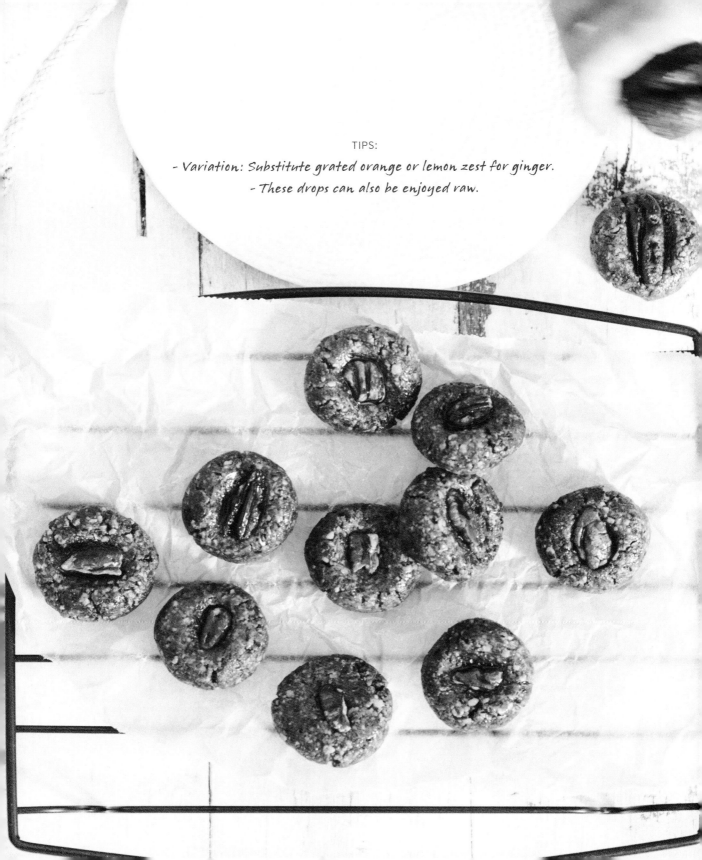

TIPS:
- Variation: Substitute grated orange or lemon zest for ginger.
- These drops can also be enjoyed raw.

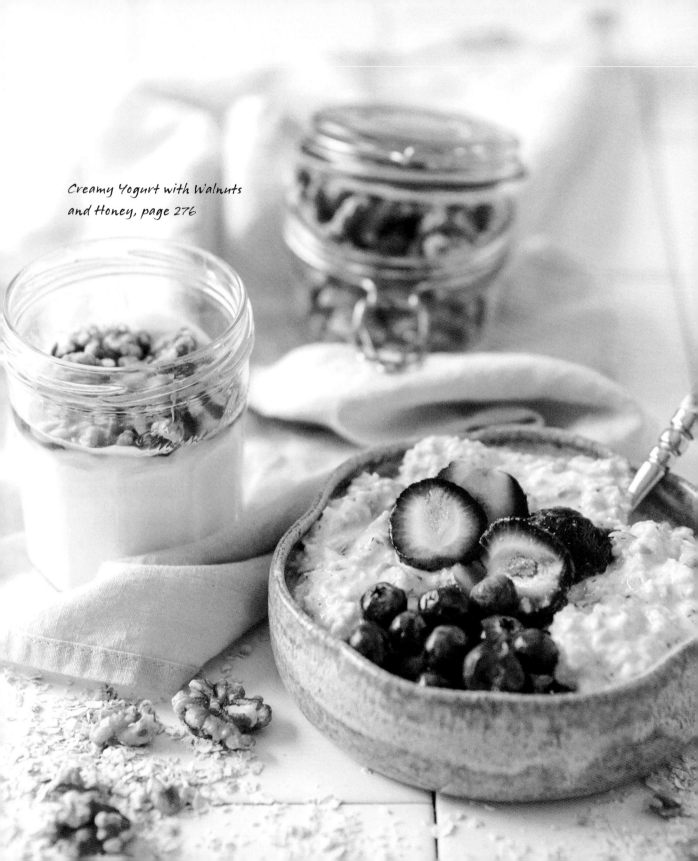

Creamy Yogurt with Walnuts and Honey, page 276

One of my all-time favourite snacks, desserts and breakfast recipes! Use canned berries when fresh berries are out of season. This recipe is high in plant protein and dietary fibre, and a good source of iron and zinc. It is very simple to make, but you need to start the night before. Bircher muesli will keep for several days in the fridge.

BIRCHER MUESLI WITH BERRIES

PREPARATION: 10 MINUTES + 8 HOURS CHILLING, COOKING: 0 MINUTES, SERVES 6

2 cups rolled oats
½ cup chopped dried peaches and dates
½ cup smashed almonds and hazelnuts
2¾ cups lite soy milk
1 green apple, unpeeled, grated
2 tablespoons honey
2½ cups mixed fresh berries (raspberries, blueberries and boysenberries)

1. Place rolled oats, dried fruit and nuts in a bowl.
2. Pour over soy milk and mix. Cover and place in the fridge for about 8 hours or overnight until the mixture becomes soft and sticky.
3. Remove from the fridge and stir in apple and honey. Serve in bowls or cups topped with berries!

TIPS:

- Vary dried fruit and nuts to your taste! There is no wrong combination.
- You can also use other nut or grain milks instead of soy. Some people prefer fruit juice but this results in a higher glycaemic load, which is undesirable for your blood sugar.

Per serve: energy 1437 kJ (343 Cal); protein 10 g; fat 11 g; saturated fat 1 g; cholesterol 0 mg; carbohydrate 46 g; sugars 24 g; fibre 10 g; calcium 210 mg; iron 2.4 mg; sodium 82 mg

Here is a delicious Cretan dessert idea. While Greeks generally don't eat sweets after meals, this nutritive dish is enjoyed during hot weather as an afternoon snack or light meal. Use a thick, Greek-style yogurt known in Greece as "strangisto," meaning strained, and a floral honey, such as from thyme, if available. The sweet-and-sour combination of the ingredients intermingled with the crunchy texture of the walnuts is wonderful! (Recipe image, page 274.)

CREAMY YOGURT WITH WALNUTS AND HONEY

PREPARATION: 5 MINUTES, COOKING: 0 MINUTES, SERVES 4

500 g (17½ oz) Greek-style reduced-fat yogurt
24 fresh walnut halves
8 teaspoons honey

1. Divide yogurt between 4 small dessert bowls. Create grooves on top with the back of a spoon.
2. Sprinkle with walnut pieces and drizzle with honey. Enjoy immediately or make in advance and refrigerate for a few hours before serving.

TIPS:

- Variation: Swap dairy yogurt for a non-dairy alternative, such as coconut or strained soy yogurt.
- For an alternative topping, try coarsely grinding the nuts. Ideally, shell nuts yourself as they will be fresher and taste sweeter. Walnuts are high in omega-3, so they are prone to oxidation and bitterness when stored at room temperature. After shelling, I usually freeze mine.

Per serve: energy 1243 kJ (297 Cal); protein 7 g; fat 15 g; saturated fat 5 g; cholesterol 16 mg; carbohydrate 33 g; sugars 28 g; fibre 1 g; calcium 134 mg; iron 0.5 mg; sodium 68 mg

I love making this compote when quinces are in season. Their sweet aroma pervades the entire kitchen. Prunes are similarly delicious and nutritious. They're exceptionally high in potassium, a good source of fibre and used as a time-honoured natural laxative. Recent research suggests prunes might also make your bones strong. Enjoy nursing a hot mug of this compote in the cool of the evening—it's like drinking tea with floating fruit! In Croatia, this compote is also enjoyed at breakfast. (Recipe image, page 279.)

APPLE, QUINCE AND PRUNE COMPOTE

PREPARATION: 8 MINUTES, COOKING: 35 MINUTES, SERVES 4

1 small quince, peeled and cored
2 medium apples, peeled and cored
12 prunes, pitted
1½ tablespoons honey
1 cinnamon stick

1. Cut quince and apples into small squares, about 2 centimetres (1 inch) in size.
2. Place in a medium saucepan with remaining ingredients and 6 cups of water. Cover and bring to boil.
3. Turn down heat to medium and simmer for about 25 minutes until the fruit has softened and starts to turn clear. Remove from stove and allow to rest for 15 minutes before serving. Discard cinnamon stick and serve compote warm or cold in a mug or bowl with a spoon. Compote can be stored in the fridge for several days. It is unsuitable for freezing.

TIP:

- The golden colour of the compote will intensify with storage, as the prunes swell up and soften further.

Per serve: energy 633 kJ (151 Cal); protein 1 g; fat 0 g; saturated fat 0 g; cholesterol 0 mg; carbohydrate 35 g; sugars 31 g; fibre 5 g; calcium 24 mg; iron 0.6 mg; sodium 9 mg

A lovely Croatian-style dessert made from whole wheat (also known as wheat berries), freshly ground pecans and dried fruit. Traditionally, this dish is served at room temperature for a dessert, snack or breakfast. The wheat berries are low GI and rich in antioxidants.

WHEAT BERRIES WITH PECANS AND SULTANAS

PREPARATION: 7 MINUTES, COOKING: 30 MINUTES INCLUDING PRESSURE COOKER, SERVES 6

1 cup uncooked whole wheat (wheat berries)
¾ cup pecans, freshly ground
½ cup sultanas
2 tablespoons honey

1. Rinse wheat berries and cook, covered, with 5 cups of water until tender. This will take 15 minutes in a pressure cooker, once at pressure (or approximately 1 hour in a conventional saucepan). Allow pressure to reduce naturally before removing lid—this will further soften grains.
2. Transfer wheat berries to a strainer over the sink, rinse, then allow to drain and place into a mixing bowl.
3. Add remaining ingredients and mix well, so honey is distributed and coats all ingredients. Serve in small bowls. Recipe keeps well in the fridge for up to 1 week. It is unsuitable for freezing.

TIPS:

- You can also pulse nuts using a food processor for a more coarse texture.
- Traditionally, this dish is not served with "extras" such as ice-cream. But you can add a dollop of yogurt or stewed fruit, if desired.

Per serve: energy 1108 kJ (265 Cal); protein 6 g; fat 9 g; saturated fat 1 g; cholesterol 0 mg; carbohydrate 37 g; sugars 18 g; fibre 6 g; calcium 31 mg; iron 4.1 mg; sodium 8 mg

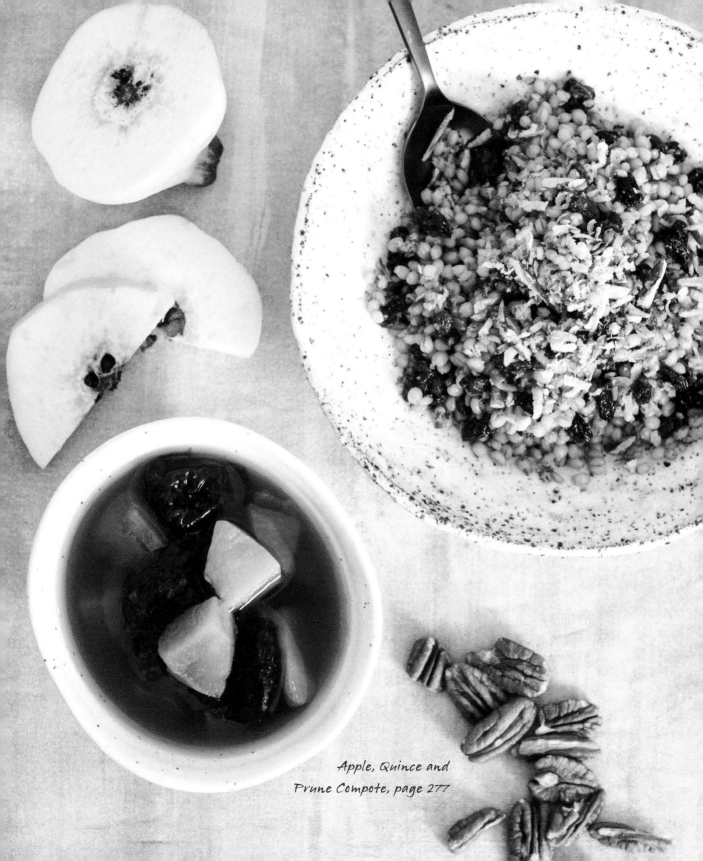

Apple, Quince and
Prune Compote, page 277

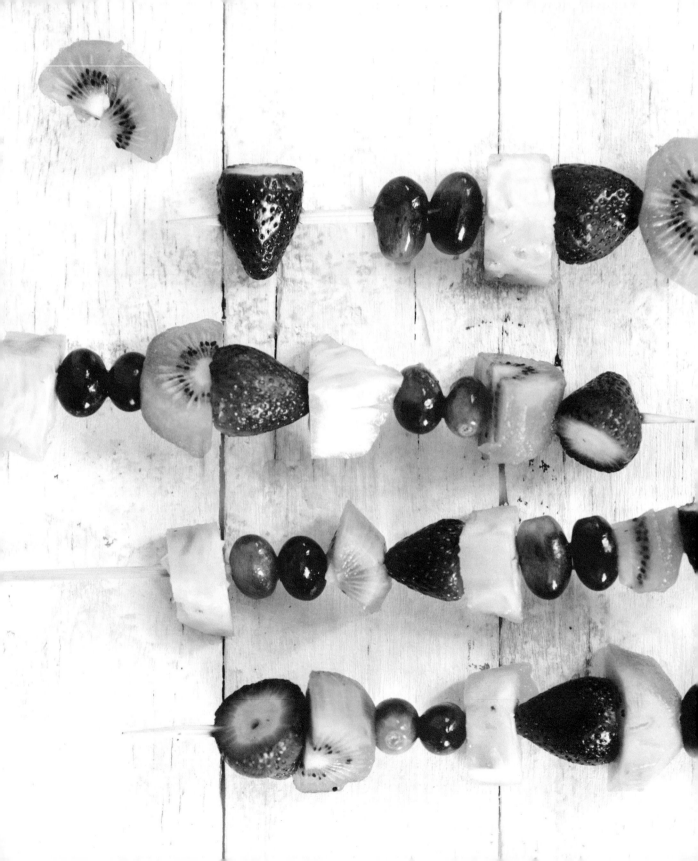

Frozen fruit is delicious as a snack or dessert on a summer's day. I saw this idea in a classy resort on the island of Mykonos, Greece, and realised it's potential for both adults and kids alike! Prepare this recipe a day ahead.

FROZEN FRUIT KEBABS

PREPARATION: 10 MINUTES + 5 HOURS FREEZING, COOKING: 0 MINUTES, SERVES 4

8 fresh pineapple chunks
16 large red grapes
8 large strawberries, hulled
2 kiwi fruits, peeled, quartered
8 long bamboo skewers

1. Prepare fruit as described.
2. Holding skewers at the blunt end, thread each with the fruit pieces through the sharp end in a sequence of your choice.
3. Place skewers on a tray, cover and freeze. Serve frozen or defrost for 30-60 minutes prior to serving, depending on the air temperature, to soften slightly.

TIP:

- Variation: Freeze other fruits such as watermelon or rockmelon (canteloupe).

Per serve: energy 284 kJ (68 Cal); protein 1 g; fat 0 g; saturated fat 0 g; cholesterol 0 mg; carbohydrate 13 g; sugars 13 g; fibre 3 g; calcium 26 mg; iron 0.5 mg; sodium 5 mg

An indulgent, easy-to-make treat that's full of goodness and only lightly sweetened! The nuts lower cholesterol and temper blood sugar levels. They're also good to stave off hunger and won't make you put on weight, especially if you swap them for other snack foods. Recent research shows we acually also don't absorb all the fat contained in nuts.

SWEET TREAT NUT SQUARES

PREPARATION: 15 MINUTES + 3 HOURS SETTING, COOKING: 5 MINUTES, MAKES 25 SQUARES

½ cup macadamia nuts
½ cup pecans
½ cup sunflower seeds
½ cup pepitas (pumpkin seeds)
½ cup LSA (linseed, sunflower seed and
   almond mixture)
1 teaspoon ground cassia
½ cup natural maple syrup
2 tablespoons natural peanut butter

1. Line a 20 x 20-cm (8 x 8-in) tin with parchment (baking) paper. When cutting parchment paper, ensure sides will reach approximately 5 centimetres (2 inches) above the slice.
2. Coarsely chop nuts on a board and place in a medium bowl. Mix in seeds, LSA and cassia, so ingredients are evenly dispersed.
3. Place maple syrup and peanut butter in a small saucepan, and stir on a low-medium heat until the mixture boils and darkens slightly, about 5 minutes. Do not overcook. Mix into dry ingredients. The mixture should be sticky.
4. Transfer mixture into the prepared tin and flatten as much as possible using a spatula. Fold sides of parchment paper over slice and cover with an extra sheet of parchment paper. Using your hands, press down firmly on the parchment paper to flatten and spread the mixture evenly.
5. Leave parchment paper in place and allow to cool to room temperature. Refrigerate overnight or for several hours until set.
6. When set, invert onto a board and cut into 25 bite-size squares or longer bars and wrap "to go." Squares can be frozen.

Per square: energy 440 kJ (105 Cal); protein 3 g; fat 8 g; saturated fat 1 g; cholesterol 0 mg; carbohydrate 5 g; sugars 5 g; fibre 1 g; calcium 16 mg; iron 0.9 mg; sodium 2 mg

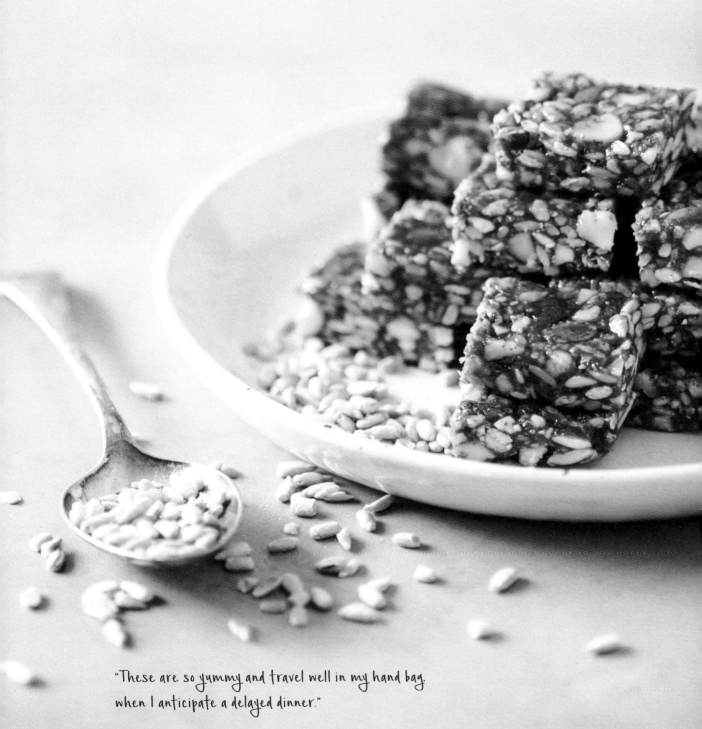

"These are so yummy and travel well in my hand bag,
when I anticipate a delayed dinner."

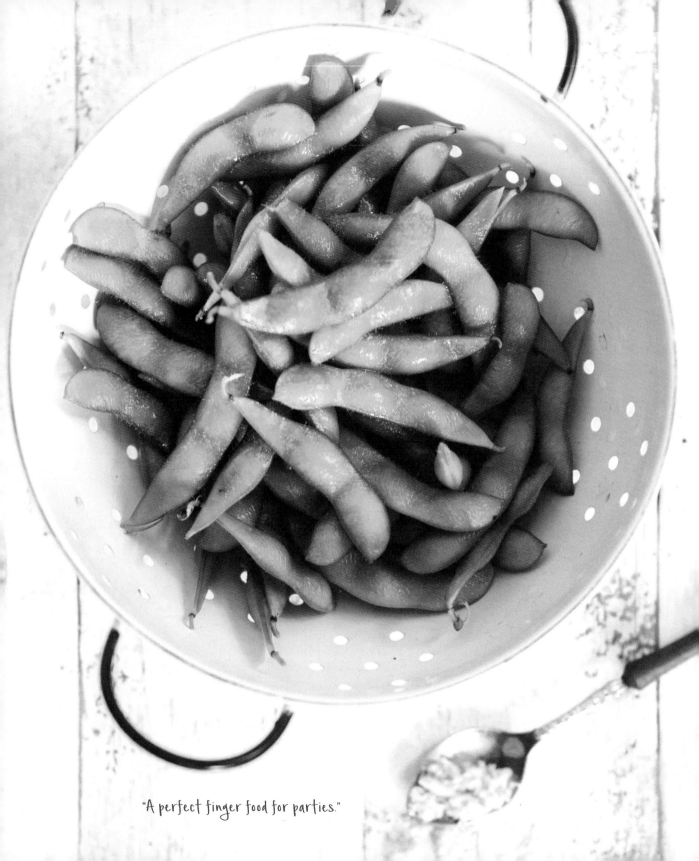

"A perfect finger food for parties."

Pronounced Eh-dah-ma-may, these immature bright green soybeans are a favourite snack idea from Japan and a handy standby to keep in your freezer. They're easy to prepare, super delicious and seriously good for you. Soybeans are high in protein and supply important phytonutrients to protect against breast or prostate cancer. They also lower cholesterol and blood sugar. Once you've tried them, you'll be hooked!

EDAMAME

PREPARATION: 1 MINUTE, COOKING: 12 MINUTES, SERVES 3

350 g (12 oz) frozen edamame in pods
¼ teaspoon salt, optional

1. Boil 6 cups of water in a medium pot. Add edamame and return to boil, then cook for 4 minutes. Note: Don't overcook edamame or the pods will start opening.

2. Drain edamame in a colander. Shock with cold water and drain again, then transfer to a serving bowl. Sprinkle lightly with salt, if desired, and serve immediately. Store leftovers in the fridge.

TIP:

– Fresh green soybeans can be difficult to source, but are available from some organic markets. You can buy frozen edamame in their pods from Asian grocery stores. Check the nutrition information panel as some edamame are already pre-cooked and salted.

Per serve: energy 321 kJ (77 Cal); protein 6 g; fat 3 g; saturated fat 0 g; cholesterol 0 mg; carbohydrate 3 g; sugars 1 g; fibre 3 g; calcium 37 mg; iron 1.3 mg; sodium 3 mg

These fresh rolls are ideal for a light entrée or snack. They are also great fun to assemble at the table with groups! The longest part is to prepare the filling and this doesn't take much more effort for additional serves. This recipe is gluten-free.

FRESH VIETNAMESE RICE PAPER ROLLS

PREPARATION: 30 MINUTES + 20 MINUTES MARINATING, COOKING: 3 MINUTES, SERVES 4

Marinade

2 teaspoons lemon juice

¼ teaspoon brown sugar

½ teaspoon gluten-free soy sauce

½ teaspoon extra virgin sesame oil

Vegetable Filling

1 cup bean sprouts

25 g (1 oz) carrot

25 g (1 oz) Lebanese cucumber

¼ small red onion

Noodle Filling

50 g (2 oz) rice vermicelli noodles, softened in hot water and drained

Herb and Salad Filling

16 large basil leaves

16 large mint leaves

15 g (½ oz) coriander (cilantro) sprigs with soft stems

30 g (1 oz) soft lettuce, torn into small pieces

16 strands of chives, for garnish

8 medium-sized (22-centimetre/9-inch diameter) rice-paper wrappers

1. Bring water to boil in a small saucepan to blanch bean sprouts.

2. Meanwhile, prepare marinade by combining ingredients in a small jar and shaking vigorously. Set aside.

3. Blanch sprouts for about 3 minutes in boiling water, then drain well. Finely slice carrot, cucumber and onion, and place in a small bowl with drained sprouts. Pour over marinade and mix to combine, then allow to marinate for 20-30 minutes.

4. Place vermicelli in a medium bowl and cover with hot water. Allow to soften for about 5 minutes, then drain and cut roughly with scissors into 5-centimetre (2-inch) pieces.

5. Meanwhile, gently wash and dab dry herb and salad filling. Set aside.

6. To prepare rolls, place warm water into a large bowl, then dip a rice-paper wrapper for 3 seconds until it just softens. Lift to drain, then place on a plate, rough side up, ready for filling. Note: Don't soak the wrapper or it will become too soft.

7. Take a small portion of each filling in turn and stack it on one end of the rice wrapper, starting with the herbs and salad (position leaves lengthwise), then noodles and vegetables. Tongs are helpful.

8. Fold bottom edge of the wrapper over the filling, pulling it in tightly, followed by the left and right edges. Roll until you have almost reached the end, then add 2 chive strands to stick out on one side and finish rolling tightly. Place roll on a serving platter.

9. Repeat steps 6 to 8 until you have used all the ingredients. Serve immediately with an Asian dipping sauce or refrigerate for several hours and enjoy later. Recipe is unsuitable for freezing.

Per serve: energy 266 kJ (64 Cal); protein 2 g; fat 1 g; saturated fat 0 g; cholesterol 0 mg; carbohydrate 12 g; sugars 1 g; fibre 1 g; calcium 21 mg; iron 0.6 mg; sodium 52 mg

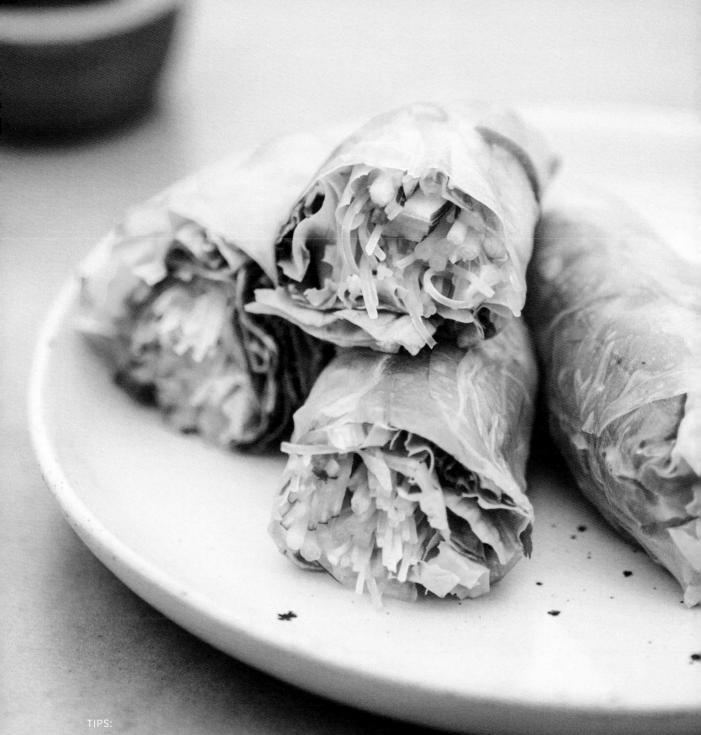

TIPS:
- Variation: For the filling, use strips of hicama,
Chinese cabbage, celery, garlic chives, fried tofu or mushrooms.
- There are 2 types of rice paper wrappers, a stiffer one for frying
(more glutinous) and another for fresh rolls. Be sure to buy the correct one!

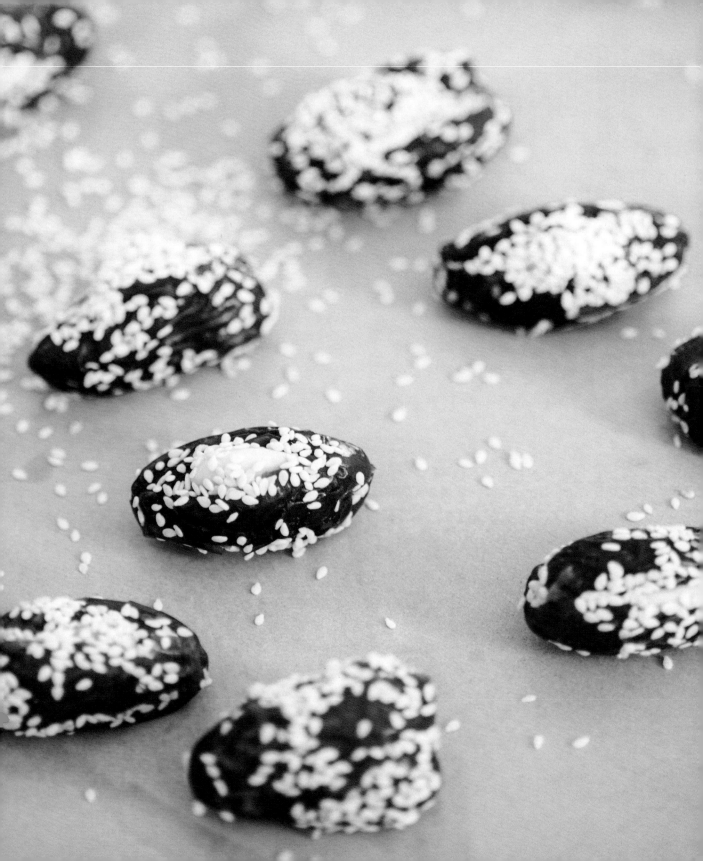

A lovely after-dinner treat or something to serve with a hot drink when guests pop around. Dates and nuts deliver many antioxidants, are high in fibre and lower elevated blood-cholesterol levels. New research shows that as much as one-third of the fat from almonds is not absorbed into the body, so the actual energy contribution of this recipe is likely to be lower than stated.

FRESH DATES STUFFED WITH ALMONDS

PREPARATION: 4 MINUTES, COOKING: 0 MINUTES, SERVES 6

12 fresh, large medjool dates
12 whole, large blanched almonds
½ tablespoon sesame seeds

1. Using a sharp knife, make a small slit on the side of each date and gently pull out the seeds with your fingers.
2. Replace each seed with an almond and press the date back together, leaving a bit of the almond slightly protruding from the crack. The dates should stick together easily.
3. Place sesame seeds in a small bowl and roll each stuffed date to coat. The sesame seeds will stick to the dates as these will be slightly sticky from being handled when removing their seeds. Store in an airtight container until ready to serve. Recipe can also be frozen.

TIP:

– Variation: Replace almonds with other nuts, such as walnuts, cashews or Brazil nuts.

Per serve: energy 521 kJ (125 Cal); protein 1 g; fat 2 g; saturated fat 0 g; cholesterol 0 mg; carbohydrate 24 g; sugars 24 g; fibre 4 g; calcium 23 mg; iron 1 mg; sodium 5 mg

An easy snack to make at home as commercial microwave popcorn often contains hidden trans fats! This recipe takes only 3 minutes using a popcorn machine or 10 minutes with the traditional stovetop method.

HOMEMADE POPCORN WITH OLIVE OIL

PREPARATION: 1 MINUTE, COOKING: 3 MINUTES, SERVES 7

½ cup popping corn
1 tablespoon extra virgin olive oil
¼ teaspoon salt

1. Switch on the popcorn machine and pour in the popping corn into the allocated chamber. Place a deep bowl beneath the chute and collect the hot popcorn. Drizzle with olive oil and sprinkle with salt. Serve hot or cold.

2. Alternatively, to make stovetop popcorn, place oil and popping corn into a 3-litre (about ¾-gallon) capacity saucepan on medium heat. Cover with lid and wait until you hear the corn starting to pop, then turn up heat and agitate saucepan continuously until all the corn has popped and you have a full saucepan. This takes about 10 minutes in total.

TIPS:

- *Make your own olive oil spray by buying a pump-action oil spritzer. Use this to better disperse oil over the popcorn if using a popcorn machine.*
- *Other popcorn flavourings include ground cinnamon, sweet paprika, lemon pepper or dried oregano.*

Per serve: energy 307 kJ (73 Cal); protein 1 g; fat 3 g; saturated fat 0 g; cholesterol 0 mg; carbohydrate 10 g; sugars 0 g; fibre 0 g; calcium 0 mg; iron 0 mg; sodium 87 mg

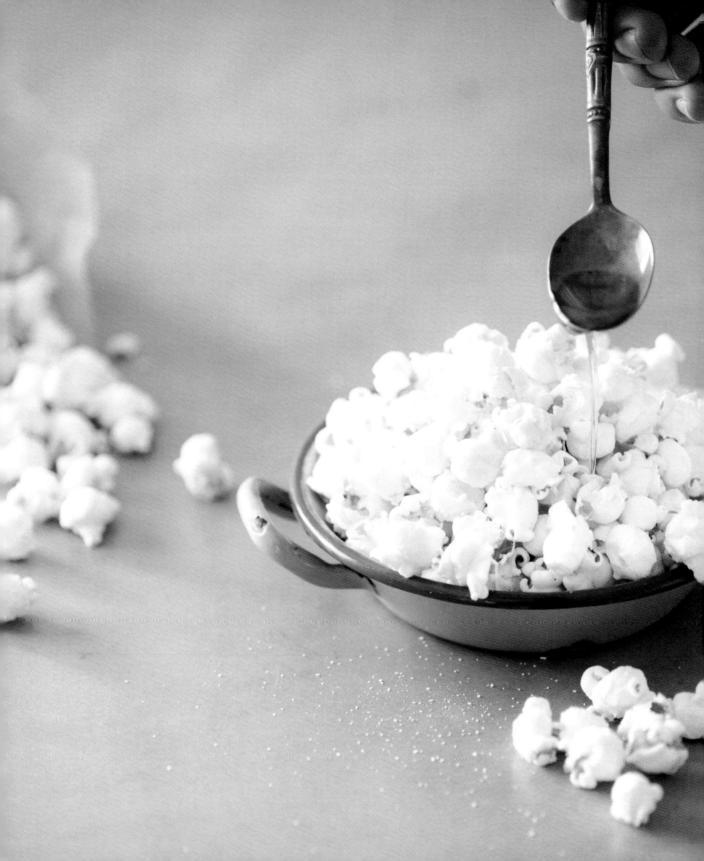

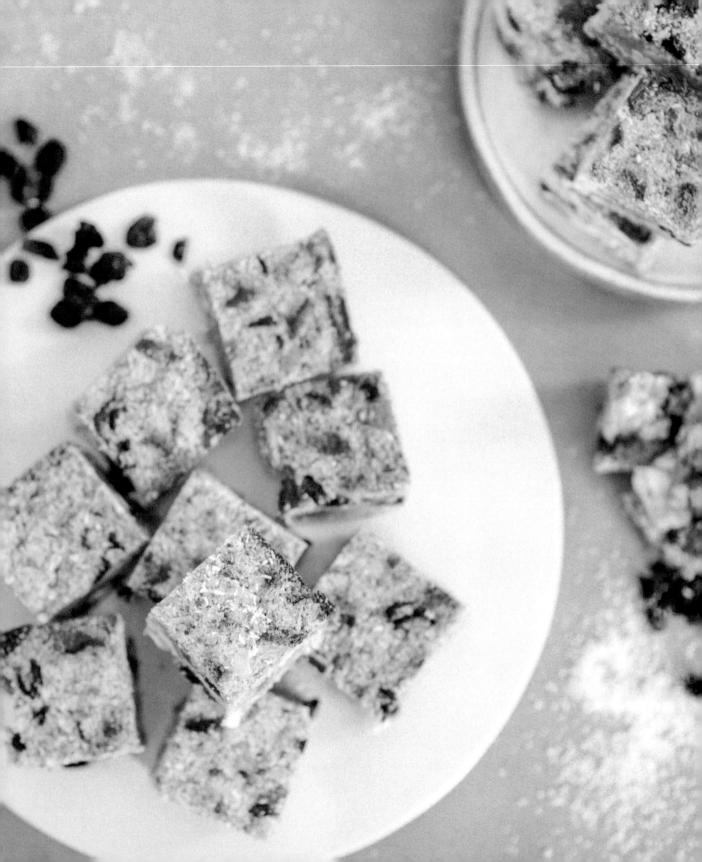

This tasty slice is perfect for peckish children and adults. A batch will last up to one week in an airtight container in the fridge—unless eaten sooner! Compared to most commercial bars and slices with large amounts of added fat and sugar, this recipe is nutritious and contains the goodness of dried fruits and wheatgerm. It is also egg-free and dairy-free.

TROPICAL FRUIT SLICE

PREPARATION: 10 MINUTES, COOKING: 35 MINUTES, SERVES 15

2 tablespoons ground linseeds
¼ cup honey
¼ cup lite soy milk
½ cup tropical juice, no added sugar
1 cup desiccated coconut
1 cup wheatgerm
¼ cup wholemeal self-raising flour
400 g (14 oz) dried fruit medley, chopped
½ cup dried cranberries

1. Place ground linseeds into a small bowl with 6 tablespoons of water, stir well and set aside for 10 minutes. The mixture will thicken and form a "linseed egg."
2. Pre-heat oven to 180°C (350°F). Line a rectangular tin (25 x 16 x 3 cm/10 x 6 x 1½ in) with parchment (baking) paper.
3. In a large bowl, using a metal spoon, dissolve honey in milk and juice, then stir in the linseed egg.
4. Fold in coconut, wheatgerm, flour, fruit medley and cranberries, until well combined.
5. Press mixture firmly into prepared tin.
6. Bake for 35–40 minutes until golden brown. Allow slice to cool in tin.
7. Remove slice from tin and place onto a chopping board, then peel off parchment paper. With a serrated-edged knife, cut into small squares. Squares can be frozen.

TIP:

- Variation: Swap cranberries with dried currants (or sultanas).

Per serve: energy 727 kJ (174 Cal); protein 3 g; fat 4 g; saturated fat 3 g; cholesterol 0 mg; carbohydrate 30 g; sugars 26 g; fibre 4 g; calcium 33 mg; iron 1.2 mg; sodium 26 mg

Yogurt makes a great snack and delicious addition to breakfasts and smoothies. This recipe uses the EasiYo yogurt maker system, available online, so it's very easy to achieve consistent results. You can also simply warm the milk to body temperature, transfer to a jar and stir in some starter culture, then allow mixture to sit on the bench until ready (the required fermentation time can be similar but depends on room temperature). Start the process before bed or early in the morning. Unlike most commercial yogurts, which contain gelatin or thickeners, the texture of this yogurt is more delicate, so it can also be used as "buttermilk" and strained to achieve a thicker texture. Soy yogurt can deliver the health benefits associated with soy protein and its natural isoflavones, including reduced risk of breast and prostate cancers, and cholesterol reduction.

HOMEMADE SOY YOGURT

PREPARATION: 4 MINUTES + 10 HOURS FERMENTATION, COOKING: 0 MINUTES, SERVES 5

3 tablespoons (60 g) any probiotic yogurt
3½ cups soy milk

1. Fill a kettle with water and bring to boil.
2. Place the probiotic yogurt (this is your starter culture) into the EasiYo yogurt jar.
3. Add 3 cups of soy milk to yogurt jar, secure lid and shake well. Add remaining soy milk and replace lid.
4. Pour boiling water into the EasiYo thermos until water line reaches the top of the red plastic insert.
5. Carefully insert yogurt jar into the thermos and screw on thermos lid until it clicks. Leave on kitchen bench to ferment for 10 hours.
6. Remove yogurt jar from thermos and refrigerate it for at least 3 hours so the yogurt firms up. Store in the fridge for up to 1 week.

TIPS:

- To avoid making yogurt in the plastic EasiYo yogurt jar that comes with the thermos, purchase an equivalent-sized 1 litre glass canister (example: Peep Canister from Maxwell and Williams).
- Variations: For a more tangy flavour, squeeze in some lemon juice before serving; for a dessert-style yogurt, stir in cinnamon or grated ginger.

Per serve: energy 407 kJ (97 Cal); protein 6 g; fat 3 g; saturated fat 0 g; cholesterol 0 mg; carbohydrate 10 g; sugars 5 g; fibre 1 g; calcium 247 mg; iron 0 mg; sodium 119 mg

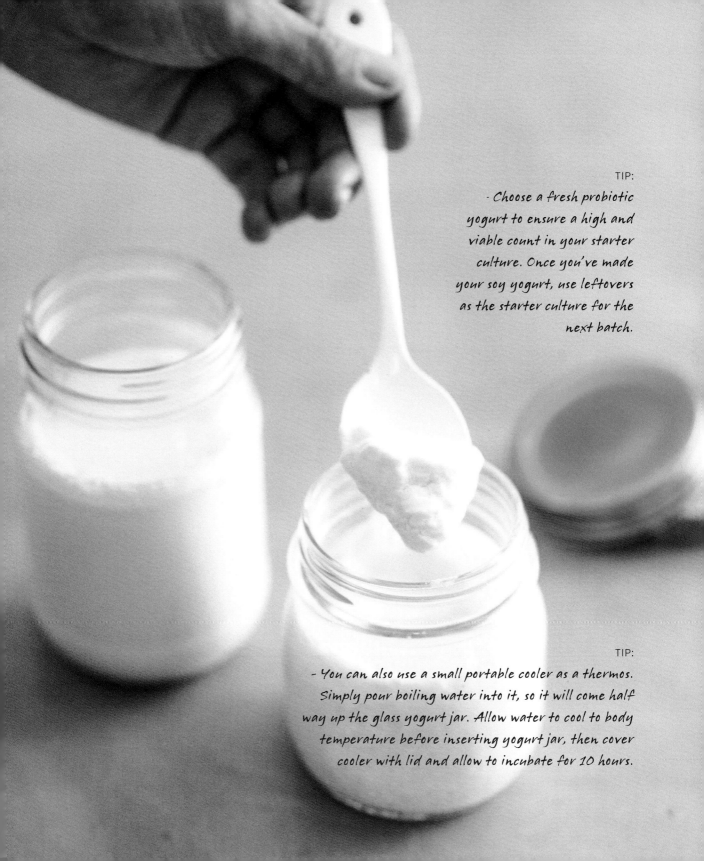

TIP:
- Choose a fresh probiotic yogurt to ensure a high and viable count in your starter culture. Once you've made your soy yogurt, use leftovers as the starter culture for the next batch.

TIP:
- You can also use a small portable cooler as a thermos. Simply pour boiling water into it, so it will come half way up the glass yogurt jar. Allow water to cool to body temperature before inserting yogurt jar, then cover cooler with lid and allow to incubate for 10 hours.

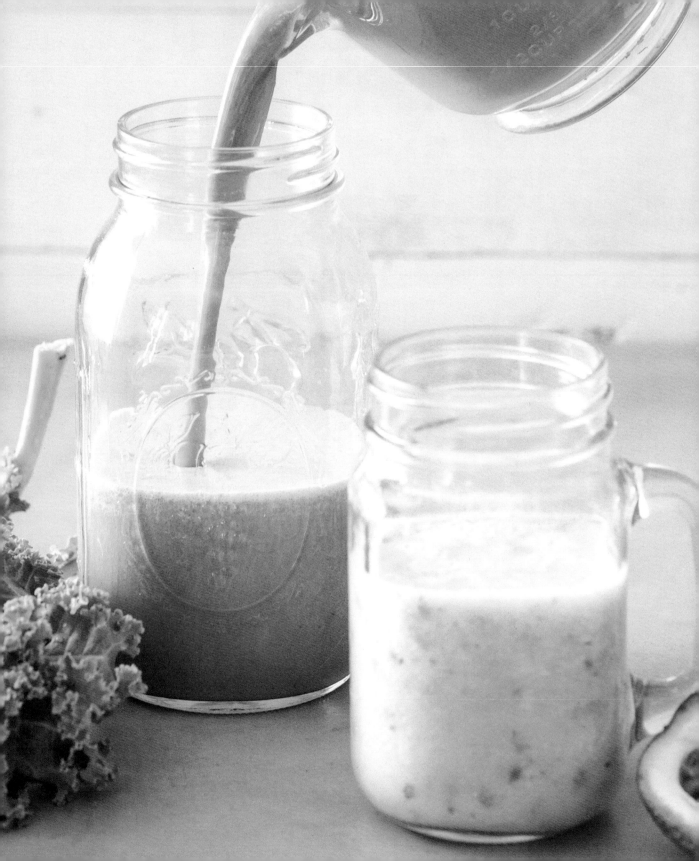

DRINKS

SIMPLE WAYS WITH WATER

About 60 per cent of your body is made up of water. So being adequately hydrated is important for you to function at your peak!

PLAIN WATER

Tap or filtered tap water is perfectly fine. You don't need to buy bottled water if your water supply is safe. Add a squirt of lime or lemon juice to flavour.

WATER INFUSIONS

Add any fruit, herb or spice of your choice to make water look pretty and taste more interesting to encourage consumption. You can also place these flavour enhancers in ice-cube trays and freeze:
• Cucumber with ginger and lemon.
• Orange with lime and rosemary.
• Strawberries with kiwi fruit and lavender.
• Raspberries with lime and mint.
• Lemon with whole cloves.

HERBAL ICED TEAS

Chill jugs of your favourite caffeine-free herbal tea, such as rosehip and hibiscus, lemongrass and ginseng, or sage. Enjoy unsweetened as a refreshing drink.

5 tips to drink more water

1. Drink 1–2 glasses of water as soon as you wake up.
2. Travel with your glass water bottle.
3. Keep a jug of water at your desk or work-station.
4. Drink before, during and after exercise.
5. Drink a glass or 2 in the evenings.

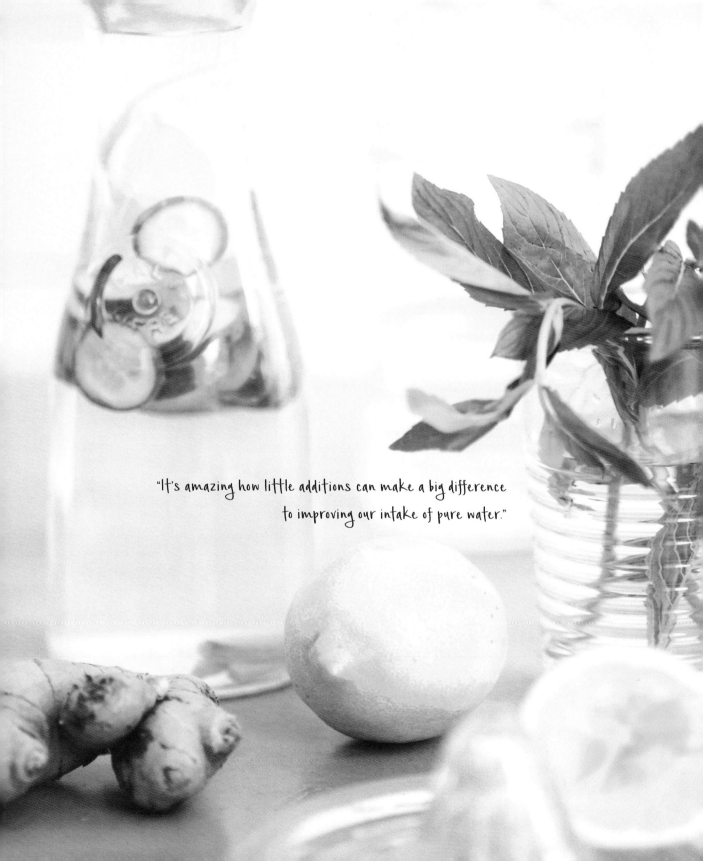

"It's amazing how little additions can make a big difference to improving our intake of pure water."

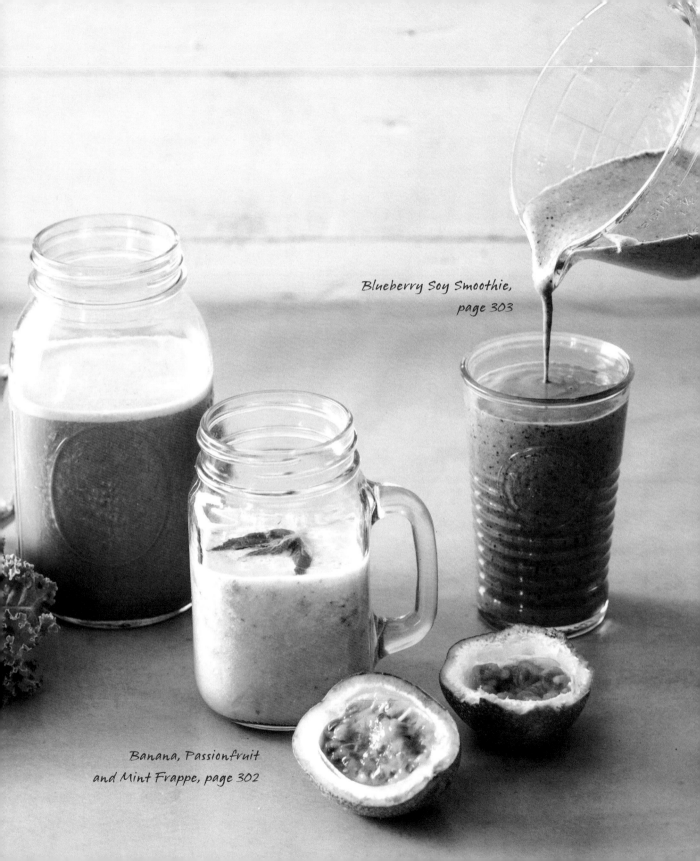

Blueberry Soy Smoothie,
page 303

Banana, Passionfruit
and Mint Frappe, page 302

There's no wrong way to make a green smoothie, but this one contains lots of greens, creating a monstrous colour that screams health protection! Raw kale is an important way to boost your immunity and add anti-cancer folate. Consumed raw, it is 10 times more effective at suppressing the growth of colon cancer cells in the test tube than heat-processed kale. Folate is important because even small deficiencies can cause as much damage to your DNA as doses of radiation well above the safe-exposure limit. The linseeds boost your omega-3 and fibre intake, plus thicken up the drink. In order to obtain a super-smooth and silky smoothie, I recommend a high-speed blender.

GREEN MONSTER SMOOTHIE

PREPARATION: 10 MINUTES, COOKING: 0 MINUTES, SERVES 2

4 kale leaves (60 g/2 oz) (top part only without the fibrous stalk)
1 cup tightly packed baby spinach leaves
10 g (⅓ oz) mint leaves (leaves from about 4 large sprigs)
1 large ripe banana, fresh or frozen
small knob of fresh ginger, peeled
1 tablespoon ground linseeds
2 cups almond milk
12 large ice cubes

1. Place ingredients into blender in the order listed and whiz until smooth. Tip: Start on low power and gradually increase speed until smooth and creamy. Smoothie is best served immediately but you can refrigerate it and consume within 24 hours. If smoothie separates during storage, simply stir again until smooth.

TIPS:

- Variations: Use other green leaves, herbs or seaweed flakes; swap ginger with fresh turmeric.
- Over-ripe bananas, peeled, chopped and frozen, are perfect for this recipe!
- For extra plant protein, replace almond milk with soy milk.
- If using organic kale, wash leaves carefully for aphids and their eggs. If infested, soak leaves in a clean sink with some vinegar and salt, then rinse well.
- To clean blender, add some warm water and a drop of dishwashing detergent, and run it for a few seconds before rinsing.

Per serve: energy 693 kJ (165 Cal); protein 4 g; fat 6 g; saturated fat 0 g; cholesterol 0 mg; carbohydrate 22 g; sugars 19 g; fibre 5 g; calcium 242 mg; iron 1.3 mg; sodium 193 mg

While I mostly avoid drinking fruit juices and prefer munching whole fruit, I might indulge on special occasions. This drink is based on a refreshing experience I had in Hanoi, Vietnam, where it can get extremely hot and humid. It was so delicious I never forgot it! Here is my re-creation. Passionfruit is a perfect way to increase fibre intake. (Recipe image, page 300.)

BANANA, PASSIONFRUIT AND MINT FRAPPE

PREPARATION: 5 MINUTES, COOKING: 0 MINUTES, SERVES 2

12 large ice cubes

1 large ripe banana

5 g (⅕ oz) mint leaves + 2 sprigs for garnish

¾ cup freshly squeezed orange juice with pulp

50 g (2 oz) pulp from 2-3 passionfruits

1. Place all ingredients, except passionfruit and garnish, in a blender and whiz until smooth.

2. Stir in passionfruit pulp until dispersed.

3. Divide between 2 tall glasses and garnish each with mint. Serve immediately.

TIPS:

- Use a high-powered blender to create the best frappe consistency at home.
- 1 large Panama variety of passionfruit can provide 50 g of pulp!

Per serve: energy 412 kJ (98 Cal); protein 2 g; fat 0 g; saturated fat 0 g; cholesterol 0 mg; carbohydrate 18 g; sugars 16 g; fibre 6 g; calcium 20 mg; iron 0.4 mg; sodium 8 mg

Smoothies are made in a matter of minutes—ideal for breakfast-on-the-go or a light meal replacement. This smoothie has a lovely lilac colour and delicious fruity flavour. Blueberries have been dubbed the brain berry because of their antioxidant benefits for memory and improved brain function. (Recipe image, page 300.)

BLUEBERRY SOY SMOOTHIE

PREPARATION: 3 MINUTES, COOKING: 0 MINUTES, SERVES 2

1 punnet (125 g/4½ oz) blueberries

1 fresh banana

1 tablespoon wheatgerm

1 tablespoon honey

1 cup lite soy milk, chilled

1. Place all ingredients into a blender and whiz for about 1 minute until smooth.

2. Pour into 2 tall glasses and serve. Smoothie will thicken slightly on standing.

TIP:

– Frozen blueberries can also be used and give the smoothie a nice texture.

Per serve: energy 733 kJ (172 Cal); protein 6 g; fat 3 g; saturated fat 0 g; cholesterol 0 mg; carbohydrate 31 g; sugars 25 g; fibre 4 g; calcium 156 mg; iron 0.5 mg; sodium 77 mg

Get inspired by the Mexicans and South Americans and sip on this drink throughout the day—straight from your water bottle. You will lift your fibre intake by 8 grams! Chia seeds are rich in omega-3 fats and water-soluble dietary fibre, so they can help lower elevated cholesterol and blood sugar, as well as keep you more full and regular! This drink is gelatinous in the mouth and the suspended seeds make for an impressive presentation.

CHIA FRESCA

PREPARATION: 3 MINUTES, COOKING: 0 MINUTES, SERVES 1

2 tablespoons chia seeds
juice of ½ lemon
2 teaspoons natural maple syrup

1. Place chia seeds directly into a large, dry water bottle and top with 2½ cups of water. Screw on lid and shake vigorously.
2. Add lemon juice and maple syrup, stir if you see any clumps, then replace lid and shake again. Allow to sit for 15 minutes until seeds swell, then enjoy at room temperature or chilled. Shake chia fresca before sipping.

TIPS:

- *Add more lemon for a tangier version.*
- *Variation: Substitute coconut water for water and lime for lemon juice.*
- *Variation: Use honey or stevia for sweetness or omit sweetener altogether.*

Per serve: energy 800 kJ (191 Cal); protein 6 g; fat 13 g; saturated fat 1 g; cholesterol 0 mg; carbohydrate 10 g; sugars 10 g; fibre 8 g; calcium 96 mg; iron 2.1 mg; sodium 11 mg

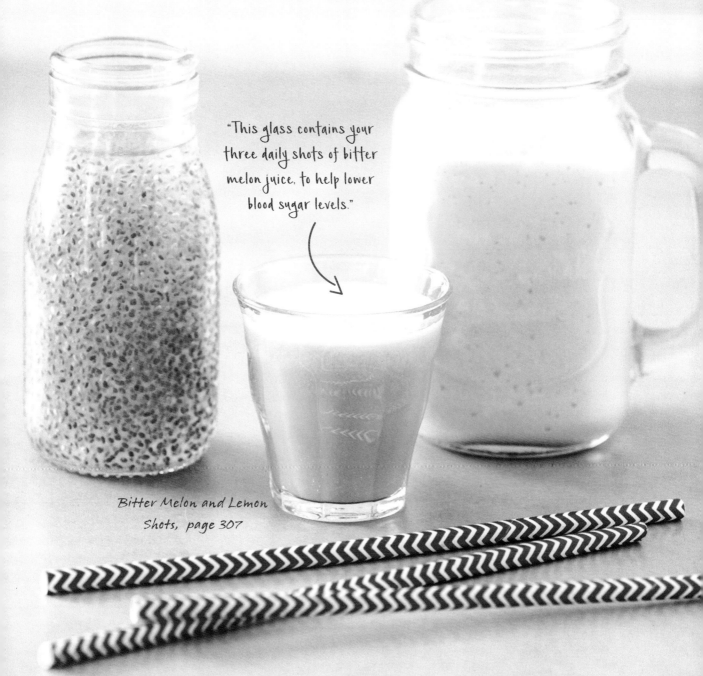

Mango Lassi, page 306

"This glass contains your three daily shots of bitter melon juice, to help lower blood sugar levels."

Bitter Melon and Lemon Shots, page 307

An Indian-inspired thick, creamy, cooling drink. It only takes a few minutes with a good blender. This lassi also provides a good source of isoflavones for breast and prostate health. (Recipe image, page 305.)

MANGO LASSI

PREPARATION: 4 MINUTES + 30 MINUTES CHILLING, COOKING: 0 MINUTES, SERVES 2

6 large ice cubes
1 cup ripe mango flesh
200 g (7 oz) mango-flavoured low-fat soy yogurt
2 teaspoons honey

1. Place all ingredients in a blender and process for about 1 minute, until smooth. Chill for 30 minutes, then serve.

TIPS:

- Add extra ice cubes, if your cubes are small or you wish to make the lassi thinner.
- Use vanilla-flavoured yogurt if mango is unavailable.

Per serve: energy 658 kJ (157 Cal); protein 4 g; fat 1 g; saturated fat 0 g; cholesterol 0 mg; carbohydrate 32 g; sugars 28 g; fibre 3 g; calcium 133 mg; iron 1.5 mg; sodium 127 mg

I designed this drink especially for people with diabetes or insulin resistance, as bitter melon has blood sugar-lowering properties. The shots are a way to slam it down fast and benefit from its "vegetable insulin," as dubbed in the scientific literature. Bitter melon is also high in vitamin C and folate. Make this recipe twice weekly and store in the fridge for everyday use. Although popular in southeast Asia, India, Africa and South America—and considered a longevity food—bitter melon is disliked by many Westerners as it has an intensely bitter flavour. The lemon significantly improves its palatability. (Recipe image, page 305.)

BITTER MELON AND LEMON SHOTS

PREPARATION: 7 MINUTES, COOKING: 0 MINUTES, MAKES 16 SHOTS

2 large bitter melons (600 g/21 oz in total)
¼ cup lemon juice (about 1 juiced lemon)

1. Wash bitter melons well and slice in half, lengthwise. Using a metal spoon, scoop out seeds and discard them.
2. Chop bitter melon roughly and place in a blender with 2 cups of water. Blend until smooth.
3. Stir in lemon juice, transfer to a flask or jug and store in the fridge for up to 5 days. The natural vitamin C acts as a preservative. Contents will settle upon standing. Simply stir or shake before pouring. Take 1 shot after each meal.

TIPS:

- Variation: Add a cucumber to lighten the flavour.
- Other vegetable juices can also be beneficial for health as they are high in phytonutrients. For example, 2 cups of beetrool juice daily has been proven to lower high blood pressure.
- To clean a bottle that has had bitter melon juice stored in it, add a small handful of rice grains together with some water and shake vigorously.

Per serve: energy 21 kJ (5 Cal); protein 0 g; fat 0 g; saturated fat 0 g; cholesterol 0 mg; carbohydrate 0 g; sugars 0 g; fibre 1 g; calcium 9 mg; iron 0.4 mg; sodium 1 mg

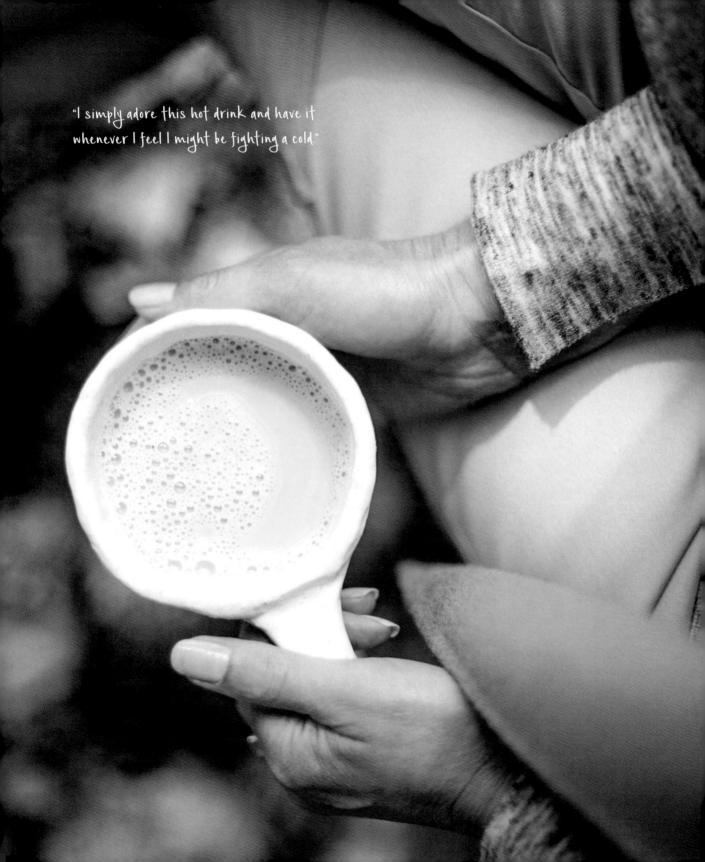

"I simply adore this hot drink and have it whenever I feel I might be fighting a cold."

A delicious bedtime drink, based on the traditional use of turmeric in India. Turmeric has potent anti-inflammatory properties and the addition of some pepper significantly enhances absorption of its active ingredient, curcumin. In some traditional medicines, turmeric is used for coughs and colds, while honey is recommended as a cough medicine by the World Health Organization.

GOLDEN TURMERIC MILK

PREPARATION: 4 MINUTES, COOKING: 8 MINUTES, SERVES 2

2 cups lite soy milk
1 teaspoon ground turmeric
pinch ground black pepper
knob of fresh ginger, sliced
4 cardamom pods, bruised
2 teaspoons honey
ground cinnamon, for garnish

1. Place all ingredients, except honey and cinnamon, into a small saucepan and bring almost to boil, stirring constantly.
2. Simmer for 2-3 minutes, then remove from heat and stir in honey to dissolve.
3. Strain, discarding ginger and cardamom pods, and serve hot in mugs with a sprinkle of cinnamon on top.

TIPS:
- *Variation: Use other plant-based milks such as almond milk.*
- *Mix in a blender before serving to make it foamier.*
- *Try adding 1 teaspoon of coconut oil for a richer taste.*

Per serve: energy 680 kJ (163 Cal); protein 8 g; fat 5 g; saturated fat 1 g; cholesterol 0 mg; carbohydrate 20 g; sugars 12 g; fibre 0 g; calcium 332 mg; iron 0.9 mg; sodium 159 mg

This warming spiced beverage is perfect for a cold winter's night. Unlike most chai lattes, it is caffeine-free so you can consume it with the assurance of a good night's sleep. Spices are medicines you can pull from your kitchen cupboard as they provide strong antioxidant, anti-inflammatory and anti-microbial properties. The drink is also lactose-free and gluten-free.

CHAI LATTE

PREPARATION: 5 MINUTES, COOKING: 5 MINUTES, SERVES 2

1 rooibos tea bag
1 teaspoon whole cloves
1 teaspoon green cardamom pods
½ stick cassia
small knob of fresh ginger, peeled and sliced
1¼ cups lite soy milk
2 teaspoons honey
ground cinnamon, for garnish

1. Place 1¼ cups of water into a small saucepan with the tea bag and spices, cover and bring to boil. Turn down heat slightly and boil for 3 minutes.
2. Mix in soy milk and honey, and bring to boil again, uncovered, being careful that it doesn't burn or boil over. Remove from heat just as it starts to foam and rise.
3. Pour into 2 tall mugs through a small strainer. Sprinkle with ground cinnamon. Enjoy immediately.

TIPS:

- Rooibos (or red bush) tea comes from South Africa and can be purchased from supermarkets and health-food stores. It is a popular caffeine-free alternative to black tea.
- For best results, use fresh spices, as spices tend to lose their volatile oils with storage.
- Store whole spices for up to 2 years. Ground spices should be used within 12-18 months. Never store spices in the fridge as the condensation will increase oxidation of their volatile oils.

Per serve: energy 469 kJ (112 Cal); protein 5 g; fat 3 g; saturated fat 0 g; cholesterol 0 mg; carbohydrate 15 g; sugars 10 g; fibre 3 g; calcium 216 mg; iron 0.9 mg; sodium 101 mg

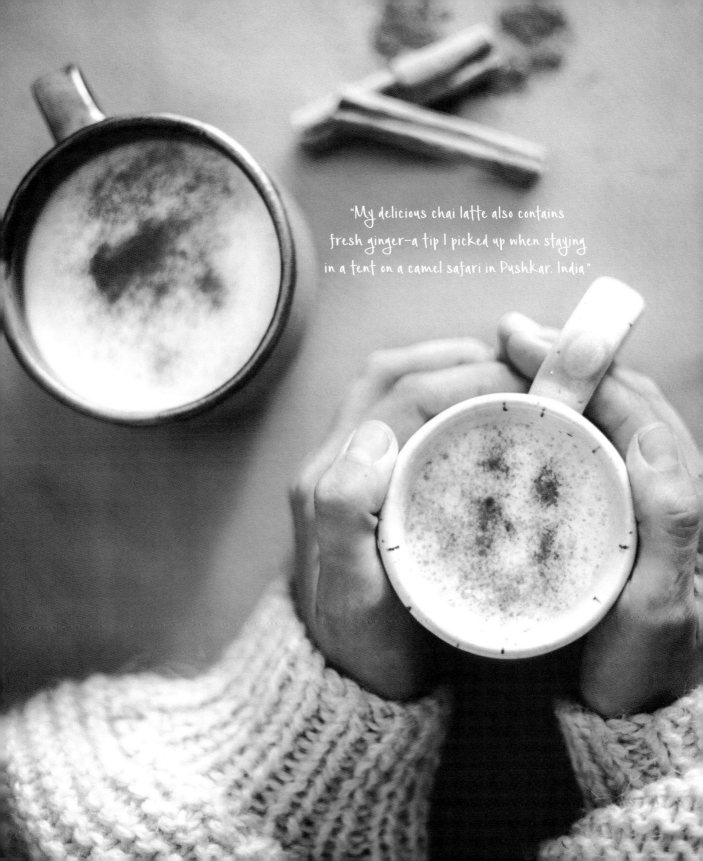

"My delicious chai latte also contains fresh ginger—a tip I picked up when staying in a tent on a camel safari in Pushkar, India."

Meal ideas that heal

Here are some examples of healing meal ideas for different occasions. Add extra food items to each idea, as per the tips in the recipes, or experiment with other combinations. They do not need to be consumed at the same time. (Recipe page numbers in brackets for easy reference.)

Weeknight meals for busy people
- *Brown Lentil Soup with Oregano (210)*
- *Warm Fava Bean Salad (118)*
- *Greek-style Pea Stew with Mint (106)*
- *Chickpea Curry with Pumpkin and Baby Spinach (142)*
- *Lentil, Olive and Semi-Dried Tomato Pasta Sauce (154)*

Kids' lunch box snacks
- *High Energy Balls (265)*
- *Tropical Fruit Slice (293)*
- *Homemade Popcorn with Olive Oil (290)*
- *Bircher Muesli with Berries (275)*
- *Fresh Vietnamese Rice Paper Rolls (286)*

Adult treats to have with a hot drink
- *Spiced Pear, Walnut and Muscatel Loaf (243) served with Cashew Nut Cream (244)*
- *Pecan and Ginger Drops (272)*
- *Fresh Dates Stuffed with Almonds (289)*
- *Chocolate Brownies with Walnuts (268)*
- *Sweet Treat Nut Squares (282)*

Fast foods at home
- *Black Bean Burgers with Fresh Salsa (102)*
- *Zucchini, Chilli and Feta Pizzas (115)*
- *Japanese Soba Noodle and Mushroom Salad (130)*
- *Tofu Burgers with Ginger, Chilli and Garlic (134)*
- *Almond and Sage Pesto (215)*

Recipes kids will love
- *Smooth Carrot and Orange Soup (204)*
- *Cashew Fried Rice (111)*
- *Mini Sausage Rolls (124)*
- *Walnut and Mushroom Meatballs in Tomato Sauce (190) served on top of Soft Yellow Polenta (189)*
- *Spaghetti Bolognaise Sauce with Cinnamon (157)*

Family desserts you can enjoy every night
- *Strawberry and Banana Mousse (232)*
- *Japanese-style Grape Jelly (247)*
- *Real Banana Ice-cream (228)*
- *Frozen Fruit Kebabs (281)*
- *Fig and Vanilla Polenta Pudding (239)*

Super supper snacks
- *Edamame (285)*
- *Apple, Quince and Prune Compote (277)*
- *Boiled Chestnuts (271)*
- *Golden Turmeric Milk (309)*
- *Homemade Soy Yogurt (294)*

Seasonal menu plans

Almost totally based on minimally refined plant foods, here are four sample seven-day menu plans—one for each season. These menu plans will give you an idea of the types of foods and dishes you could enjoy for different occasions to significantly boost your intake of natural plant foods. They also show you how to achieve dietary variety. (Recipe page numbers in brackets for easy reference.)

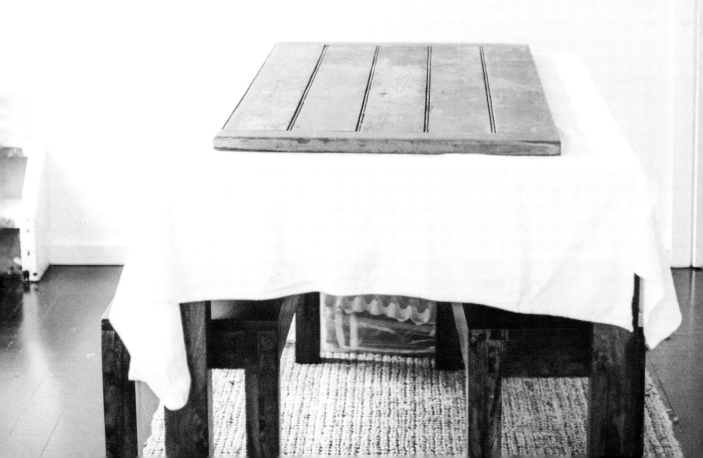

Summer

Meal	Sunday	Monday	Tuesday	Wednesday	Thursday	Friday	Saturday
BREAKFAST	Scrambled Tofu with Tomato (123) + Baked Yellow Banana Peppers with Yogurt Sauce (35) + wilted spinach	Natural muesli + ground linseeds + almonds + strawberries + soy milk	Whole grain bread + fresh avocado + sliced tomato + dried oregano	Chia seed porridge + seasonal fruit	Green Monster Smoothie (301)	Wheat Berries with Pecans and Sultanas (278)	Bircher Muesli with Berries (275)
LUNCH	Village-style Vegetable Stew (137) + wholemeal spelt and sunflower sourdough bread	Japanese Soba Noodle and Mushroom Salad (130)	Barley wrap with Sunflower Seed Sour Cream (218) + strips of firm tofu + Fresh Beetroot, Carrot and Mint Salad (38)	Fluffy Bulgur Pilaf with Eggplant (93) + Tabbouleh (58)	Bruschetta topped with Black-eyed Bean Salad with Lemon and Shallots (127)	Sandwich with Roasted Red Capsicum, Walnut and Pomegranate Dip (219) + veggie burger + rocket	Oven-baked Capsicums Filled with Eggplant and Barley (80) + Fresh Daikon Salad with Lemon (70)
DINNER	Warm Fava Bean Salad (118) + wholemeal Lebanese bread	Lentil, Olive and Semi-Dried Tomato Pasta Sauce (154) + wholemeal penne	Szechuan-style Eggplant and Wood Ear (166) + steamed whole grain rice and black-eyed bean combo	Spiced Chickpeas with Silverbeet and Lemon (112)	Okra in Fragrant Tomato Sauce (151) + Butter Bean and Thyme Mash (87)	Kale and Kidney Beans with Garlic and Chilli (114)	Lasagne with Roasted Vegetables (186) + Fresh Kale, Avocado and Pomegranate Salad (62)

Note: Items in capitals refer to recipes in this cookbook (page numbers in brackets).
For dessert or snack ideas, see pages 226 and 266.

Autumn

Meal	Sunday	Monday	Tuesday	Wednesday	Thursday	Friday	Saturday
BREAKFAST	Crispy Multigrain Waffles with Warm Strawberry and Rhubarb Sauce (258)	Soft Yellow Polenta (189) + chia bran + soy milk	Cinnamon Spiced Quinoa with Dried Fruits + Homemade Soy Yogurt (294)	Multigrain porridge with cinnamon + walnuts + sunflower seeds + stewed fruit + soy milk	Sprouted grain bread + ABC spread + Apple, Quince and Prune Compote (277)	Millet with Macadamia and Currants + soy milk	Wholemeal Lebanese bread + zataar mixed with extra virgin olive oil + sliced cucumber + sliced tomato + mint leaves
LUNCH	Sweet Potato, Red Lentil and Lemon Soup (195) + crusty bread	Roasted Vegetable Salad with Creamy Orange Tahini Dressing (67)	Pita pocket bread + Creamy Hummus (216) + Walnut and Mushroom Meatballs (from recipe, 190) + mixed salad	Bruschetta topped with Eggplant Salad with Mint and Red Capsicum (42)	Tangy Lentil Soup with Silverbeet and Zucchini (207) + soy and linseed bread	Cashew Fried Rice (111)	Oven-baked Chickpea Casserole with Crispy Eggplant Topping (183) + Shaved Savoy Cabbage with Lemon Dressing (51)
DINNER	Zucchini, Chilli and Feta Pizzas (115)	Chickpea Curry with Pumpkin and Baby Spinach (142) + steamed whole grain and wild rice combo	Yellow Split Pea Soup with Leek and Thyme (209) + whole grain bread	Pasta with Creamy Mushroom Sauce and Baby Spinach (156) + Konnyaku Noodles (168)	Tofu Skewers with Indonesian Satay Sauce (161) + Steamed Baby Bok Choy with Garlic Sauce (61) + Chinese Glass Noodles with Bean Shoots (78)	Roasted Vegetables on Couscous with Moroccan Dressing (140)	Tofu Treasure Chests (165) + Exotic Bulgur Wheat with Amaranth Leaves (89)

Note: Items in capitals refer to recipes in this cookbook (page numbers in brackets). For dessert or snack ideas, see pages 226 and 266. "Cinnamon Spiced Quinoa with Dried Fruits" and "Millet with Macadamia and Currants" are recipes from The Breakfast Book by Sue Radd.

Winter

Meal	Sunday	Monday	Tuesday	Wednesday	Thursday	Friday	Saturday
BREAKFAST	Ful Medames (172) + diced tomatoes + diced onions + wholemeal pita pocket bread	Porridge with cinnamon + walnuts + chia seed + blueberries + soy milk	Dark rye toast + Creamy Hummus (216) + sliced tomato + dried oregano	Soft Yellow Polenta (189) + ground linseeds + soy milk	Multigrain porridge + almonds + sunflower seeds + Caramel Date Sauce (230) + soy milk	Millet with Macadamia and Currants + soy milk	Carrot, Rosemary and Zucchini Muffins
LUNCH	Crispy Eggplant Cutlets with Paprika and Garlic Sauce (152) + whole grain bread + Shaved Fennel, Pink Lady and Arugula Salad (44)	Whole grain bread roll + Creamy Hummus (216) + Zucchini and Shallot Fritters (126) + mixed green leaves + sliced tomato	Creamy Celeriac and Cauliflower Soup (197) + Wholemeal spelt and sunflower sourdough bread	Bulgur with Brown Lentils and Caramelised Onion (84) + watercress, cucumber and tomato salad	Pasta Sauce with Eggplant, Red Capsicum and Currants (158) + wholemeal penne	Tofu Burgers with Ginger, Chilli and Garlic (134)	Indian Potato, Cauliflower and Tofu Curry (145) + Three-Bean Dal (146) + steamed whole grain rice
DINNER	Black Bean Burgers with Fresh Salsa (102)	Brown Lentil Soup with Oregano (210) + soy and linseed bread	Spaghetti Bolognaise Sauce with Cinnamon (157) + wholemeal spaghetti + Sicilian Orange and Fennel Salad (52)	Greek-style Pea Stew with Mint (106) + steamed whole grain rice and red quinoa combo	Cannellini Bean and Carrot Soup with Parsley (201) + wholemeal spelt and sunflower sourdough bread	Walnut and Mushroom Meatballs in Tomato Sauce (190) + Soft Yellow Polenta (189) + salad of green leaves	Barley Risotto with Porcini Mushrooms and Sage (83) + Kohlrabi, Green Apple and Mint Salad (47)

Note: Items in capitals refer to recipes in this cookbook (page numbers in brackets). For dessert or snack ideas, see pages 226 and 266. "Millet with Macadamia and Currants" and "Carrot, Rosemary and Zucchini Muffins" are recipes from The Breakfast Book by Sue Radd.

Spring

Meal	Sunday	Monday	Tuesday	Wednesday	Thursday	Friday	Saturday
BREAKFAST	Crispy Multigrain Waffles with Warm Strawberry and Rhubarb Sauce (258)	Bircher Muesli topped with papaya and passionfruit	Soy and linseed bread + almond spread	Multigrain porridge + ground linseeds + pepitas + prunes + soy milk	Wholemeal spelt and sunflower sourdough bread + tahini + sliced banana	Chia seed porridge + seasonal fruit	Wheat Berries with Pecans and Sultanas (278)
LUNCH	Black-Eyed Bean Salad with Lemon and Shallots (127) + Greek Potato Salad (94) + Authentic Greek Salad (56)	Bitter Melon Fritters (121) + Wild Rice Salad with Wasabi Dressing (77)	Barley Salad with Cherry Tomatoes, Feta and Pine Nuts (129)	Whole grain Roll with natural peanut butter + mixed salad	Black Bean, Orange, Coriander and Mint Salad (120)	Sprouted Bean, Avocado and Red Papaya Salad (32)	Baked Giant Lima Beans in Tomato Sauce (162) + Greek-style Beetroot with Lemon and Olive Oil (48) + Wilted Endive with Lemon and Olive Oil (64)
DINNER	Lemony Chickpea Soup (203) + crusty seeded bread	Almond and Sage Pesto (215) + Kelp Noodles (101)	Mediterranean Braised Green Beans with Tomato (133) + olives + whole grain sourdough bread	Steamed Silken Tofu with Garlicky Soy Sauce (105) + Braised Chinese Broccoli with Ginger and Garlic (73) + steamed red rice	Persian Split Pea, Lime and Tomato Curry (147) + steamed millet and white quinoa	Creamy Coconut, Potato and Vegetable Curry (169) + steamed red and whole grain rice combo	Moroccan Tagine with Vegetables and Chickpeas (179) + steamed white quinoa

Note: Items in capitals refer to recipes in this cookbook (page numbers in brackets).
For dessert or snack ideas, see pages 226 and 266.

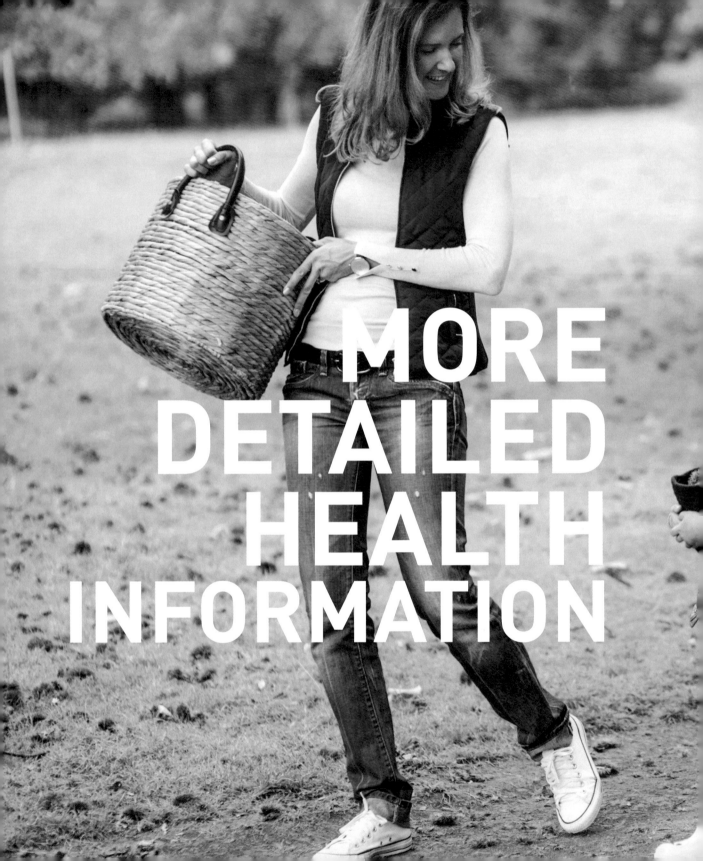

MORE
DETAILED
HEALTH
INFORMATION

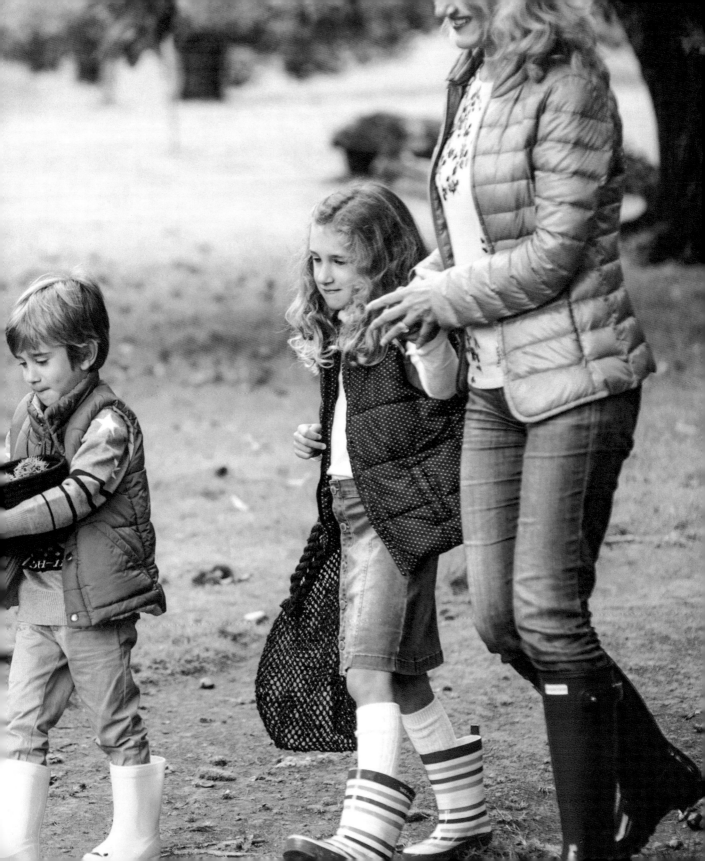

Why a single meal matters

What has always fascinated me is that after only a single meal, you will switch on or turn off thousands of genes in your body, either suppressing or promoting processes such as inflammation, oxidative stress and insulin resistance. These processes are well established as initiating and progressing disease.

Silent disease processes at a glance

Chronic systemic inflammation: Uncontrollable, widespread inflammation in your body affecting multiple organs, which does not switch off. Initially a natural defence mechanism triggered by your immune system, inflammation can be perpetuated by influences from your diet and other lifestyle habits so that it becomes chronic. Chronic systemic inflammation is recognised as a driver for chronic disease and is related to poor health outcomes including diabetes complications, atherosclerosis, and decline in memory and brain function.

Oxidative stress: The trauma your body experiences when the balance between the level of free radicals (causing damage to the DNA, fats and proteins) and your body's antioxidant defence systems is disturbed. Your body's innate antioxidants work to mop up free radicals so they can't cause harm. These can be helped by an antioxidant-rich diet. Oxidative damage to your cells is irreversible and contributes to heart disease, cancer and aging.

Insulin resistance: A condition in which your body does not respond normally to the hormone insulin that it produces, resulting in spikes in blood sugar and insulin levels leading to type 2 diabetes. Frequent high insulin levels are now also linked to many other diseases including heart disease, and breast and bowel cancers.

In your blood vessels

A small study of healthy volunteers showed that, within just hours of eating a fatty fast-food meal, their arteries' normal ability to relax was reduced by half! While one unhealthy meal can impair blood-vessel function, when that internal inflammation starts to calm down—after five or six hours—many people go on to stress their arteries with another unhealthy high-fat hit. It is not difficult to see why people who eat unhealthy diets remain in a chronic state of inflammation as they perpetuate this process one meal at a time.

In your lungs

It's not only your arteries that are affected. Shortly after eating a single pro-inflammatory meal, the effectiveness of anti-asthma medication in the lungs is also reduced. A study from the

University of Newcastle (in Australia) showed that four hours after feeding a high-fat, high-calorie fast-food meal compared with a low-fat, low-calorie meal (low-fat yogurt) to stable asthmatics, there was a significant increase in inflammation in the airways and a reduced ability of the bronchodilator medication (Ventolin) to work properly.

In your intestines

Your microbiota starts to alter within one day of changing your diet. This can be positive or negative. Since we are outnumbered by the bugs that live within our intestines—there are 10 times more bacteria than the number of cells in your entire body—we should be eating in a way that promotes a good balance between beneficial and harmful colonies. More than 20 years ago, few people imagined a colon could play such a major role in overall health. It turns out that reducing risks or managing almost every chronic condition relies on good gut health as this is critical for our immunity. Indeed, your gut contains 70–80 per cent of your body's immune cells!

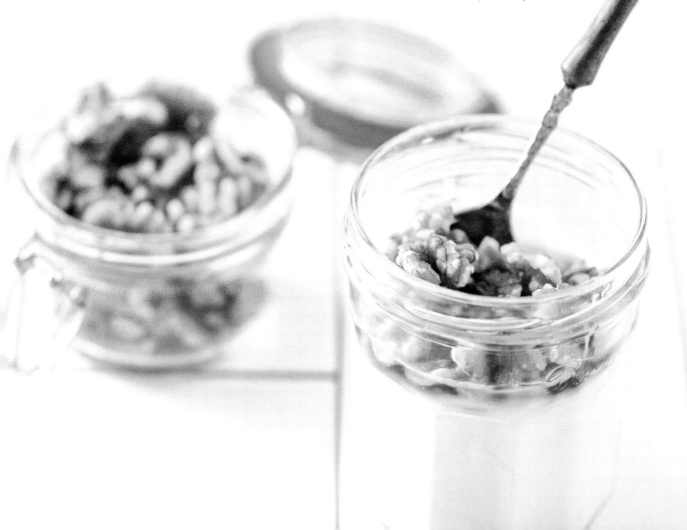

While *probiotics* can aid digestion and may offer some protection from harmful bacteria, their effect is transitory unless you keep taking them. What you do need is to regularly eat *prebiotic* foods. These are high fibre and will provide ongoing foodstuff for healthy microbes (microscopic organisms) to live off. My recipes are loaded with various types of fibres and prebiotic ingredients!

Microbiota: Previously known as microflora or gut flora, microbiota is the collection of bacterial communities and other microbes, including yeasts and viruses that live in your digestive tract. They are important for regularity, immune function and weight control. Your microbiota can be manipulated by antibiotics, probiotics, prebiotics and even a faecal transplant! Regularly eating foods rich in prebiotics will increase their diversity, which is considered vital for good health.

Microbiome: The collective genes of your microbiota (akin to the human genome, which includes all our genes) studied using DNA-sequencing. The microbiome is critically important because it is the bacterial genes that provide instructions for what the bacteria should make (known as metabolites) from the foods you feed them. These metabolites signal multiple organs in your body. Some metabolites are nasty, promoting inflammation and disease, while others are soothing, reducing inflammation and boosting your immune system. While your genome is fixed for life, your microbiome changes over time.

Dysbiosis: When harmful bacteria in your gut overwhelm the good bacteria resulting in a "bad bacterial mix," responsible for most intestinal disorders. Endotoxins produced by the bad bacteria can cause intestinal permeability (leaky gut) and cross the gut wall into the bloodstream to cause damage at various sites in the body. Tip the scales in the right direction by eating significant amounts of prebiotic foods (and dark green leafy greens), which act as a fertiliser for good bacteria to grow.

Prebiotics: Types of fermentable fibres and starches from plant foods that pass through your intestines undigested and end up as the food source for the growth and activity of beneficial bacteria. Prebiotic foods include wheat, oats, polenta, soybeans, lentils, chicory root, Jerusalem artichoke, leeks, onions, banana, almonds, honey and many more.

Probiotics: Health-promoting live microbial supplements that, when ingested, feed on the prebiotics. Bacteria with probiotic properties are also found in certain yogurts, but not all yogurts or fermented foods contain probiotics. Probiotics might assist with conditions such as diarrhoea, inflammatory bowel disease, asthma, type 1 diabetes, allergy, irritable bowel syndrome and colds/flu.

Whatever way you look at it, if you want to live longer and reduce the risks of increasingly common lifestyle diseases, every meal matters. Eating a diet heavily based on animal foods and lacking fibre results in dysbiosis and disruption of a healthy microbiome. On the other hand, more and more research suggests that the best way to feed a hungry microbiome is by eating plenty of natural plant-based meals.

Keeping your biological clocks in sync

To reduce chronic disease risk, consider what time of day or night you eat, so you can keep your body clocks in rhythm. Scientists have discovered you have more than 20 biological clocks in your body, with the master clock in your brain. You have clocks in your liver and even in your gut. The food you choose to eat and the timing of your meals is a major regulator of these clocks. According to research on circadian rhythms (known as chronobiology), your body is designed to work on a 24-hour cycle. It has multiple and complex regulatory pathways to ensure everything runs at optimal times. All these processes are co-ordinated by your body clocks, which exist inside your genes.

For example, your body's insulin levels are optimised to handle carbohydrate foods best early in the day. This is why everyone is more insulin-resistant when eating carbohydrates in the evening—whether you are diabetic or not—and nibbling late at night is a bad idea! So it's no surprise that late-night eating has been repeatedly linked with obesity and other health problems.

Even the contractions in your gut that propel food through the digestive tract are more frequent around 8.30 am, whereas they cease by around 10.30 pm. Your body clocks regulate these muscular contractions. Therefore, we should be eating most earlier in the day to help keep our body clocks in sync. If we eat at the wrong times, we upset our natural biorhythm, putting our clocks out of sync, and disease can strike early.

Every meal you eat can make a difference. Effects are immediate inside your body and within your cells. The sooner you start the better. But it's never too late to start receiving benefits!

Focus on foods, not nutrients

If your diet has been focused on a single nutrient target, such as tallying up 200 grams of daily protein to bulk up, you might be missing the point. We are now certain that health and disease outcomes depend almost entirely on the foods you eat and your entire dietary pattern, not on individual nutrients. The quality of your everyday calories is more important than any single nutrient.

Think of the low-fat message. Recent evidence suggests low-fat diets might increase the risk of haemorrhagic stroke. It all depends on what the bad fats in your diet are replaced with. Swap them with good fats from nuts and extra virgin olive oil or low-glycaemic whole-grain carbs and you will lower your risk of heart attack and stroke. Replace them with calories from refined carb foods, like white rice and sugary drinks, and you bring on more harm than by eating saturated fat.

There is no evidence that the harmful effects of dietary animal fats also apply to olive oil, nuts, seeds or avocado.

One large study from Denmark that followed healthy people for 12 years showed replacing saturated fat with high GI carbs (page 346) significantly raised the risk of heart attack. The finding doesn't mean butter or cream have been given a clean bill of health. Rather, refined carbs are now known to be even more harmful than saturated fat. Refined carbs are particularly injurious to overweight people because they already have underlying insulin-resistance problems, so their body simply can't cope.

Ultra-processed carbohydrate foods, often marketed as "low fat," are therefore detrimental. Unfortunately, "low fat" claims still feature prominently on many food labels because they sell product. The question is, if the fat has been removed, what has it been replaced with?

While the type of low-fat diet recommended by the American Heart Association can lower an elevated cholesterol, research shows a high-fat Mediterranean diet and a total plant-based (vegan) diet is effective at lowering your actual risk of heart disease. Some raw-food enthusiasts also follow healthy high-fat diets because of their liberal use of whole plant foods, including nuts and seeds, rather than copious amounts of refined vegetable or coconut oils.

Some nutrients require attention in most diets, such as sodium (limit), trans fat (avoid), and vitamin B12 in vegans and people aged 50 and older. But, by eating a *variety* of natural plant-based foods, most nutrients will usually take care of themselves.

How nutrients speak to your genes

According to a study of Danish twins, only about 10 per cent of how long you live is dictated by your genes, the other 90 per cent is determined by your lifestyle. The exciting field of nutrigenomics is uncovering numerous interactions between the nutrients in the food you eat and the expression of your genes. These interactions can either promote disease processes or block them and protect you from chronic illness. What you eat is even more critically important if your genes aren't perfect—and that applies to most of us.

One example of a beneficial gene-nutrient interaction is the way phytonutrients called indole-3-carbinol and isothiocyanates (derived from cruciferous vegetables such as broccoli, rocket and radish) talk to your genes, telling them to boost your internal detox mechanisms to reduce your risk of cancer. Due to a common polymorphism—a slightly different form of a gene that doesn't work quite as intended—half of the population lacks an important detox enzyme in their liver, called Glutathione S-transferase. This predisposes them to an increased risk of cancer.

However, according to nutrigenomics research, if these people eat broccoli three times per week, they can greatly compensate for the missing enzyme and reduce their raised cancer risk by 50 per cent. Even people who don't lack Glutathione S-transferase but regularly enjoy broccoli seem to benefit from a 20 per cent reduced cancer risk, suggesting that isothiocyanates are powerful in boosting our internal detox mechanisms by speaking to various influential genes.

The important message: Your genes do not determine disease on their own. They function by being activated or silenced and your diet plays a critical role in this process, previously underappreciated.

The power of diet versus drugs

Research urges that up to 90 per cent of chronic diseases are preventable with a healthy diet and lifestyle. These measures can be more effective than any therapy your doctor can offer. But, like conventional medicine, you need to take lifestyle medicine every day for best results.

CHOLESTEROL

Many people can avoid cholesterol-lowering medication by basing their diet on a portfolio of unique cholesterol-lowering plant foods and ingredients, including soy, nuts, viscous fibres and plant sterols. This is called the Portfolio Diet (page 336). If already on medication, research shows this eating style will make your medication more effective, so your doctor might be able to reduce the dose and reduce risks of side effects. Clinical trials suggest reductions in bad cholesterol of up to 30 per cent are possible, depending on how well you comply with this diet.

But cholesterol is only half the heart-disease story. Inflammation and other processes discussed in this cookbook (page 322) make up the other half. Fortunately, the same plant wholefoods help everything change for the better.

HEART ATTACK

Even if you have already had a heart attack, the Lyon Diet Heart Study showed that, by adopting a Mediterranean-style diet, you could reduce your risk of having a second heart attack by 50 per cent. People following this diet were also found to have fewer cancers and a significant decrease in all causes of premature death. The diet worked better than medication or the American Heart Association-recommended low-fat diet to which it was compared.

The PREDIMED study from Spain found a 30 per cent reduction in first heart attack risk by following a Mediterranean diet to which additional fat was provided in the form of nuts (30 g/1 oz per day) or extra virgin olive oil (4 tablespoons per day), as compared to a lower-fat diet. Not all fat is bad. Natural plant fats, used in the recipes in this cookbook, can have medicinal effects.

Anti-inflammatory food swaps

PRO-INFLAMMATORY FOOD		ANTI-INFLAMMATORY FOOD
White bread	→	Whole-grain seeded bread, sourdough
Potato crisps	→	Unsalted, unroasted nuts
Refined vegetable oil high in omega-6 (example: safflower oil)	→	Unrefined oil high in omega-9 or omega-3 (examples: extra virgin olive oil, flaxseed oil, chia seed oil)
Red meat	→	Legumes, nuts, fish (salmon, tuna, sardines)
Minced meat	→	Textured vegetable protein (TVP) or vegetarian mince, chopped mushrooms, chopped/ground nuts
Processed meats	→	Soy luncheon slices, soy bacon
Lollies, sweets	→	Dried fruit, 85% dark chocolate (not produced using the Dutching process)

INSULIN RESISTANCE AND DIABETES

If you have insulin resistance (example: polycystic ovarian syndrome (PCOS)) or are pre-diabetic, improving your food choices, moving more each day and, if overweight, achieving modest weight loss is about twice as effective at preventing type 2 diabetes as the commonly prescribed medication—Metformin—according to well-known research from the Diabetes Prevention Program. You would be foolish not to give lifestyle medicine a go. And every doctor should be prescribing this first.

Harnessing lifestyle medicine

While there is a place for more drastic measures when necessary, we have become too reliant on drugs and surgery. Many people miss out on the great benefits afforded by simple lifestyle improvements. Adding more natural plant foods to every plate could help you defer or avoid many health problems. Here are a few examples.

HEART DISEASE

Your heart is very forgiving. Research shows adults can undo their heart-disease risks by improving their lifestyle. One interesting study tracked 5000 young adults over a period of 20 years to see if adopting a greater number of healthy habits could influence the thickening and calcification of two major arteries in their body supplying blood to the brain and the heart. The scientists discovered a link with less clogging of the arteries for each positive lifestyle change. But giving up healthy lifestyle habits, such as no longer following a healthy diet, was associated with more arterial thickening and hardening. Such changes are a strong predictor of heart attack and stroke risk in middle age. Adulthood is not a "safe place" to abandon healthy habits, but to continue to improve them.

In people at high risk of heart attack and stroke, a Mediterranean-style diet, supplying 30 grams (1 oz) of nuts daily, was able to delay the hardening and plaque accumulating in the main artery that supplies blood to the brain, compared to a lower-fat diet without additional nuts, which allowed blocking of this artery to progress, according to data over a two-year period from the PREDIMED study.

The sooner you can get your family started the better. A small study from the Cleveland Clinic found that nine measures of heart and blood-vessel disease were improved in very overweight children after just four weeks on a total plant-based diet (in this case low fat, with proportionally lower calories). These included Body Mass Index (BMI), cholesterol, systolic blood pressure and CRP, a broad marker of inflammation in the body. Yet, in a second group of children counselled to follow a healthy omnivorous dietary pattern recommended by the American Heart Association, only four of these measures improved.

CANCER

Cancer cases are forecast to increase by 75 per cent during the next two decades, according to the International Agency for Research on Cancer. Treatment alone is not enough; preventive measures are essential. Research published in the *American Journal of Clinical Nutrition* on more than 500,000 people followed up for 13.6 years found those who adhered more closely to the American Cancer Society cancer-prevention guidelines had a significantly lower risk of developing cancer or dying from it, and a reduced risk of death from any cause. The researchers concluded that after giving up smoking, sticking to a set of healthy behaviours relating to diet, alcohol, body weight and physical activity is paramount.

Dr Dean Ornish, founder of the Preventive Medicine Research Institute in California, wanted to find out if lifestyle changes over a one-year period, including a total plant-based diet, could make some difference to low-grade prostate cancer in men who chose to forego medical treatment and its undesirable side effects. Dr Ornish found that men who renovated their diet and lifestyle experienced a 4 per cent drop in their PSA (prostate specific antigen) level, whereas those in a "usual care" group, who didn't receive intensive lifestyle advice, had a 6 per cent rise, suggesting their disease was progressing. Further, serum from the men who received lifestyle medicine blocked the growth of prostate cancer cells in a test tube eight times more powerfully compared to serum from the "usual care" group.

Later follow-up of the men in this study also showed those who made comprehensive lifestyle changes had a significantly improved relative length of their telomeres. Why is this important? Telomeres exist on the end of your chromosomes inside your genes and telomere shortening in humans is a marker of disease and aging. If we could prevent telomere shortening, we'd be able to stop getting old!

How many pills are you popping?

A large US study comparing vegetarians with non-vegetarians found non-vegetarians have twice the odds of being on aspirin, sleeping pills, tranquilisers, antacid, pain medication, blood-pressure medication, laxatives and insulin.

So, if you or I were a cancer survivor or facing another life-threatening disease, we would all want top-quality blood coursing through our body to help slow disease. The "secret" is a natural plant-based diet. Advances in radiation, chemotherapy and surgery may continue to make progress in treating cancer. But plant-based diets will be essential in the future as the safest way to reduce the risks and impacts of cancer.

The good news is your body has a remarkable capacity to heal itself, much faster and more effectively than previously thought. Dr Ornish pioneered much of the work in this area, showing that simple, low-cost lifestyle interventions are just as powerful—or more powerful—as drugs or medical devices for some diseases. The recipes in this cookbook will show you how to make healthy eating happen for life.

"The Lifestyle Heart Trial" was the first to show that intensive lifestyle changes, including a low-fat vegetarian diet, can reverse moderate to severe coronary heart disease. After just one year, people taking the prescribed "lifestyle medicine" experienced an average 4.5 per cent relative improvement in the blockage of their coronary artery. After five years, the results were even better, with a relative improvement of 7.9 per cent. In contrast, over a five-year period, the average blockage worsened by 5.4 per cent in people who did not make lifestyle improvements.

Why popular diets don't work (especially for health)

In comparison to some popular diets, my cookbook is not aimed merely at weight loss without regard for your long-term health. Instead, it is a prescription for wellness.

If you're after big and permanent results on the scales, go as plant-based as you can manage. One large population study from the United States found that people following a vegan diet weigh 15–20 kilograms (30–45 pounds) less on average compared to their omnivorous friends, without any calorie restriction or keeping of a food diary.

Other population studies comparing vegetarians with non-vegetarians have similarly found the more people switch to a plant-based diet, the lower their BMI and the less weight they gain over a five-year period. Adding more animal-based products into the diet over this time, however, was linked with weight gain.

Which diet is best for natural weight loss?
When comparing the efficacy of five diets ranging from vegan to omnivorous (non-vegetarian), a clinical trial published in the journal *Nutrition* found the greatest weight loss at six months was achieved among people on a total plant-based (vegan) diet. This occurred despite minimal contact with dietitians.

The problem with most popular weight-loss diets is that they are only a temporary diversion from normal eating habits. They are also unsustainable because constantly restricting calories in an obvious way can make you feel deprived and hungry. Worse still, some diets might shift weight but risk your health. This seems to be the case for high-protein diets based on liberal amounts of animal foods like meat, according to research from Harvard University tracking more than 120,000 people for at least 20 years.

That is why I advocate a minimally processed plant-based diet for good. Soon after swapping to my recipes, people tell me things like "I can't believe I'm losing weight because I'm eating more than ever" and "I'm going to the toilet every day now." Their blood test results also testify to a reduced disease risk and that makes their doctor happy.

The problems with going paleo

Paleo diets have received a lot of media attention recently, based on the belief that our genes are best suited to the diets of a hunter-gatherer lifestyle, which were not necessarily optimal. (Optimal diets allow for survival to old age without disability.) The advice to avoid ultra-processed foods is sound. But it is dangerous to tell people to forgo all legumes and whole grains! Research has proven such foods are important to protect us against chronic disease.

The modern paleo diet promotes meat, fish, seafood, eggs, vegetables, and nuts and seeds, with or without fruit. For some people, this has been taken as a license to eat slabs of meat, including processed meats like sausages, bacon and salami. Yet, eating meat without the protective effect of beans and whole grains on your microbiota is risky.

Paleontologists believe cavemen got protein from snails, brain, liver, kidney and other game meats, which are more nutrient dense and contain much less saturated fat than modern meats. Interestingly, anthropological experts state that traditional diets varied greatly depending on geography, climate and season. They believe that many paleolithic diets did include starchy foods like grains and seeds of grasses. Even experts who emphasise the role of hunting and meat suggest that some 50 per cent of calories in the traditional paleolithic diet came from gathered plant foods. Given the energy density of meat relative to most plants, this would translate to a diet that is, by volume, mostly plants!

Scientific evidence to support benefits for the modern paleo diets is poor. It comes from a few short-term studies with small numbers, and the feedback from study participants has mostly been that it is unsustainable.

What's good for you is good for the planet

Plant-based diets have ancient origins and are now also recognised as a greener way of eating for a healthier planet. If you decide to eat a plant-based diet, you are personally choosing to be responsible for lower greenhouse gas emissions, and less water, land and pesticide use. Increasingly, a meat-based, dairy-rich diet has been identified as an environmental hazard. Modern agricultural methods, particularly the factory farming of animals, produce more greenhouse gas emissions than all our transport methods combined.

Buying locally produced food can be helpful but researchers suggest a dietary shift away from red meat and toward more plant foods is most effective. They calculate that switching the food calories of less than one day in the week from red meat and dairy to a vegetable-based diet will achieve more for greenhouse gas reduction than sourcing all your food locally!

Foods defined as "non-core" in the "Australian Guide to Healthy Eating" should also be reduced. Think biscuits, cakes, pastries, crisps and soft drinks. They are energy-intense to produce and usually come wrapped in large amounts of plastic packaging. Modelling released by Australian researchers in 2012 showed discretionary foods accounted for 29 per cent of diet-related greenhouse gas emissions in Australia, almost as much as the 33.9 per cent emissions attributed to the meat and alternatives food group.

Finally, for planetary health it's also important that we eat more with the seasons and contemplate what to do with leftovers to reduce our kitchen food waste. See my "Seasonal menu plans" for ideas (page 315).

Defining plant-based diets

There are many types of plant-based diets, from the modern to the traditional. For example, traditional Mediterranean, Asian and African diets limit the frequency or quantity of meats and dairy due to culture and availability but are not strictly vegetarian.

What plant-based diets share in common is this: the majority or all that fills your plate on a daily basis comes from plants. This doesn't mean eating chips and drinking cola. Healthy plant-based meals focus on a variety of vegetables, legumes and unrefined grains, with some nuts and seeds, while whole fruit is usually enjoyed as a snack or dessert.

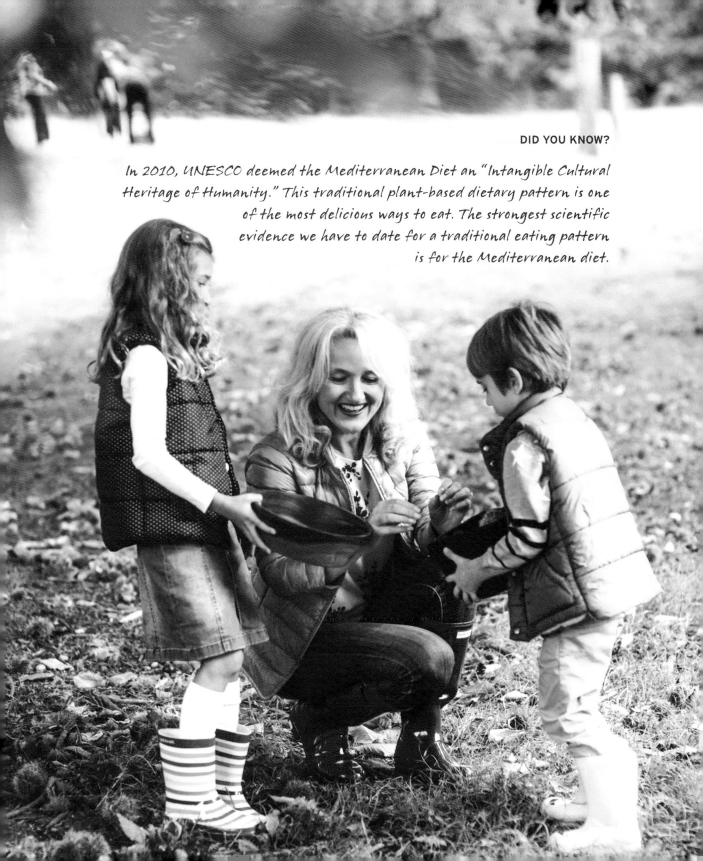

In 2010, UNESCO deemed the Mediterranean Diet an "Intangible Cultural Heritage of Humanity." This traditional plant-based dietary pattern is one of the most delicious ways to eat. The strongest scientific evidence we have to date for a traditional eating pattern is for the Mediterranean diet.

The most common types of plant-based diets today are:

SEMI-VEGETARIAN diets restrict red meat, poultry and fish to less often than once per week, but there is no limit on eggs and dairy.

PESCO-VEGETARIAN diets are basically vegetarian in nature but with some fish and seafood once or more per month. Red meat and poultry is consumed less than once per month.

LACTO-OVO VEGETARIAN diets exclude red meat, poultry and fish altogether but may incorporate variable amounts of eggs and/or dairy.

VEGAN diets are 100 per cent plant-based, meaning no meats, dairy or eggs. Other foods such as honey and materials like leather might also be avoided, if the motivation for veganism is animal welfare rather than purely health.

MACROBIOTIC diets usually include no meat, poultry, eggs or dairy but fish and seafood is consumed up to several times per week. These diets are centred on whole grains, such as brown rice, with plenty of vegetables and some beans or soy products.

RAW FOOD diets avoid cooking with heat but use other innovative preparation techniques to make foods more palatable and digestible. Most commonly, they are vegan and include 75 per cent or more raw food by weight (page 372).

Plant-based diets designed for research

Several plant-based diets have been designed specifically for research purposes so health outcomes could be clinically tested.

The Dietary Approaches to Stop Hypertension Diet (known as the DASH Diet) was set up to study the effects of plant-based eating on blood pressure. Later, researchers also discovered the DASH Diet can benefit blood sugar, cholesterol and digestive health. The DASH Diet involves eating daily at least nine serves of fruits and vegetables, about three serves of low-fat dairy and using plant proteins–such as legumes and nuts or seeds–for main meals four to five times per week, while limiting the amount of red meat.

Plant-based diets are richer in potassium and magnesium, which help counter harmful sodium from salt. You can expect improvements in your blood pressure, without even dropping your sodium intake!

The Portfolio Diet brings together clinically therapeutic amounts of four key cholesterol-lowering foods and ingredients: soy protein, nuts and seeds, viscous dietary fibre and plant sterols. While each of these foods can lower high cholesterol in its own right, their collective effort is much more powerful and has been proven to rival that of a starting dose of a first-generation statin medication!

In my Nutrition and Wellbeing Clinic in Sydney, we use both the DASH and Portfolio Diets therapeutically with great success. These diets are ideal if you wish to avoid (or postpone) taking life-long medication. An experienced dietitian or nutritionist can tell you which foods to eat to follow these diets, while the recipes in this cookbook will show you how.

8 Swaps for Eggs and Dairy

INSTEAD OF THIS	TRY THIS
Eggs*	Chia seeds, ground linseeds, psyllium husks, nut paste, pureed fruit or vegetable (example: apple, banana, pears, prunes, pumpkin), rolled oats, silken tofu, breadcrumbs, tomato paste, cooked lentils, chickpea flour (besan), brown rice flour, arrowroot flour
Dairy milk	Fortified soy milk, rice milk or almond milk
Dairy yogurt	Soy or coconut yogurt (see page 294 for Homemade Soy Yogurt)
Cream for dessert	Cashew Nut Cream (page 244)
Cream for pasta sauce	Tahini (see page 156 for Creamy Mushroom Sauce)
Sour cream	Sunflower Seed Sour Cream (page 218), strained Homemade Soy Yogurt (page 294)
Cottage or ricotta cheese	Blend of extra firm and silken tofu
Cream or feta cheese	Almond Cream Cheese Topped with Herbs (page 224)
Mayonnaise or creamy dressing	Dressing made with silken tofu and turmeric or tahini (see page 67 for Creamy Orange Tahini Dressing)

Note: Eggs serve various functions in cooking, such as to bind, moisten, thicken, flavour, colour and leaven. It is difficult to find one substitute to provide all these functions, so you will need to experiment with various options or combinations. If you require leavening, you can use commercial egg replacers or some baking powder.

Are all plant-based diets equal?

Simply opting for meat- or dairy-free won't instantly make your diet healthy. What you *do* eat is important. You should include more whole, unrefined plant foods—and not only fruit and vegetables. You need to learn to use lesser-known foods, such as legumes and whole grains. The primary reason for this cookbook is to teach you how to do that.

The word "diet" tends to conjure up restrictive regimes for weight loss. But it comes from the Greek word *"diaita,"* meaning a way of life. While any calorie-restricted diet can help you lose weight, the focus should never be only on calories without regard to food quality. What I love about plant-based diets is that they can cut your disease risk and better manage existing medical conditions, while helping you shed excess body fat at the same time—without making you feel you're "on a diet."

Regardless of which plant-based approach you choose, you should never feel hungry again. My recipes will also help you re-discover the pleasures of eating at home more.

Your health results can be further enhanced if you add regular physical activity, adequate sleep, rest and relaxation. Don't forget to stand up for just three minutes, every half hour, while reading this book. It's easy to do if you're in the kitchen!

What's the most alkalising diet?

The internet is awash with advice on foods to eat and foods to avoid to alkalise your diet. But a total plant-based diet (vegan) is the most alkalising dietary pattern, eliminating the need for confusing and contradictory lists of acid- and alkaline-forming foods. This is true even if you include some healthy whole grains, such as whole wheat and brown rice, because it's your total diet that counts, not occasionally drinking a green juice.

Loading your plate with mostly natural plant foods and limiting meats will shift your body's acid-base balance in an alkaline direction. This is particularly important if you already have a decline in your kidney function.

One study of 1500 people with impaired kidney function who were followed for 14 years found a meat-rich diet, which is highly acidic, appears to triple the risk of kidney failure, according to the *Journal of the American Society of Nephrology*. Researchers believe a healthy diet, rich in fruit and vegetables, could be a way to avoid or delay the high cost and the suboptimal quality of life that dialysis brings.

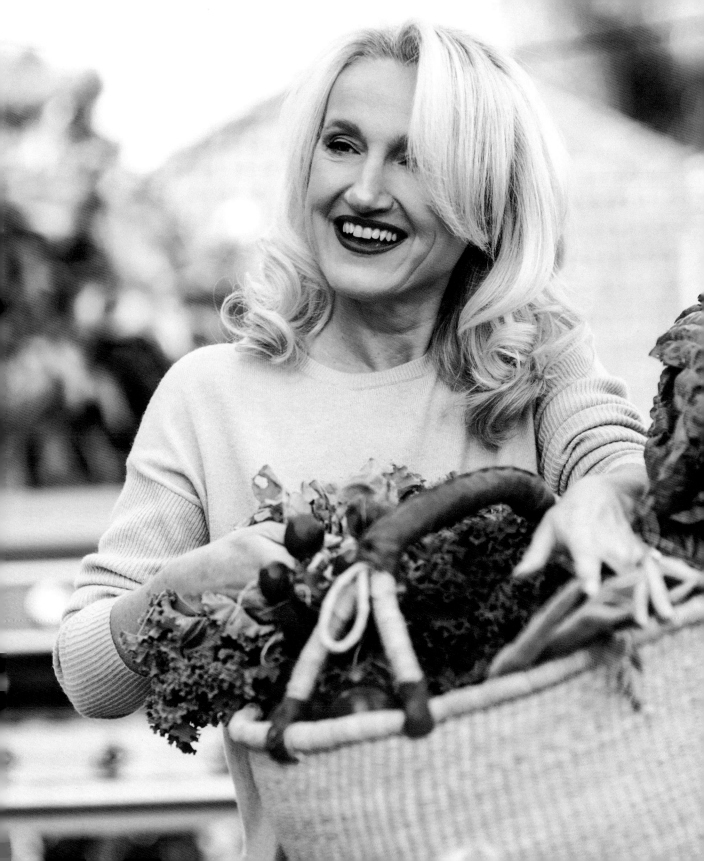

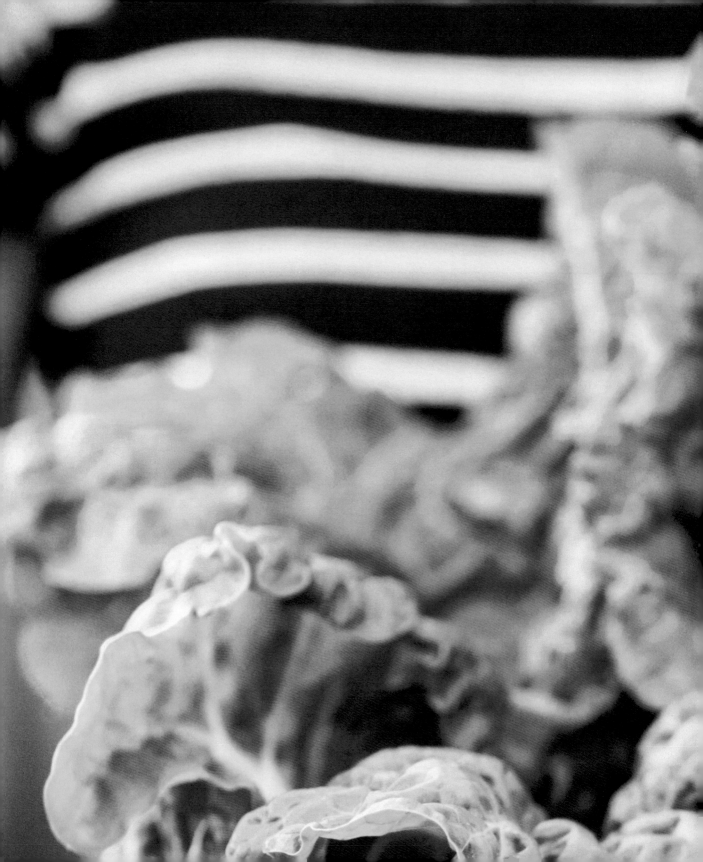

HELPFUL NOTES ON VARIOUS FOODS

Eat more of these foods

VEGETABLES AND SALADS

Pile these on, to fill at least half of your daily plates. Include a variety of intense colours and flavours. At least some should be raw or fresh. I try to include a salad with most meals.

Wild or bitter dark leafy greens (examples: endive and chicory) and those from the cruciferous family (examples: broccoli, kale, watercress and rocket) are especially worthy, as they deliver unique cancer-fighting phytonutrients. While 70 per cent of people genetically dislike bitter vegetables, you can reduce their bitterness so they taste great by drizzling with extra virgin olive oil and lemon juice.

The entire onion family, including leeks, garlic and shallots, is important as they can protect your heart and add to your anti-cancer arsenal. Try to include onion daily in some form. In Mediterranean cultures, they use it as the basis for most dishes.

Adding one extra daily serve of any vegetable or fruit can help improve lung function, especially important if you have asthma or emphysema. And eating your vegetables with their skin on is always best. While I have given specific examples, please be clear on one thing: all vegetables are useful and their high total intake best promotes health and wellbeing.

Health authorities often promote five serves of vegetables daily as realistic and beneficial. But many studies suggest that even higher amounts might be better. One study of more than 65,000 British people found that eating seven portions of fruits and vegetables each day is linked to a 42 per cent reduced risk of dying prematurely compared to eating less than one portion! Vegetables seemed to give the most protection, followed by salads and then fruit. Achieving high intakes of vegetables regularly is easier if you adopt a plant-based diet.

If you lack vegetables in your diet and are thinking about topping up with extracts and powders, these will never provide all the same benefits as eating the wholefoods. The thousands of phytonutrients and fibres present in plant foods also work best in concert, like members of an orchestra. Taking high doses of antioxidants in pills might even cause cancer, according to some research.

You can learn about new vegetable varieties over time. I always discover new types when I visit different countries—and find out how to cook traditional recipes using more vegetables. If you try my delicious Village-style Vegetable Stew (page 137), Succulent Eggplant and Tomato Bake (page

180) and Mediterranean Braised Green Beans with Tomato (page 133), you will see it's not difficult to eat enough vegetables, if you make them the main event in your meals.

PLANT PROTEINS

Legumes of all kinds (examples: dry beans, lentils, edamame and more)—as well as foods made from these (example: lentil burgers)—should satisfy about one-quarter of your food plate. You can also source plant protein from nuts and seeds used in savoury dishes or eaten as snacks (examples: Mini Sausage Rolls (page 124), trail mix).

Plant protein is linked with lower rates of multiple chronic diseases, including heart disease, type 2 diabetes and cancer. This is probably because high-protein plant foods contain a different mix of amino acids compared to animal foods, while supplying fibre and some unique phytonutrients not found in high levels even in fruits and vegetables. Plant protein foods are also filling, so you can eat fewer calories yet feel satisfied.

Nuts contain high levels of arginine, an amino acid that makes blood vessels relax and remain flexible as you age. The combination of nutrients in nuts also tones down inflammation, which is a key to fighting chronic disease. Like soybeans, nuts supply plant sterols, which help lower high blood cholesterol.

Most importantly, enjoying nuts could be an easy strategy to save lives. In 1992, scientists first published the astounding finding that eating nuts five times a week was linked to a 50 per cent reduced risk of heart attack. As other large-population studies confirmed this finding and clinical trials showed that nuts successfully lower cholesterol, their superfood status was assured and nuts migrated from the "avoid" to the "include" lists of heart foundations around the world.

The largest clinical trial in the world—called PREDIMED from Spain—found that eating a handful of nuts each day as part of a Mediterranean diet can reduce the risk of developing type 2 diabetes, diabetic retinopathy, and both classical and emerging cardiovascular risk factors.

Nuts are a "food as medicine" now prescribed by health professionals around the world. Some people are still afraid of eating them for fear of weight gain but the data consistently shows nut lovers tend to be thinner and suffer less from obesity. Clinical studies have found nuts can help dampen your appetite and improve insulin sensitivity. Their fat content is not all available for absorption into the body because it is enclosed by plant cell walls that are not completely broken down even with thorough chewing. One study found the calories available to the body from walnuts, for example, are actually around 20 per cent less than expected. In the future, the calorie contents of nuts will need to be revised.

What are activated nuts?

These nuts have been soaked, then dehydrated at low temperature to produce a texture akin to roasted nuts. Soaking nuts enables their antioxidants and other nutrients to be more readily available to the body. However, there is currently no research proving that activated nuts have superior health benefits over regular nuts.

In a nutshell, the best way to consume nuts is in their raw state as chemicals, called acrylamide and AGEs (page 380) form on nuts roasted at high temperatures. For example, formation of acrylamide on almonds begins when the internal temperature of the nut reaches around 130°C (265°F). Commercial nut roasting typically occurs at temperatures between 140-180°C (280-355°F).

If you have trouble chewing nuts, soak them in water or use their pastes. The Lebanese have a tradition of offering soaked almonds on tables at wedding parties as a fertility symbol. Soaked almonds also taste sweeter!

Legumes stimulate the growth of good bacteria in your intestines and promote their diversity. Such bacteria are important to ferment dietary fibre and indigestible carbohydrates, and make short chain fatty acids, like propionate and butyrate, which are important for health. These end products can help lower cholesterol, slow the generation of new fat cells and even protect against bowel cancer. To boost your production of propionate and butyrate, eat more fibre from legumes and resistant starch from foods like polenta.

Australians don't eat enough legumes and should increase their intake by 470 per cent, according to dietary modelling that underpins the Australian Dietary Guidelines!

Legumes also have the lowest GI (page 346) of any food group. Besides providing quality protein, a recent study showed beans contain the best carbs to beat even whole grains! If you have an irritable bowel, sprouted legumes are better tolerated. As for the flatulence factor, this depends on which legume you use, how it's prepared and whether your gut has adapted to eating beans. Soaking legumes for at least 18 hours in water removes up to 90 per cent of their oligosaccharides, which are responsible for gas formation. Other traditional remedies might also be helpful.

3 ANTI-FLATULENCE TIPS

1. **Chew fennel seeds, or sip fennel or cumin tea, after eating.**
2. **Add a strip of kombu (seaweed) when soaking and cooking legumes.**
3. **Use asafoetida in your cooking to flavour food, as they do in India.**

Adding some nuts or seeds to a dish that contains carbohydrates can tone down the blood sugar and insulin spikes that result after eating such a meal. This is clearly beneficial if you have diabetes or insulin resistance, but it can also help those with acne and polycystic ovarian syndrome (PCOS).

Scientists now believe keeping blood insulin from soaring could be important for all of us to protect against various chronic diseases. For example, the Nurses Health Study of 75,000 women followed over 30 years found women who ate two or more serves of nuts per week had a 35 per cent lower risk of pancreatic cancer. The researchers believe this might be because nuts help to regulate insulin levels, among other mechanisms.

Adding nuts is especially important if you choose to eat refined carb foods. While I don't recommend white bread for regular use, smearing it with some natural peanut butter will reduce the insulin rise your body experiences afterwards. Many traditional societies have intuitively added nuts, seeds or legumes to dishes containing refined carbohydrate (examples: lentil dal served with basmati rice, baklava).

Eating beans regularly and including a handful (30 g/1 oz) of nuts or seeds on most days is important for good health. Here are some ways to do this:

1. *Try my Pakistani-style Dal with Green Chilli (page 175).*
2. *Make Tofu Skewers with Indonesian Satay Sauce (page 161) for a barbecue.*
3. *Cook up Baked Giant Lima Beans in Tomato Sauce (page 162) on the weekend for the week ahead.*
4. *Create my popular Black-eyed Bean Salad with Lemon and Shallots (page 127) while on vacation—you can now buy canned black-eyed beans for easy use.*
5. *Swap tofu for chicken in your chicken salad—it cooks like chicken.*
6. *Toss sprouts through your salads or use them to fill sandwiches.*
7. *Make Walnut and Mushroom Meatballs with Tomato Sauce (page 190) and serve on top of Soft Yellow Polenta (page 189) for a dinner party.*
8. *Swap ham and cheese in your sandwich for a nut or seed paste with sliced banana.*

Why soy is so special

Including foods made from soybeans (examples: tofu, soybean sprouts, miso and soy milk) from an early age might be one of the best ways to reduce your family's risk of hormone-dependent cancers, such as breast and prostate cancers. Soybeans are rich in isoflavones and other phytonutrients, which work through multiple pathways (both hormonal and non-hormonal) to block cancer-cell growth.

Several population studies on women (from different ethnic backgrounds) who have had breast cancer show better survival rates and less cancer recurrence among those who eat more soy foods, compared to those who avoid them. Rather than interfering with or blocking cancer medication as once feared, these studies suggest soy might increase the efficacy of anti-cancer drugs like Tamoxifen. Unfortunately, many women might be missing out on soy as previous hypothetical concerns have resulted in scaremongering. Yet no human studies have ever shown that soy causes cancer.

WHOLE GRAINS

Include grains that are unrefined or minimally processed and foodstuffs made from them. Knowing they are an excellent source of good carbohydrates, you can enjoy ancient grains like spelt, pseudograins such as quinoa and more modern varieties like pearled barley. Wheat has been unfairly represented because some people are intolerant to its fructan and/or gluten content. For most people, the real problem is that they consume wheat as highly refined products (examples: biscuits or pizza) rather than in its intact form (examples: wheat berries or cracked wheat). See my list of useful whole grains to keep in your pantry on page 17.

Intact, cracked or rolled whole grains (rather than finely milled flour) provide a slower release of sugar into your bloodstream, meaning they are low GI compared to starchy foods made from refined white flour, like white bread and muffins. This is the quality you need, if you are trying to lower insulin resistance and control your weight. Unlike refined grains, whole grains also fill you up more, so you will stop eating sooner.

What is GI?

Glycaemic index (GI) is a system originally developed in 1981 by Professor David Jenkins from the University of Toronto to rank carbohydrate foods according to how quickly or slowly they raise blood sugar levels in people with diabetes. Low GI foods (where the GI is less than 55) are slow acting, whereas high GI foods (GI greater than 70) are fast acting. It's important to include some low GI foods at each meal for better blood sugar and insulin control in all of us.

Whole grains are very high in fibre and some contain resistant starch. Australian CSIRO researchers now recognise resistant starch as critically important for intestinal health as it acts like a type of dietary fibre. Resistant starch also exists in certain foods that don't rate extremely high on the fibre scale (example: cooked and cooled polenta). When dished up with beans and greens, such as in rural African diets, high resistant-starch foods have been linked with the lowest rates of gut problems recorded, including constipation, haemorrhoids and even bowel cancer!

Including dense and grainy breads (rather than light and fluffy smooth white breads) and other whole grains regularly will help you with regularity. Being able to easily evacuate your bowels on a daily basis is a sign of a good diet and reduced risk of bowel cancer. Passing a bowel motion only every few days shows that you are not getting enough fibre and could benefit from eating more whole grains and beans. Note: If your bowels suddenly become sluggish, check with your doctor as there can also be other medical causes.

Research shows eating three or more serves of whole grains each day is linked to a reduced risk of heart attack and stroke, type 2 diabetes, weight gain and colorectal cancer.

Like legumes, whole grains dampen inflammation in various parts of your body, such as your lungs. They're ideal if you have asthma or need to eat anti-inflammatory foods for arthritis or multiple sclerosis.

I love to use whole grains as a basis for salads or side dishes to replace refined grains like white rice or pasta made from white flour. Try my delicious Freekeh with Aromatic Spices and Pine Nuts (page 91) or Barley Risotto with Porcini Mushrooms and Sage (page 83) and you'll see why. See also easy ways to prepare a range of whole grains using a rice cooker on page 76.

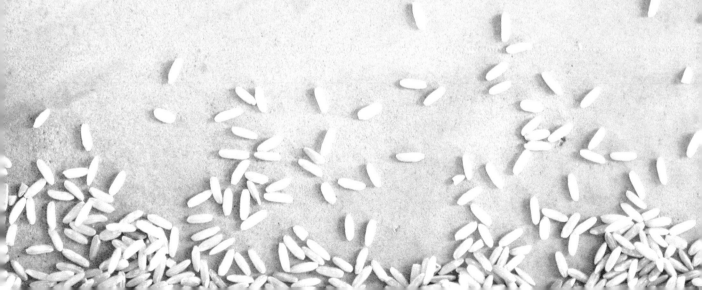

Low GI Carb Food Swaps

INSTEAD OF THIS	TRY THIS
Rice Bubbles or cornflakes	Porridge, Bircher muesli
Mashed potato	Creamy Cauliflower Mash (page 86), soft cooked dal or Butter Bean and Thyme Mash (page 87)
White or wholemeal bread	Grainy seeded bread or rye/wholemeal sourdough
White rice, especially jasmine and arborio	Red rice, brown basmati rice, pearled barley, buckwheat or quinoa
Pasta salads	Legume salads

Dairy or fortified plant alternatives

Health authorities generally recommend 2–4 serves of calcium-rich foods daily to get enough calcium. Everyone knows these include dairy milk and yogurt, but few people appreciate that calcium can also be obtained from plants and fortified plant-based foods.

Have you tried soy milk?

If using alternatives to cows milk on a regular basis, it's important to check food labels and pick a brand enriched with calcium and vitamin B12, especially if you are a low dairy consumer or don't eat meat.

There are many healthy plant sources of calcium, such as firm tofu (which can provide 300–500 mg per half cup, depending on setting agent), legumes, tahini (especially unhulled), dried figs, almonds, Asian greens and low-oxalate green vegetables (examples: bok choy, broccoli and kale). While low-oxalate greens contain less calcium than milk, 40–60 per cent of their calcium content is absorbed compared to only 30–32 per cent taken up from dairy or soy milk. The contribution of calcium from plant foods also adds up during the day. Plant-food sources of calcium have been used by many populations throughout the world who traditionally consumed little or no dairy.

Why not try tahini (sesame seed paste) to make a delicious silky smooth dressing? See my recipe for Roasted Vegetables with Creamy Orange Tahini Dressing (page 67). Or use it to whip up a creamy sauce for pasta such as my Pasta with Creamy Mushroom Sauce and Baby Spinach (page 156). How about spreading your breakfast toast with almond butter rather than margarine? You can also chiffonade and massage kale to create a gorgeous raw salad with flavours reminiscent of bubblegum—check out my Fresh Kale, Avocado and Pomegranate Salad (page 62).

Have you tried nutritional yeast?

Some people miss parmesan when they give up dairy. Nutritional yeast can add a subtle cheese-like flavour to foods and dissolves well in pasta sauces, soups and casseroles. It is not the same as brewer's or baker's yeast, both of which taste bitter. Nutritional yeast comes in flakes and powder. For greater versatility, buy the flakes in a shaker from health-food stores.

FRUIT

Whether fresh, frozen or dried, you should include fruit two to three times over the day. This is nature's original dessert and snack food!

Eating a variety of brightly coloured fruits over time will supply you with an enormous range of phytonutrients. It's no wonder fruit has been linked to protection against stroke and heart attack, while cakes, cookies and sweets will promote inflammation and oxidative stress processes immediately after eating them, silently but surely making you sick on the inside!

You don't need to buy the most expensive fruit to benefit. Commonly available choices, including apples and oranges, also guard health. A modelling study from Oxford University published in the *British Medical Journal* suggests prescribing an apple-a-day to everybody over 50 would prevent or delay deaths to the same extent as putting folks on statin medication, yet carry none of the side effects of this drug!

Citrus fruits are ideal to indulge in over winter. They might reduce the risk of certain cancers, such as stomach cancer, by up to 50 per cent, according to a report from Australian researchers. While most people know oranges are an excellent source of vitamin C (one orange provides double the recommended daily intake), few realise oranges contain more than 170 different phytonutrients to help prevent oxidation in your body, block inflammation, slow down aging and help maintain your skin's healthy glow! Many of these phytonutrients are found in the white pith, which is why it's important to eat a whole orange fruit, rather than downing some strained orange juice at breakfast.

Some so called "superfruits" contain exceptionally high antioxidant levels. For example, the deep red, blue and purple pigments of raspberries, blueberries, cherries and the Queen Garnet plum signal their very high contents of anthocyanins (antioxidants that lower inflammation and protect against diabetes, heart disease and arthritis). Berries are also very low GI (page 346) and low in calories. When berries are not in season, you can eat frozen or dried berries so you don't miss out. More exotic (and often more expensive) fruit choices marketed as superfoods include pomegranate, noni, acai, mangosteen, goji, Inca berry and cranberry. The problem is that the rankings of superfruits change according to the analytical test used. There is also no test available yet to compare their antioxidant potency inside the human body.

If you limit your fruits to only one or two varieties, you will be missing out. There are literally thousands of phytonutrients in plant foods and they're not all found in one species, no matter how exotic it might sound. Long-term studies show that diets rich in colourful (including commonly available) fruits and vegetables best protect against chronic disease. No single food can do it all.

Dried fruits can add extra sweetness, while delivering antioxidants and viscous fibres, mostly preserved in the drying process. While you need to be careful with dental caries in children, especially if you give them fruit leathers, it's smarter to get your sugar hit from these natural sweets than from processed sweets. I like to use dried fruits as a replacement for refined sugar in desserts and to make porridge and other whole grains taste even better at breakfast. See my recipe for Caramel Date Sauce (page 230).

Always eat the skin on fruit, if it's edible, and enjoy fruit whole rather than juicing it and discarding the fibre. This will have a lower impact on your blood sugar levels. Drinking more than one glass of fruit juice daily can also make you gain weight just like soft drink! Studies with apples show there are more polyphenolic phytonutrients in the skin than flesh. Apple with its skin intact more powerfully blocks the growth of liver and colon cancer cells in the test tube.

Eating seasonal fruit for dessert is one of the best habits you can teach your kids—and it will reduce your risk of heart attack at the same time. In many Mediterranean and Asian countries, fruit is served to conclude a meal. I was offered a small bunch of fragrant grapes from the dessert trolley at a fancy restaurant in Bologna, Italy. Watermelon slices automatically arrived after my main meal in a restaurant in Athens and orange wedges were shared as part of my dining experience in a Chinese restaurant in Beijing.

If you are after something fancier to serve guests, try my Strawberry and Banana Mousse (page 232) or Sour Cherry Sago (page 262). My recipes for Sweet Endings (page 226) are based on wholefoods to help you make every mouthful count.

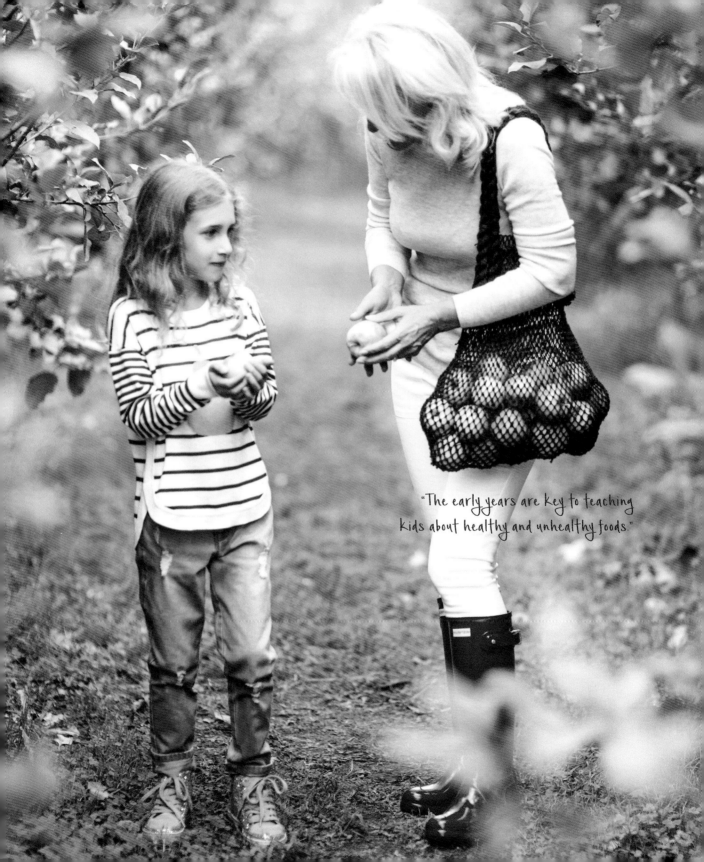

"The early years are key to teaching
kids about healthy and unhealthy foods."

MUSHROOMS

Generally thought of as a vegetable, mushrooms and fungi belong to their own food kingdom. I love mushrooms for their meaty texture and earthy flavour due to the naturally high glutamate content. When using mushrooms in recipes, you can get away with less salt, yet achieve a robust flavour.

Mushrooms are very low calorie (eating them has been linked with a lower BMI), low carb, high fibre (good for satiety) and gluten-free. They are also one of the foods that can supply beta glucan (which lowers elevated cholesterol) and an antioxidant called ergothioneine, which your body can't make. Ergothioneine is used by the body as an important "back up" when other internal antioxidants become depleted.

You can now buy "Vitamin D mushrooms." These are useful for any plant-based diet because vitamin D is not usually found in non-animal-based foods. However, despite previous marketing campaigns suggesting otherwise, mushrooms are *not* a good source of active vitamin B12 for the human body. If you are vegan or a vegetarian, enjoy mushrooms but make sure you also include other fortified food sources of vitamin B12 and/or take a supplement.

What excites me most about mushrooms is their food-as-medicine potential. Mushrooms contain some unique phytonutrients that might boost immunity. They seem to do this by encouraging a greater diversity of the microbiota in your gut. Mushrooms might be helpful for autoimmune diseases, such as rheumatoid arthritis and lupus, because of their anti-inflammatory and immune-modulating effects. Some animal studies show mushrooms might delay cognitive decline and the onset of dementia. Newer research shows vegetables, legumes and mushrooms are also linked with a lower risk of gout. Mushrooms are currently being studied for their anti-cancer properties, especially with regard to breast and prostate cancer.

The good news is that these benefits don't only apply to more exotic varieties but to the common white button mushrooms as well. You also don't need to eat buckets of mushrooms to gain protection. Just one mushroom daily, on average, is linked with a more than 50 per cent reduced risk of breast cancer in a study comparing the food intakes of women with and without cancer.

Want a creative way to include more mushrooms in your meals? Try my Walnut and Mushroom Meatballs in Tomato Sauce (page 190). I like to make the balls ahead in bulk and freeze them for when required.

HERBS AND SPICES

I adore herbs and spices, not just for their amazing flavours, colours and aromas, but because they add significant health benefits to every mouthful. Since ancient times, herbs and spices have been the basis for almost all medicines, until synthetic drugs were developed in the 19th century.

We now know that the antioxidant level in a modest serve of herbs and spices is higher than in many fruits and most vegetables. So learning to season your meals with herbs and spices is a smart idea. For example, researchers from Australia's Southern Cross University have shown that adding herbs like oregano, rosemary, mint and garlic to an olive oil and lemon juice dressing can triple the antioxidant value of a simple salad.

Combinations of herbs and spices seem to be even more potent. This is how they are traditionally used in countries like India, where up to 60 herbs and spices might appear together in one blend! The word "masala" literally means a mixture. So *garam masala* is a mixture of spices used in Indian cookery, like Arabic seven spices is a blend used in the Middle East.

FOUR SALT-FREE SEASONINGS

1. **Dulse granules or blended seaweed flakes.**
2. **Splash of lemon juice or vinegar.**
3. **Fresh and dried herbs (examples: oregano, basil).**
4. **Nutritional yeast seasoning.**

Herbs and spices contain thousands of phytonutrients that cleverly influence the expression of your genes so you can better fight chronic diseases. And studies on their antioxidant and anti-inflammatory effects show these properties do not disappear after cooking and digestion. Here are a few examples:

Cassia (the common form of cinnamon) might help improve your body's sensitivity to insulin. This is important if you have diabetes, metabolic syndrome or PCOS. It might also provide benefits for a fatty liver. As little as 1 gram daily (¼ teaspoon) has been shown to lower blood sugar levels by 18-29 per cent in people with type 2 diabetes. Trials have used 1-6 grams with varying results. Avoid high doses (more than 6 g or 1½ teaspoons) per day, especially through supplements, as this could be toxic to your liver. I use ground cassia when making porridge, a hot drink or dessert, and include a quill when cooking whole grains, such as my Fragrant Buckwheat and Quinoa Pilaf (page 92) or Spaghetti Bolognaise Sauce with Cinnamon (page 157).

Ginger can boost your immune system and helps reduce inflammation. Several ginger phyto-nutrients have also been shown to have anti-cancer effects. Traditionally used for nausea (with benefits shown for 1 gram per day of standardised ginger extract) and stomach ailments, in test tube studies, ginger has more recently been found to kill all 19 disease causing *Helicobacter pylori* bacteria species, which cause stomach ulcers. You will see ginger in many of my recipes. In my Culinary Medicine Cookshops, I show people how they can easily make fresh ginger tea in a hotel room while travelling, how to peel it with a metal spoon as they do in Indonesia, and to freeze leftovers so there is no waste.

Oregano is one of the richest sources of polyphenols among herbs. While it has been grown and used for centuries in the Mediterranean as both a culinary herb and medicine, oregano has been shown by modern science to contain several antioxidants with anti-inflammatory, blood sugar and blood-fat lowering properties. If there is one herb I would not leave home without, it is oregano. I use dried oregano extensively in my recipes. It adds tremendous flavour to plant-based dishes. Fresh oregano is less commonly used by cooks but Lebanese people make a salad entirely from its leaves.

Rosemary contains significant quantities of several antioxidants with anti-tumour properties. One of these—rosmarinic acid—holds promise for Alzheimer's disease, as it seems to prevent the deposit of amyloid plaque in the brain—as well as the plaque in your arteries—and might contribute to its breakdown. Rosemary has traditionally been touted for memory. When added to beef patties prior to high-temperature cooking, this intensely scented herb significantly reduces the formation of cancer-causing chemicals called HCAs (page 379).

Turmeric provides anti-inflammatory, antioxidant and anti-cancer properties. It is found in almost every Indian spice box and consumed on a daily basis in various Asian communities. Two types of turmeric powder exist with variable contents of the primary active ingredient called curcumin. Madras, the bright yellow one more commonly sold in shops contains 1.5-1.8 per cent curcumin, whereas the darker yellow Allepey boasts 3.5-4 per cent curcumin. Curry powder is generally low in curcumin. In his book on the "Blue Zones" of the world, with the longest living people, Dan Beuttner quotes a study that found turmeric is one-fifth as powerful as Cisplatin, one of the most effective chemotherapy drugs! Scientists have discovered that turmeric can damage cancer cells in more than 100 ways, with potential to block all the necessary stages of cancer growth and development.

A 2012 study suggests that taking curcumin supplements might help delay or prevent development of type 2 diabetes in people at high risk. Another recent study showed that taking just 1 gram turmeric daily can improve working memory (critical for planning, problem solving and reasoning) in older people with early-stage diabetes.

Turmeric is also looking promising for Alzheimer's disease (the most common type of dementia), symptoms of arthritis, inflammatory bowel disease, and possibly even liver fibrosis and cirrhosis, psoriasis, burn pain and wounds. Based on the existing research, the University of Maryland Medical Center suggests 1–3 grams of dried, powdered turmeric root per day is needed if you want to gain health benefits. You can drink a shot of turmeric each day by mixing ¼ teaspoon of the powder into some soy milk. Or try my delicious Golden Turmeric Milk (page 309). Stir a pinch of ground turmeric into tea and sip it throughout the day, like the centenarians do in Okinawa. Don't forget to add a knob of fresh turmeric to your blender when making green smoothies.

Black pepper, while not a strong antioxidant in its own right, the phytonutrient responsible for pepper's pungent zing, called piperine, significantly increases the bioavailability of the active ingredient in turmeric and appears to stop cancer cells from growing and dividing. Piperine can improve the bioavailability of phytonutrients in turmeric and green tea by more than 1000 per cent, which testifies to the benefits of using combinations of herbs and spices. Pepper also has anti-microbial and anti-inflammatory effects.

While herbs and spices are useful for the entire family and vitally important for anyone with chronic disease, their food-as-medicine potential still seems largely unknown in Western countries. My recipes show you various ways to use them, so you can get more power on your plate.

SEAWEED

Also known as "sea vegetable," seaweed has been identified as a novel way to add flavour to food and reduce chronic disease risk. Seaweeds come in different colours, tastes and textures, although they mostly look green when cooked. Seaweed is generally not part of the modern diet, but has been eaten in some traditions for thousands of years. In Asia, even today, seaweeds of various types, together with soy and fish are thought to be one of the keys to longevity.

Studies on humans eating seaweed are limited, but a few link higher seaweed intake to lower rates of certain cancers. Edible seaweeds contain some unique proteins and polysaccharides (carbs) not found in terrestrial plants, and an alternative source of omega-3 fats (eicosapentaenoic acid or EPA) to oily fish. Seaweeds are generally rich in minerals like iron and calcium, and boast polyphenol phytonutrients (including phlorotannins) and an abundant iodine content.

While Japan is still the leading producer and exporter of sea vegetables, Canada, France, Portugal, Scotland and Australia also produce supplies for human consumption as a fast-growing and sustainable food source.

Getting enough iodine

Iodine is important for your thyroid gland to function properly. Inadequate levels of iodine during pregnancy can result in mental retardation, loss of IQ and learning difficulties for your child. While fish and other seafood, dairy and iodised salt have been the major sources of iodine in the past, we are no longer getting adequate amounts of iodine from these sources.

You can easily obtain extra iodine by eating some seaweed from time to time. Why not try seasoning some of your dishes with a crumbled or powdered nori sheet instead of salt? Or buy a seaweed shaker with dulse or mixed granules. Just one teaspoon of some ground seaweeds can supply you with your daily dose of iodine, iron and magnesium! You can also enjoy wakame in soup. See my easy Miso Soup with Wakame and Silken Tofu (page 198). I also occasionally add a strip of dried kombu (a brown kelp) when making stocks, stews or boiling dry beans to enrich recipes with minerals and reduce the flatulence factor from legumes. And I love to use agar agar (derived from seaweed) in desserts (page 247) instead of animal-derived gelatine. Raw foodists eat noodles made from kelp (page 101) as these can simply be re-hydrated and don't require cooking. Just don't go overboard so you don't get too much iodine, which is also harmful.

EXTRA VIRGIN OILS

Extra virgin (unrefined), cold-extracted oils are always the best choice. Look for such oils derived from olive, macadamia, avocado, peanut, mustard seed, chia seed and flaxseed. Refined vegetable oils (example: canola) lack phytonutrients so they are akin to eating white bread. Most refined polyunsaturated oils and margarines also provide large amounts of omega-6 fats, which might promote inflammation in your body if not counterbalanced with adequate omega-3.

To stay well and better fight chronic disease, use unrefined oils rich in omega-9 or omega-3 fats, as listed above and illustrated in my recipes. These oils are not chemically processed, so retain their anti-inflammatory phytonutrients as nature intended. While omega-9 fat is not omega-3, it is complementary rather than being antagonistic in its actions inside your body. By contrast, omega-6 fats will compete for the same enzyme in your body that processes plant sources of omega-3 into the anti-inflammatory omegas found in fish.

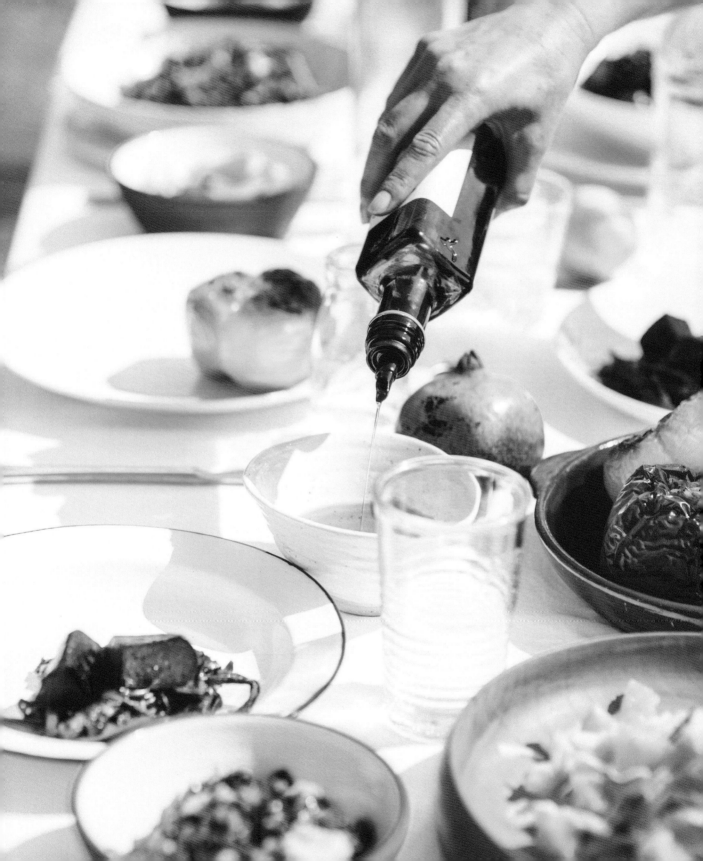

To further boost the omega-3 content of your diet, swap some of the oils used to dress your salads, vegetables and pasta for flaxseed or chia seed oils. They have a stronger taste and should always be stored in the fridge. They should also be consumed raw and never heated.

The scoop on olive oil

For everyday cooking, I use extra virgin olive oil. I buy it in large cans and decant a smaller amount into a small dark glass bottle, which I store in my kitchen cupboard. For wider flavour profiles, you can also try macadamia, avocado or pungent mustard seed oil. I prefer extra virgin olive oil as an "all-rounder" because it has stood the test of time, is widely available and integrates well with most flavours. Extra virgin olive oil has been used for centuries with good results. Multiple studies confirm its amazing health properties to reduce chronic disease.

Extra virgin olive oil reduces oxidation in your body (protecting your cholesterol, DNA and cell membranes) and tones down inflammation as well as your sugar, insulin and blood-pressure levels. The latest research suggests it does most of this by positively influencing your microbiome (page 324). The peppery taste from a good-quality extra virgin olive oil high in polyphenols, which provides a burning sensation in the back of your throat, is due to *oleocanthal*. This phytonutrient is a natural anti-inflammatory agent. It works like the medication Ibuprofen by inhibiting COX2 enzymes in your body, which lead to inflammatory pathways!

Will olive oil make you fat?

Studies generally show people who regularly use extra virgin olive oil as their main fat in the diet tend to have a lower body weight and gain less weight over time. One study found patients who used extra virgin olive oil as part of a weight-loss program did better than those given a low-fat diet.

Some people incorrectly liken canola oil to extra virgin olive oil as if the two will provide the same effects inside the body. Extra virgin olive oil is not only a healthy omega-9 monounsaturated fat, it also contains more than 40 types of phytonutrients, including polyphenols, tocopherols (vitamin E), plant sterols and squalene (a tumour inhibitor for UV protection), which scientists now consider the secret to its health-giving properties.

Certain varieties of fresh extra virgin olive oils pack a punch with up to 2500 mg polyphenols per kilogram! (Australian extra virgin olive oils contain around 300 mg per kilogram, on average.) The only oil that even comes close to this level of polyphenols is extra virgin coconut oil at an average of 50 mg per kilogram.

As always, fresh is best, so you can't beat locally produced oils. With storage of oil over time, as well as heating during cooking, the phytonutrients from even the best oils will be lost. For example, polyphenols, tocopherols and squalene are reduced by around 30 per cent with cooking. Even so, extra virgin olive oil will still provide your body with more of these phytonutrients than any refined oil such as lite olive oil, canola or sunflower oil.

How to choose olive oil

When choosing olive oil, look for the year of processing on the label. A good extra virgin olive oil will last 18 months, if stored correctly. In the European Union (EU), however, legislation allows manufacturers to declare the year of packaging instead, so by the time European olive oil reaches Australia, for example, it might already be quite old. Much extra virgin olive oil is also blended—a bit of new for flavour with a bit of old from surplus stores—which is why there is no harvest date provided in the EU.

Never buy refined olive oils, called "light" or pomace, if you are seeking optimal health. They are devoid of phytonutrients, so they lack both taste and nutrition. Interestingly, even refined olive oils can withstand frying temperatures better than refined seed oils, as measured by greater resistance to oxidative deterioration. "Pure olive oil" is refined olive oil mixed with a small quantity of extra virgin olive oil to restore some colour and flavour. For the highest polyphenol levels, meaning maximum health potential, seek fresh locally produced extra virgin olive oil and store this safely in your kitchen.

The odds of being diagnosed with heart disease in modern-day Greeks who use olive oil exclusively in their food preparation and cooking are 49 per cent lower as compared to those who use it in combination with other fats or oils, according to the Cardio2000 study.

Can you cook with olive oil?

Contrary to popular opinion, you can safely cook, even fry, with extra virgin olive oil. Extra virgin olive oil does not oxidise easily as it is a monounsaturated fat and has a high amount of vitamin E. Vitamin E helps stop fats in oils and nuts from going rancid (oxidising). Rancid oils are oils that have used up their vitamin E.

Extra virgin olive oil holds up as well as or better than other vegetable oils. According to long-standing research, the smoke point of olive oil increases as the level of free fatty acids decreases. This means that, if you buy a top-quality extra virgin olive oil with a low free fatty acid level, you can cook foods at higher temperatures (up to 220°C/430°F). Incidentally, the ideal temperature for frying is 180°C (350°F).

While I avoid deep frying, when I sauté foods like eggplant, I always use extra virgin olive oil as they do in the Mediterranean, ensuring I don't heat the pan too much to bring the oil to its smoke point.

What is the smoke point?

Smoke point is the temperature at which a cooking oil or fat begins to break down, resulting in the formation of enough unhealthy chemicals so that a bluish smoke becomes visible. It's important not to heat any oil above its smoke point. The smoke point of olive oil depends on its quality. The higher the quality, the higher the smoke point.

How much olive oil should you use?

Use extra virgin olive oil generously on your food and in cooking. Research shows it also helps you eat more vegetables and legumes. As a guide, Professor Mary Flynn, an American dietitian and researcher of olive oil, recommends you add at least 1 tablespoon of extra virgin olive oil per cup of vegetables.

After decades of "low-fat" recommendations, it might be surprising to hear that you can't get the maximum cancer-fighting carotenoids out of vegetables and into your body without eating fat. In the famous PREDIMED study (the largest randomised controlled trial in the world), markers of inflammation in the body and blood pressure reduced significantly in people following the Mediterranean diet supplemented with extra virgin olive oil. Those consuming the most extra virgin olive oil enjoyed a 35 per cent reduction in risk of cardiovascular disease (particularly stroke) and a 50 per cent reduction in the risk of developing type 2 diabetes, compared to people following a lower-fat diet. Each 10 gram increase in intake of extra virgin olive oil per day lowered cardiovascular risk by 10 per cent and premature death risk by 7 per cent.

Early researchers on the Mediterranean diet (in the 1960s) described Cretan food as "swimming in olive oil"! Having visited this beautiful Greek island, and eaten at a couple of its heritage restaurants, I can vouch for this description and how a good extra virgin olive oil can help you to eat more plant foods.

The main thing to remember is that extra virgin olive oil is not only a food but also a medicine. Benefits start at 2–3 tablespoons per day, but traditional and active Mediterranean lifestyles include more.

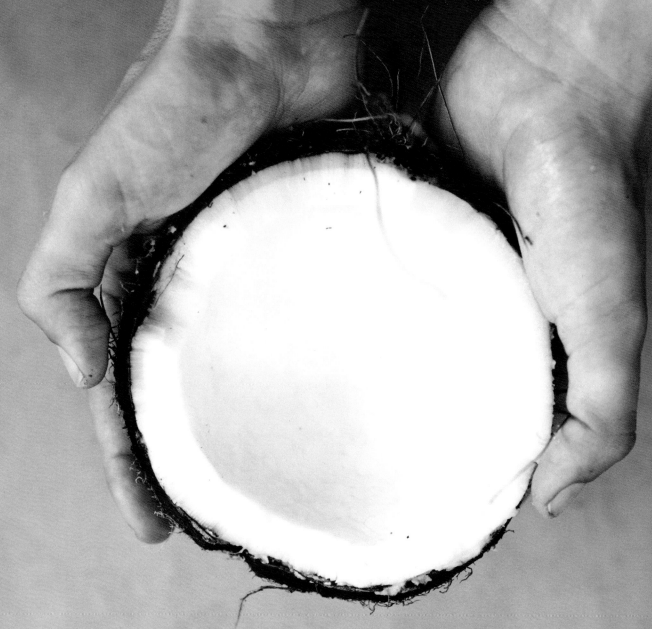

Is coconut oil healthy or hype?

Despite multiple marketing claims and testimonials touting that it is a miracle cure for everything from Alzheimer's disease to diabetes, there is very little scientific evidence to back the unrestricted use of coconut oil within a Western lifestyle. Used within a traditional context (mostly as coconut flesh and milk rather than oil) as part of a diet rich in fish and vegetables and including physical activity, it does not seem to raise heart-disease risk. But change that diet by adding meat, eggs and refined carbohydrates, and heart-disease rates start to escalate. Research in Indonesia has shown that rates of heart disease are increasing as diets are being Westernised, despite the continued use of a similar amount of coconut. If you love coconut, choose the less-refined products, such as the milk or some cream, as part of a plant-based diet.

PURE WATER

Research shows that being dehydrated by only 1-2 per cent (lacking as little as 400 ml of fluid) can make you feel tired and less alert. Yet pure water (which you can freely source from the tap in most developed countries and filter if desired) can help prevent fatigue, keep your skin moist, and enhance physical and mental functioning. Getting enough water will also help your bowels move, reduce the risk of kidney stones and may even prevent overeating, since many people mistakenly confuse hunger for thirst.

The latest evidence suggests pure water is also critically important to protect against some more serious diseases. Drinking at least six glasses of water daily, as compared to one glass, cuts the risk of bladder cancer by half in men, according to one observational study from Harvard University. Drinking at least five glasses daily, as compared to two or less reduces the risk of dying from heart attack by 40-50 per cent, according to research on a large population of Seventh-day Adventists published in the *American Journal of Epidemiology*. Surprisingly, other fluids like juices or tea were not protective.

The National Health and Medical Research Council in Australia recommends drinking at least eight cups of fluid each day if you are woman. If you are a man who is physically active, drink at least 10 cups daily. Based on the available research, now linking water deficiency to chronic disease, I would suggest pure water for at least five of your daily fluid cups.

To check whether you are drinking enough water, examine the colour of your urine. If you are well hydrated, it should be fairly clear. A dark yellow colour suggests you are not drinking enough (unless you are taking a supplement of riboflavin, which colours it yellow, or there is some other dietary influence).

Spilling the beans on coffee

Despite the realisation that it contains antioxidants, coffee hasn't suddenly become a health food. While some studies suggest mild benefits at high doses for conditions like Parkinson's disease, liver cirrhosis or liver cancer, and type 2 diabetes, these are yet to be proven. No health authority is recommending you join the coffee culture anytime soon. There is good evidence that high doses of caffeine increase anxiety, irritability and reflux symptoms, and will speed up your heart rate and contribute to poor sleep. Caffeine also provides withdrawal symptoms such as headaches and fatigue when you reduce consumption. Further, some researchers suggest the performance bonus gained by regular caffeine users might only be a reversal of their withdrawal symptoms, rather than a direct benefit.

Unfiltered coffee and all espresso-based coffees can raise your LDL cholesterol (the bad one). But even filtered coffee can cause homocysteine and other inflammatory risk factors for cardiovascular disease to rise in your bloodstream. Alarmingly, within 30 minutes after just one cup, even healthy people will experience a reduction in the ability of their blood vessels to dilate normally, although they can't feel this. Chronic coffee ingestion has been shown to increase stiffness of the aorta, the main artery in your body. Yet de-caffeinated coffee may help relax blood vessels.

The story on coffee is not straight forward. It's not a single food so it is difficult to study and the results may depend on your genes. Based on current evidence, I believe it's safer to avoid or limit consumption of coffee and other highly caffeinated beverages. If you are seeking something to perk you up, drink green tea. This contains lower levels of caffeine, no acrylamide (page 380), and has generally been linked to improved blood-vessel function and other potential health benefits, without apparent health risks. Or you could go for a walk in the sunshine or have a chat with a friend!

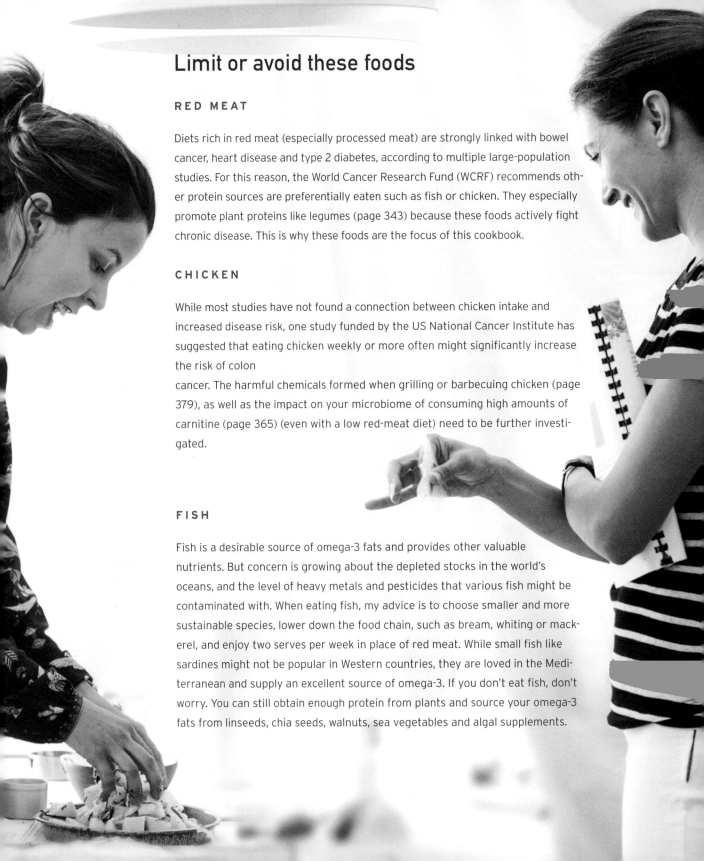

Limit or avoid these foods

RED MEAT

Diets rich in red meat (especially processed meat) are strongly linked with bowel cancer, heart disease and type 2 diabetes, according to multiple large-population studies. For this reason, the World Cancer Research Fund (WCRF) recommends other protein sources are preferentially eaten such as fish or chicken. They especially promote plant proteins like legumes (page 343) because these foods actively fight chronic disease. This is why these foods are the focus of this cookbook.

CHICKEN

While most studies have not found a connection between chicken intake and increased disease risk, one study funded by the US National Cancer Institute has suggested that eating chicken weekly or more often might significantly increase the risk of colon
cancer. The harmful chemicals formed when grilling or barbecuing chicken (page 379), as well as the impact on your microbiome of consuming high amounts of carnitine (page 365) (even with a low red-meat diet) need to be further investigated.

FISH

Fish is a desirable source of omega-3 fats and provides other valuable nutrients. But concern is growing about the depleted stocks in the world's oceans, and the level of heavy metals and pesticides that various fish might be contaminated with. When eating fish, my advice is to choose smaller and more sustainable species, lower down the food chain, such as bream, whiting or mackerel, and enjoy two serves per week in place of red meat. While small fish like sardines might not be popular in Western countries, they are loved in the Mediterranean and supply an excellent source of omega-3. If you don't eat fish, don't worry. You can still obtain enough protein from plants and source your omega-3 fats from linseeds, chia seeds, walnuts, sea vegetables and algal supplements.

Why meat might be harmful

It's not just the fat in meat that could be harming your health, as previously thought. A diet rich in meats of any type might be problematic in various previously unforeseen ways.

Three reasons scientists think meat might cause cancer and other health problems:

1. Overabundance of iron, which increases oxidation products inside your body that attack your DNA.
2. Formation of toxic chemicals (example: PAHs, HCAs) with certain cooking methods (page 379), which can cause harmful changes to your DNA.
3. Increased animal protein arriving in your gut leads to noxious bacterial fermentation products (examples: ammonia, N-nitroso compounds, sulphides) linked with cancer and other health problems, including inflammatory bowel disease.

Red meat, chicken, fish and dairy all contain carnitine. If you have certain types of bacteria living in your gut, these can act on the carnitine you swallow (from food or supplements) and, through various bodily processes, lead to the generation of trimethylamine N-oxide (TMAO). TMAO is now recognised as a highly predictive risk factor for rapidly clogging up arteries, even in people without classical risk factors such as high cholesterol.

By eating a lot of animal-based products, you could be unintentionally promoting the growth of harmful bacteria and the products they make in your gut. Yet people who eat plant-based diets seem to be protected as they have a greater diversity and predominance of good bacteria in their intestines. For example, vegans who were fed carnitine or beef steak in a test diet did not make TMAO because vegans lack these sinister bacteria since they don't regularly eat meat or other carnitine-rich animal foods.

Your usual diet has a major influence on determining the types of bacteria that take up residence in your intestines. A change in your diet—for better or worse—can make a difference to your gut bacteria in as short a time as a day.

One study by a cardiologist in the United States looking at how blood flows in the coronary artery that feeds the heart found a high-protein, low-carb omnivorous diet impairs blood flow. After following this diet for 12 months, there was a 5–10 per cent increase in the extent and severity of coronary artery disease, plus an increase in various other risk factors. Conversely, the arteries of patients who ate a low-fat, high-carb vegetarian diet were found to be "opening up."

More than 17 studies of populations from different countries have consistently found high-protein, low-carb diets are linked with an increased risk of premature death.

If you love eating lots of meat and feel you will struggle to reduce your exposure, my suggestion is to start with one meat-free day each week. Why not adopt Meat-Free Mondays? Such movements are growing in popularity around the world.

EGGS

It's now known that saturated fat from your diet is much more important in raising blood-cholesterol levels than dietary cholesterol from egg yolks. But the story on eggs is not just about their impact on your blood cholesterol. Dietary cholesterol might still promote inflammation and oxidative stress resulting in dangerous plaque build up inside your arteries, especially if you already have diabetes. As noted above, if you have certain bacteria residing in your gut, regularly consuming rich dietary sources of carnitine (meats and dairy) (page 365), and also choline (from eggs), can result in the formation of TMAO within the body. TMAO is known to rapidly promote atherosclerosis without registering a blip in your cholesterol level! A number of studies have also linked moderate egg consumption with a significantly increased risk of men dying from prostate cancer. So the research on the impact of egg consumption on your health is far from over.

Independent Canadian scientists have warned that eggs should therefore not be eaten indiscriminately without considering your genetic predisposition, overall food habits and risk of heart attack. Short-term studies showing cholesterol doesn't rise in people with diabetes using eggs for protein (as compared to meat proteins), within the context of a 30 per cent calorie-restricted diet, do not prove eggs are safe for people with diabetes longer term, when eating usual Western diets. I recommend limiting eggs to no more than two per week if you have pre-diabetes, diabetes, risk factors for heart attack and stroke, or a raised PSA (warning sign for possible prostate cancer). Don't forget to count eggs used in cooking and recipes. If you are young and perfectly healthy, you might get away with more eggs with no apparent harm. But nobody has conducted long-term studies to prove that eating multiple eggs each day is safe even in younger healthy people. Such an intake might have negative effects on their microbiome.

Plant-based wholefood egg alternatives are the smartest solution as they can actively help relax your blood vessels and prevent or reverse chronic disease because of what they do contain (example: soy protein in tofu). Try my Scrambled Tofu with Tomato (page 123) for breakfast or a light meal. Use "chia egg" to bind and thicken recipes. While it's not easy to replace the many functional properties of eggs in cooking and baking, page 337 provides some egg-swap ideas.

DAIRY PRODUCTS

Dairy has been widely promoted in Western societies for its calcium to improve bone health and reduce fracture risk. Yet large-population studies and randomised clinical studies have failed to find convincing evidence that dairy actually prevents osteoporosis. And then there are the risk factors. Many people avoid full-cream milk for fear of saturated fat. But it's the lactose and type of protein, as well as other hormonal factors that exist in dairy, that scientists are becoming increasingly interested in. These components are of relevance even if you drink skim milk.

Some scientists believe the lactose in milk (or more specifically galactose, derived from the digestion of lactose in your body) might induce internal changes that mimic natural aging. When fed to animals, galactose promotes oxidative stress, chronic systemic inflammation, degeneration of the nervous system and a decreased immune response. These processes not only drive heart disease and cancer but are underlying mechanisms for age-related bone loss and osteoporosis. Population studies suggest similar mechanisms might operate in humans who have high intakes of milk. Yet fermented dairy products, such as yogurt (in which most of the lactose has been converted to lactic acid), are not linked to increased fracture risk nor early death and seem to be protective. Research also shows including three serves of low-fat dairy per day as part of a plant-based diet lowers high blood pressure (page 336). And dairy, generally, has been linked to a reduced risk of metabolic syndrome and type 2 diabetes.

However, the consequence of a lifetime exposure to hormonal factors from dairy, designed to promote rapid growth in a calf, on hormone-dependent chronic disease in humans has not been well studied. Yet several studies in men have linked high milk intakes with an increased risk of metastatic prostate cancer (a hormone-dependent disease). And high milk intakes are known to raise blood levels of insulin-like growth factor 1 (IGF-1), which has been repeatedly linked with a higher risk of developing prostate cancer. In its latest review of 32 studies, the World Cancer Research Fund concluded that high intakes of total dairy (from milk, cheese, low-fat milk, skim milk) but not supplemental calcium or non-dairy calcium might raise the risk of prostate cancers as a group.

A large ongoing population study in the United States, led by Dr Gary Fraser, is comparing health outcomes in people following five distinct dietary patterns: omnivorous, semi-vegetarian, pesco-vegetarian, lacto-ovo vegetarian and vegan (see page 336 for diet definitions). The latest results show that, while overall cancer rates were reduced by only 8 per cent in the two vegetarian groups combined, there was a 35 per cent reduced risk of prostate cancer and a 34 per cent lower risk of all female cancers combined (cancers of the breast, vagina, cervix, endometrium, uterus and ovary) in the vegans (dairy- and egg-free) as compared to the omnivores.

Until further research is available, you and your family might want to diversify your calcium food sources or opt for plant-based choices entirely If you choose the right foods, you can get enough calcium from plant foods (page 348).

The traditional Asian diet has been applauded for its low risk of chronic diseases including osteoporosis. It did not include dairy products. In the traditional Cretan Mediterranean diet, loved for both flavour and health promotion, cows milk was not consumed. Goat and sheep milk was reserved for children, while moderate amounts of yogurt and soft, fermented cheeses (example: feta) made from these milks, were eaten by adults. Interestingly, such milks are known to contain A2 beta-casein and higher omega-3 levels, compared to modern cows milk.

If you are interested in fermented foods, these can still be obtained from a dairy-free diet. You can buy or make plant-based yogurt and kefir from nut or grain "milks" and take a dairy-free probiotic supplement. If you miss the idea of cheese, why not try the delicious new artisan "nut" cheeses that are starting to appear at farmers' markets or make my scrumptious Almond Cream Cheese Topped with Herbs (page 224)?

SUPPLEMENTS

Thanks to innovative marketing, many people take some sort of supplement and the industry is big business. Yet no health authority has ever suggested you can replace nutritious wholefoods with pills and powders and get the same benefits. The latest scientific reviews have concluded that most supplements do not prevent chronic disease or early death and their use is not justified. They might even cause harm. Supplements also have no clear benefits in well-nourished individuals.

However, there are exceptions. Supplements might be helpful if you are deficient or unable to obtain adequate amounts of certain nutrients through your diet. For example, vitamin B12 does not naturally exist in plants, so it is important that you take a supplement and/or use fortified foods if you are vegan or follow a low-dairy, low-egg vegetarian diet. And a vitamin D supplement may be useful if you are one of the increasing number of people found to be deficient due to a lack of sun exposure.

When considering a supplement, a balance of risks and benefits for your body should be undertaken together with a qualified health professional. The safest approach to guard against illness is to base your diet on a diverse range of nutrient-rich plant foods. As the World Cancer Research Fund recommends, everyone should "aim to meet nutritional needs through diet alone."

Avoid these foods

ULTRA-PROCESSED SNACK FOODS AND FAST FOODS

Snacking on biscuits or puffed and extruded packet foods throughout the day (or night!) or grabbing a pepperoni pizza on the weekend has become so common place that many people hardly give it a second thought. Market research suggests some people spend more money on snacks than they do on fruits and vegetables combined! The reality is that discretionary foods have now displaced vegetables in the diet to the peril of our health.

While most people might accept that fast food and processed snacks may contribute to their risk of heart disease, cancer, fatty liver and obesity, few consider the effects on their children, as if they were somehow immune. Perhaps they choose to turn a blind eye due to pester power.

As 70 per cent of food preferences are established at an early age, the best way to positively influence your child is to be a good role model by eating well yourself!

If you want to give your child the best start in life, don't add crisps or mini-cookies to their lunchbox. There are many delicious and natural snacks (see my list of easy snacks on page 269). Avoid buying sweet muffins, instant noodles and chocolate bars for after-school or late-night munchies. See my wholefood recipe ideas for treats you can make at home instead (page 266).

SUGARY DRINKS

If you're looking to lose weight or improve your wellbeing, it's a smart idea to avoid sugary drinks. These include soft drinks, colas and sodas, cordials, sports drinks, energy drinks, vitamin waters, iced teas, non-alcoholic cider, ginger beer and fruit-flavoured drinks.

Sugary drinks are strongly linked with weight gain and obesity in both children and adults. Studies also link sugar-sweetened beverages with type 2 diabetes, heart attack and stroke, cancer, gout and early onset of menstruation in girls, as well as about 180,000 premature deaths worldwide each year.

Most authorities now recommend you limit your intake of all drinks containing rapidly absorbed sugars to a maximum of one glass per day. Even less is probably better. See my simple yet refreshing ways with water on page 298.

ALCOHOL

Whatever the type of alcoholic beverage, convincing evidence now exists that drinking alcohol regularly—even in small amounts—significantly raises the risk of cancer of the mouth, pharynx, larynx, oesophagus, bowel (in men) and breast (in women). You're also likely to have a thicker waistline at any age, as alcohol is a significant and easy-to-down source of calories. And if you're interested in preserving your grey matter, some studies suggest that alcohol can promote harmful oxidation and inflammation in the brain.

But what about the belief that red wine is good for the heart? Cancer Council Australia says this is misguided. In a 2011 Position Statement warning how alcohol raises the risk of cancer, they state that the previously reported role of alcohol in reducing heart-disease risk in light to moderate drinkers appears to have been overestimated.

Even if alcohol were to offer a modest benefit for the heart, researchers think this might be limited to women aged 55 years or older. There are also safer ways to reduce your heart-attack risk, such as by not smoking, eating nuts regularly and being physically active. Dr David Nelson, director of the Cancer Prevention Fellowship Program at the US National Cancer Institute, says while we talk a lot about tobacco and poor diets, alcohol is often missed as a cause of preventable diseases and deaths. "Alcohol causes 10 times as many deaths as it prevents worldwide," according to Dr Nelson.

When push comes to shove, health authorities agree there is actually no safe level of alcohol consumption. The risks increase for any amount you drink on a regular basis. In a 2015 editorial for the *British Medical Journal*, Professor of Health Policy at Curtin University in Australia, Mike Daube, wrote that the previously touted benefits of moderate drinking "are now evaporating."

Is "organic" worth it?

It's difficult to prove organic food is better if you only compare its vitamin and mineral content. After reviewing multiple studies, the UK's Food Standards Agency concluded there was no nutritional difference between organic and conventionally grown produce. But the story becomes more interesting when phytonutrients, like antioxidants, are considered.

ANTIOXIDANT BOOST

Several smaller studies found higher levels of phytonutrients in organic strawberries, apples, tomatoes and ketchup. After scrutinising 344 studies, a review published in the *British Journal of Nutrition* in 2014 concluded there are statistically significant and practically meaningful differences in the antioxidant content of certain foodstuffs, with a range of antioxidants being between 19 and 69 per cent higher in organic crops. According to these researchers, this would be like adding 1–2 extra serves of fruits and vegetables to your daily diet.

Plants produce high levels of phytonutrients for their own protection against diseases from viruses, bacteria and moulds. When they are conventionally grown (with pesticides), their need to resist such invaders is reduced. So they make fewer phytonutrients. But let them grow naturally, and their innate defence mechanisms kick in and phytonutrient levels go up.

Many studies link phytonutrient-rich diets (these are plant-based by necessity) with the lowest rates of chronic disease in people. Eating more plant foods, especially those grown organically, is a sure way to boost your personal phytonutrient intake.

CHEMICAL-FREE FOOD

Organic foods have another advantage. They lack pesticide, herbicide and insecticide residues, which might turn out to be harmful for humans. While these chemicals have been individually approved for use by authorities, nobody knows for sure the effect of consuming a cocktail of them over a lifetime, even at low doses. Exposure to pesticides and farming chemicals has been linked to an increased risk of cancer, depression, Parkinson's disease and ADHD.

From a human health point of view, I believe this is the most important reason why organic trumps conventional produce and it is worth the extra cost. It's also much better for our environment. Fortunately, studies show that when people switch to eating organic foods, there is a measurable drop in the pesticide levels in various parts of their body. This has been demonstrated in both adults and children.

Based on the annual US "Dirty Dozen" lists compiled by the Environmental Working Group (which names and shames the most pesticide-laden produce in America), it is the thin-skinned fruits like apples, berries, grapes and peaches, as well as leafy greens like spinach and kale, tomatoes, potatoes and celery, that might be particularly important to buy organic.

Eating large amounts of any types of fruits and vegetables, regardless of how they are grown, should still be your top priority. Some data exists to argue that certain phytonutrients, even from conventionally grown produce, might help counteract some of the negative effects of pesticides. Studies on vegetarians who generally eat larger amounts of fruits and vegetables (most of which have not been organically grown) also found higher levels of salicylic acid in their blood, protecting against heart attack and stroke, and probably also fighting bowel cancer. (You might be more familiar with salicylic acid as the active ingredient in aspirin.)

The bottom line is organic food is not a luxury. It's how food is supposed to be. Learn to grow your own if you can. Or buy it from farmers' markets if you don't have a green thumb. Most importantly, eat more plants of any kind.

The benefits of going more raw

Raw foodists claim they have better stamina, sleep and digestion, clearer skin and enhanced concentration levels. Some research suggests *raw plant-food diets* might offer therapeutic properties over and above cooked plant-food diets for chronic diseases like fibromyalgia, rheumatoid arthritis, heart disease, type 2 diabetes, cancer and obesity. If confirmed, these results will challenge orthodox nutrition thinking.

Incorporating more fresh foods like salads and fruit into your diet, at the expense of ultra-processed foods, might also be effective at slowing down aging. What we do know for sure from research is that when a Western-style cooked diet is resumed the benefits from having eaten a raw plant-based diet seem to disappear. It seems you need to keep up the fresh food instalments.

TYPES OF RAW-FOOD DIETS

Some people report that they feel energised by including just one raw meal daily, like a large smoothie for breakfast or a massive salad at lunch. Others opt for a more aggressive approach aiming to reverse serious disease. They go raw for two meals per day, saving one meal occasion for healthy cooked plant foods so they can eat with their family and friends.

But going 100 per cent raw requires considerable dedication and some training plus special equipment like a dehydrator. You need to know how to "uncook" recipes so you can still gain pleasure from eating, especially where texture is concerned. When done well, raw food meals such as Mexican tacos (where crispy shells are made in a dehydrator from softened linseeds) and raw lasagne (with 'walnut meat' and young coconut flesh used for pasta layers) can actually taste delicious! Check out an organic, raw-foods cafe if you get the chance. And try my scrumptious Almond Cream Cheese Topped with Herbs (page 224) or Raw Thai Green Curry (page 98).

RAW FOOD SWAPS

INSTEAD OF THIS	TRY THIS
Thickeners	Dates, linseeds, chia seeds, psyllium husks
Stock	Dried mushrooms, miso
Bread	Lettuce, cabbage leaves, dehydrated crackers from seeds and sprouts, uncooked sprouted grain breads
Butter	Avocado, nut and seed pastes, extra virgin olive oil, extra virgin coconut oil
Chocolate	Raw cacao powder, carob powder
Cooked onion/garlic	Onion/garlic powder, asafoetida
Cooked tomatoes	Re-hydrated sun-dried tomatoes
Flour	Dried almond meal, ground nuts and seeds
Meat	Ground nuts and seeds, dried or fresh mushrooms
Pasta or rice	Spiralised or finely chopped vegetables—examples: zucchini linguine, Raw Yellow Rice (page 100), Kelp Noodles (page 101)
Milk, cheese and cream	Nut milk, nut cheese or pate, Cashew Nut Cream (page 244)

BONUS NUTRIENTS FROM FRESH FOODS

Like cooked meals based on unrefined plant foods, raw plant-food meals are free from trans fats and cholesterol, they have little or no saturated fat (unless coconut is largely used), and they provide ample amounts of fibre, plant sterols and phytonutrients. But raw plant-food diets are usually lower in calories (partly, because cooking unlocks calories from foods) and provide less or no refined carbohydrates. This is a bonus if you're looking to slim down fast or get a grip on your blood sugar and insulin levels. Including more raw plant foods each day can also bump up your intake of disease-fighting phytonutrients and help reduce your exposure to harmful chemicals formed using modern, high-temperature cooking methods (page 379). Have you tried my popular Green Monster Smoothie (page 301)?

People following a raw plant-food diet have been reported to have a greater diversity of bugs in their bowels than omnivores who eat cooked food. This is considered desirable for immunity and to reduce chronic disease risk. But this is also true of vegetarians and vegans, and may simply be a result of munching on more unrefined plant foods.

ANTI-AGING POTENTIAL

The central dogma in research on aging has been that calorie restriction (by 30–50 per cent of usual intake, and preferably supplemented with micronutrients) can extend lifespan. Yet even without cutting calories, emerging studies suggest limiting the intake of protein in your diet, as compared to carbs, might also extend life. This discovery fits well with many large studies that consistently report that high-protein diets appear to cut life short.

A high-protein Western diet, especially one supplying ample branched chain amino acids like *leucine* (found in high amounts in milk and meat) might over-activate mTORC1, a protein complex in your mitochondria. Mitochondria are the energy centres of each cell in your body and they influence everything from your growth and development to your body composition, reproduction and aging. Like sugars and refined high-GI starches from unhealthy foods, these branched chain amino acids are also key signals for insulin to be released in your body. High insulin levels appear to be a growth factor for cancer and increase the risk of diabetes and cardiovascular disease, as well as promoting premature aging!

So experts in aging research suggest you eat less protein (especially from dairy and meat) and avoid high-GI carbohydrates (page 346) to prevent your insulin levels from shooting up, if you want to live longer. Raw plant-food diets (and even unrefined cooked plant-based diets) offer a way to do this naturally.

Fast facts about fasting

Total or periodic fasting can induce changes in your body linked with the slowing of aging and chronic disease. Fasting appears to work by giving the mitochondria in your cells a rest and re-focusing your body on repair mechanisms, rather than constantly fuelling growth and development. People choose to fast in various ways, either by avoiding food totally or restricting its amount or type for a given period. While most people report benefits, fasting is not suitable for everyone, especially children, pregnant women, diabetics on insulin and those with an eating disorder. Fasting is also best done under the supervision of a healthcare professional if you are on medication.

VALUE OF FOOD ENZYMES

For many years, a hypothesis has been promulgated about the value of food enzymes in raw plant foods. Yet scientific research has found these enzymes play only a minor role in human digestion since they generally don't survive the acidic conditions of the stomach to make it to the small intestine where most digestion occurs. However, a few recent studies have suggested that plant enzymes might play a unique role in activating important phytonutrients before digestion even starts. These types of phytonutrients are known to fight serious diseases like cancer.

MYROSINASE

The enzyme myrosinase occurs in raw broccoli (and other uncooked cruciferous or brassica family vegetables) and is pivotal in converting dormant phytonutrients in these vegetables, called "glucosinolates," into their active anti-cancer forms known as "isothiocyanates." There are many types of individual isothiocyanates, but the best known is sulforaphane.

Unfortunately, myrosinase is fenced within the cells of cruciferous vegetables. So you need to first chew or chop these veggies for myrosinase to be released so it can work on the glucosinolates. This needs to occur before cooking as myrosinase is progressively destroyed by heat. However, once the individual anti-cancer phytonutrients like sulforaphane are formed, they are heat-resistant and can withstand cooking.

Sulforaphane is promoted as an anti-cancer supplement. You can source it naturally in highest amounts from broccoli sprouts.

Would you get more sulforaphane and other isothiocyanates by eating your cruciferous veggies raw? The answer is yes. That is why it is so important to regularly include fresh salads, such as from cabbage (page 51) or daikon (page 70), with your meals or to drink some green vegetable juice made with kale a few times per week. Researchers have estimated that the level of sulforaphane in humans is three times higher after consuming raw or lightly cooked broccoli (steamed for up to 3 minutes until it turns a bright green) as compared to fully cooked broccoli where the myrosinase has been inactivated.

If you prefer soft-cooked or even mushy cruciferous vegetables, here is a tip to still benefit from the potential sulforaphane. Eat another raw cruciferous vegetable at the same time. For example, while you might like to tenderly cook broccoli for your favourite pasta dish, if you eat a fresh rocket or watercress salad (page 68) at the same meal, you will not miss out! Being raw, the additional cruciferous vegetable will share its active myrosinase enzyme. Alternatively, use the "chop-and-hold" technique: cut the broccoli into small pieces and allow it to sit for 40 minutes prior to cooking so that sulforaphane can be fully formed before the enzyme is destroyed by heat.

But even if you forget to do this, there is one last-minute trick. Simply sprinkle your cooked broccoli with mustard seed powder or add some wasabi or horseradish to your plate. Research shows these cruciferous species can also donate their myrosinase, so that sulforaphane can still be made from the dormant glucosinolates in your cooked broccoli, as if you were eating it raw!

Blanching broccoli before freezing is not a smart idea as it destroys myrosinase, just like cooking. Commercially produced frozen broccoli, which is usually blanched, has been shown to lack the ability to form the cancer-fighting sulforaphane!

ALLINASE

Allinase is a plant enzyme that occurs in raw garlic. Like myrosinase, it is also progressively destroyed by heating. But if you crush (or chew) garlic before cooking, you break down the cell walls within the clove, allowing the allinase to get in contact with a sleepy phytonutrient called "alliin." Allinase then quickly gets to work converting alliin into a medicinally active and pungent form known as allicin, which garlic and garlic supplements are famous for!

Allowing garlic to stand for just 10 minutes after breaking it up allows sufficient conversion of alliin to allicin. It's also a good idea to eat some garlic raw as cooking destroys the active ingredient allicin as the temperature increases. Have you tried my amazing Almond and Sage Pesto (page 215)? Note: Australian garlic is a particularly rich source of alliin.

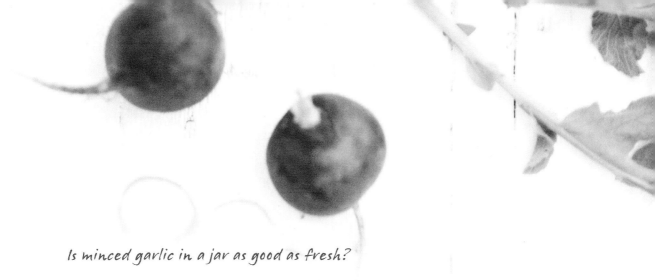

Is minced garlic in a jar as good as fresh?

While it is convenient, commercially minced garlic has an inferior flavour, is not usually grown locally and contains various additives, such as acidity regulator (acetic acid or phosphoric acid), sugar and salt. It also likely contains less allicin than what you can extract by crushing fresh garlic before you need it, since this phytonutrient is fragile with storage. Research from Japan showed crushed garlic loses about half its allicin content within six days when stored in water or in less than one hour when stored in vegetable oil at room temperature!

However, while the anti-inflammatory and anti-blood clotting effects of garlic involve allicin, there are other antioxidants present in garlic, so using jarred minced garlic is not totally useless. Just be sure to enjoy some fresh garlic (in your salad or scraped on bread) as well!

Are raw-food diets risky?

There are certain risks in adopting a raw-foods diet, depending on how raw you go and whether you take supplements. For example, a lack of vitamins B12 and D, and a variable intake of protein and calcium have been reported. Low bone-mineral density has also been found among raw foodists in one study. If you're keen on raw-food eating, it's important to make dietary changes gradually under the guidance of a qualified health professional.

Totally raw diets are not recommended for children, pregnant or breastfeeding women and fragile elderly people. But adding more raw recipes into your weekly menu can be enjoyed by everyone. Try my delicious Foamy Gazpacho soup (page 202), perfected when I visited Spain. Sit down to the popular Sprouted Bean, Avocado and Red Papaya Salad (page 32) or serve my Blood Orange, Pomegranate and Chia Seed Pudding (page 240) at a party. Even replacing that packet of potato crisps with a juicy apple for an afternoon snack will boost your health. You don't have to eat raw all the time to benefit.

MINIMIZING HARMFUL CHEMICALS

Clever cooking methods

Scientists are increasingly realising the way food is cooked might also be important for wellbeing. Modern high-heat and dry-cooking methods produce various chemicals in food that may cause your body harm.

10 TIPS TO REDUCE NASTY CHEMICALS IN YOUR FOOD

1. Go more raw and include fresh foods at meals and snacks (examples: salads, fruits).

2. Use moist cooking methods for most dishes (examples: soups, stews and curries). Steam your vegetables or slow-roast potatoes, so they are succulent, not dry. Try my delicious Roasted Lemon Potatoes (page 82). Although wok cooking involves higher temperatures, it is quick so less chemicals can form.

3. Avoid smoked and processed meat, chicken and fish of all types. The chemicals from smoked foods are hazardous and cured or preserved meats can damage the lining of your bowel.

4. Minimize firing up the barbecue. If you use it, increase the proportion of vegetables and mushrooms on the hot plate and marinate animal-protein foods with spices or wrap them in banana leaves.

5. Minimize use of the grill, dry frying, deep frying and dry roasting, especially for meats. While we all like to eat browned foods and crispy textures, these are a clue that more chemicals have formed during cooking. If you must grill or fry meats, flip frequently to prevent browning and trim any charred or blackened bits before eating. Avoid making gravy from drippings as it will be high in AGEs (page 380).

6. Avoid processed and extruded snack foods, cookies, biscuits, crackers and dark toast. These foods hide acrylamide (page 380). Never store your potatoes in the fridge (or freezer) before cooking. Fast-food chains do this, knowing it makes their fries more crispy, but it also boosts acrylamide formation.

7. Drink tea when you need a hot drink (there are many herbal and non-caffeinated varieties) in preference to coffee and other roasted-grain beverages. Acrylamide is formed during roasting of the coffee beans and grains.

8. Avoid or limit high-fat cheeses (examples: Brie, parmesan and cream cheese). Choose ricotta or cottage if you eat dairy. Or make your own plant-based "cheeses" from unroasted nuts and seeds (roasting significantly increases their content of AGEs). Try my delicious Almond Cream Cheese Topped with Herbs (page 224).

9. Avoid or limit butter, margarine, mayonnaise and chemically refined cooking oils (this includes most vegetable oils in the supermarket not labelled "extra virgin"). Such spreads and oils contain high amounts of AGEs without the balancing anti-inflammatory phytonutrients found in whole plant foods, like nuts or extra virgin oils. It's best to cook with extra virgin oils, like olive oil (page 359), but avoid extreme temperatures.

10. Never warm foods in plastic containers, or wash these in the dishwasher, as they will leach more chemicals.

Chemicals that can form during cooking

An introduction to the most-studied harmful chemicals that can form in your food during cooking:

Heterocyclic amines (HCAs) and **polyaromatic hydrocarbons (PAHs)** are formed at significant levels in all types of red meat, chicken and fish if cooked using high or dry heat, such as grilling, frying and barbecuing or if the food is smoked. This means even flame-grilled chicken breast fillets and smoked salmon will supply these chemicals to your burger or bagel. PAHs can also form in vegetable-based foods (example: smoked tofu) but at significantly lower levels. HCAs do not form in plant foods.

Regularly eating foods with HCAs and PAHs has been linked to an increased risk of cancers of the stomach, bowel, prostate and pancreas. So use safer cooking methods, which I have outlined, and protect yourself by loading the grill with more veggies and eating plant meals more often.

Advanced glycation endproducts (AGEs) are naturally present in highest amounts in animal foods like steak and high-fat cheese, before any cooking occurs. Unprocessed plant foods, such as fruits and grains, contain the lowest levels. However, cooking and processing results in the formation of new AGEs in all foods, especially if high-heat and dry-cooking conditions are used. Dry heat promotes AGEs formation by as much as 100-fold across all food categories, compared to the uncooked state! While many people may think "yum" when they see a browned or crispy food surface, those roasted, toasted and fried foods usually deliver the highest amounts of AGEs. High heat processed nut products (examples: peanut butter made from roasted nuts, roasted pecans) and grain products (examples: cookies, ready-to-eat breakfast cereals and rice crackers) can supply significant quantities if you eat them regularly.

AGEs promote chronic low-grade inflammation and oxidative stress (page 322). They have been linked to multiple conditions, including cataracts, Alzheimer's disease, heart and kidney disease, and accelerated aging. Animal studies show a diet high in AGEs speeds up the onset of diabetes complications, damaging the blood vessels, eyes, kidneys and nerves! The good news is that cutting AGEs in the diet by even 50 per cent of usual intake has been shown to be very beneficial in animal studies. A small study in healthy overweight Australians showed switching them from a high- to low-AGEs diet improved their insulin sensitivity, meaning they would be less likely to develop diabetes and heart disease. Another study in people with existing type 2 diabetes found swapping the cooking method (from fried to steamed) of even a single meal fed to them reduced their AGEs intake by more than 80 per cent and improved the functioning of their blood vessels compared to the high-AGEs meal. Eating foods low in AGEs may be particularly important for people with diabetes, since this condition already makes the body generate more AGEs internally.

Acrylamide forms in carbohydrate-rich foods prepared at high temperatures, such as when you fry, toast, bake and roast. For example, significant levels have been found in crispy French fries and hot chips, dark-brown toast, cookies, roasted coffee beans and ready-to-eat breakfast cereals. Even chocolate contains acrylamide, produced when the cacao beans are roasted (one of the reasons I prefer to use raw cacao powder). Usually, the crispier or more browned the food is, the higher the acrylamide level.

While evidence for the negative health effects of acrylamide is inconsistent and based mainly on animal studies, quite a few studies have linked acrylamide exposure in humans with higher risks of ovarian, endometrial, kidney, breast and mouth cancers.

As acrylamide exists in foods that make up around 40 per cent of a typical American diet, much of the food industry focus has been on finding ways to reduce it forming, rather than removing these foods from the marketplace. Adding vitamin C-rich foods such as lemon juice and rosemary extract can lower the levels of acrylamide formed in carb foods. Try my delicious low-acrylamide Roasted Lemon Potatoes (page 82).

What about the microwave?
Some people worry about the microwave, but there is no clear scientific evidence of harm specifically from using the microwave to cook food. Still, more research should be done. I'm particularly interested in the combined effects of all sources of radiation now pervasive in our modern lifestyle—think laptop, mobile phone, wireless networks or regularly flying in an aeroplane. As far as nutrient-retention is concerned, studies suggest microwaving food can reduce levels of some nutrients but preserve others due to the shorter cooking time and lower water usage. If you find the microwave convenient, make sure you use glass or ceramic dishes and never warm your food in plastic containers or touching plastic film.

Chemicals from containers and cookware

Some chemicals from the environment can migrate into your food. Here are three examples. While the material below might cause serious concern, you can drastically reduce your intake of these chemicals if you follow the guidelines in this cookbook.

Bisphenol A (BPA) is used to make clear, heat-resistant, polycarbonate plastics such as drinking bottles, cups and containers. It is also found in the lining of most cans to keep them from rusting. The concern with BPA: it is a well-known "endocrine disruptor," meaning it can imitate hormones, turn one hormone into another, and generally interfere with the functioning of hormones in your body.

Many studies have linked chronic exposure to BPA—even at low levels—to breast and prostate cancers, obesity, heart disease, high blood pressure and diabetes. While the long-term health concerns are unproven, scientists have called for replacements to be used in the manufacture of containers that store food and drink. A small study published in the journal *Environmental Health Perspectives* found that levels of BPA in human urine can drop substantially after just three days of switching to fresh foods and eliminating the use of plastics and canned food packaging.

Eating soy foods appears to protect against the harmful effects of BPA on fertility, according to a 2016 study of women undergoing IVF treatment published in the Journal of Clinical Endocrinology & Metabolism.

Perfluorooctanoic acid (PFOA) is released when commonly available non-stick cookware is heated to a high temperature (example: Teflon, although this is only one well-known brand). PFOA is another type of endocrine disruptor. It can also cause flu-like symptoms in humans. While human studies are limited, many health problems have been identified in animals exposed to PFOA, including infertility, immune suppression, elevated thyroid hormone levels, liver problems, cancer, and negative effects on the brain and nervous system. PFOA has been detected in the blood of 98 per cent of American adults and 100 per cent of newborns.

Research tracking women of childbearing age found those with higher blood levels of PFOA also took longer to get pregnant. Two recent studies reviewed by the European Food Safety Authority reported babies born to mothers exposed to PFOA during pregnancy had a reduced birth weight. A Danish study showed that the daughters of women exposed to PFOA during their pregnancy had triple the risk of being obese at age 20! While these associations are highly concerning, we need more research to properly understand the effects of PFOAs in the human body.

It's not only non-stick pans and baking trays that can release PFOA. Like many synthetic chemicals, PFOA can come from various sources. This includes non-stick sandwich makers and popular meat grills, as well as food packaging. Reduce your exposure by switching to safer cookware and bakeware options (page 20).

What about new generation non-stick cookware?
Many newer brands of cookware claim to be PFOA-free. But independent scientific data on these products is lacking and their longer-term health effects are poorly understood and difficult to predict.

One example of this type of non-stick cookware are products made with "diamond crystals," which is actually titanium oxide. The type of titanium oxide used in such cookware appears to be in the form of nanoparticles, which are being increasingly used in multiple consumer products, including sunscreen and cosmetics. But there is increasing concern that exposure to these nanoparticles may be toxic to your lungs and brain.

Preliminary research in people with inflammatory bowel disease suggests nanoparticles might be a transporter in the gut for endotoxins from bacteria to pass through the lining of your intestines (leaky gut). Until more clinical trials are conducted in humans, you might wish to err on the side of caution and invest in cookware with a history of safe use (page 20).

Phthalates are manufactured chemicals found in a large variety of consumer products, not only as possible contaminants in your food. They're used to make plastics more pliable, even those plastics that are BPA-free. Most plastics, including food packaging, vinyl flooring and even medical devices will contain phthalates. They are also used in cosmetics and personal-care products, including perfumes, soaps, lotions, deodorants, fake tans, hairsprays and shampoos, as well as in dishwashing detergents and air fresheners. A clue to their presence in personal-care products is the word "fragrance" or "parfum" in the ingredients list. But it can often be difficult to tell if phthalates are present in products since they don't have to be declared.

Phthalates have been linked with adverse health effects since the 1940s, especially on male reproductive development, but the research has mostly been with animals and remains inconclusive. In humans, phthalates appear to be able to alter the timing of labour, reduce semen quality and may even induce endometriosis.

One study published in the journal *Environmental Health* found that an infant eating a typical Western diet is consuming twice as much phthalates as the US Environmental Protection Agency considers safe! Meats (especially poultry), dairy (cream and cheese), cooking oils and butter have been consistently identified as the most significant dietary sources. Some types of phthalates are attracted to fat, so they migrate from storage and packaging plastics into high-fat foods.

Eliminating all phthalates and other endocrine disruptors from your environment is almost impossible. But, according to research, healthful changes in what you eat and how you store food can make a difference in the levels of phthalates that get into your body. In modelling various diets to identify which are associated with the lowest chemical exposure, US researchers found a high fruit and vegetable diet contained the lowest levels of phthalates, whereas a high meat and dairy diet provided the greatest amounts and was deemed unsafe for infants and adolescents.

My suggestion is to remove as many plastics from your kitchen as you can, screen your personal-care products to ensure they are "fragrance"-free (this does not apply to natural essential oils) and eat a diet focused on plant foods, including more fresh produce rather than shelf-stable meals that have been sitting in packaging on supermarket shelves. See my safer food storage tips on page 20. Note: Phthalates should not be confused with phthalides, which are beneficial phytonutrients found in celery!

Hormones from animal foods

Some scientists have cautioned that exposure to estrogens from eating animal foods (meat, milk, eggs) should also be considered when assessing the total impact of hormone-like substances on our health. This may be especially relevant for more susceptible groups such as infants and pre-pubertal children. Estradiol (the main type of estrogen) is 10,000 times more potent than any environmental (synthetic) estrogen, so you don't need much for it to have an effect.

One potential concern is dairy milk. The milk from modern milking cows is known to contain higher levels of estrogens than in the past because cows are kept pregnant during most of their lactation period! But how much of a risk this poses to human health is controversial. One group of Japanese researchers has linked cows milk consumption by pre-pubertal children to the early onset of puberty.

While more research is needed on various diets, some data is already showing total estrogen levels are lower in the blood and urine of younger women who eat low, rather than high, amounts of meat.

Hints for reading food labels

While most food ingredients in your trolley should come from the fresh-food section (mainly or all plants), it's important to know what to look out for when buying packets, cans and boxes or if you wish to include some animal products.

Food label tips for processed foods

Look for:

- Low-fat products with less then 3 g of total fat per 100 g. (This benchmark does not apply to nuts, seeds, avocado, other whole plant foods, fish or extra virgin oils.)
- High-fibre products with at least 3 g of fibre per serve.
- Low-salt products with less then 120 mg of sodium per 100 g.
- Low-sugar products with less then 5 g of sugars per 100 g.
- Organic foods that meet the above criteria.

Product-specific nutrition benchmarks

FRUIT AND VEGETABLES:

- All seasonal fresh fruits and vegetables, preferably locally grown.
- When buying canned or frozen produce, look for "no added salt" and "no added sugar" options and/or BPA-free cans.

BREADS, GRAINS AND CEREALS:

- Whole grain and low GI.
- At least 4 g fibre per serve (preferably 7 g).
- Less than 400 mg sodium per 100 g.
- Less than 15 g added sugars per 100 g in cereals, unless dried fruit is listed before sugar in the ingredients list.

OILS AND SPREADS:

- Choose extra virgin oils, including olive, macadamia, avocado, chia.
- Avoid chemically refined oils, such as light olive oil, canola, sunflower, grapeseed, rice bran.
- Prefer antioxidant-rich wholefood spreads, such as fresh avocado, hummus, baba ganoush and natural nut pastes, rather than processed yellow-fat spreads.
- Avoid animal or processed fats that appear solid at room temperature.

NUTS AND SEEDS:

- All unsalted, raw nuts and seeds, preferably in their shell.
- Natural nut and seed pastes or butters (not made from roasted nuts).

DAIRY PRODUCTS AND ALTERNATIVES:

- For dairy milk, less than 2 g total fat per 100 g
- Cheeses are usually high in fat and will not meet the above criteria, so look for soft white unripened varieties (example: ricotta) with the least saturated fat and sodium per 100 g.
- Less than 10 g sugars per 100 g.
- For milk alternatives, at least 250 mg calcium per 250 ml. Addition of vitamins B12 and D is an advantage.

MEAT AND CHICKEN:

- Avoid all processed meats (examples: sausages, bacon, salami).
- If you eat meat, limit to 455 g cooked weight, lean red meat per week, even if grass-fed, organic, Halal or Kosher.
- If you eat chicken, choose free-range skinless fillets, and avoid wings, nuggets, and charcoal chicken (highly browned, cooked over a direct flame).

LEGUMES AND FISH:

- All dry and canned legumes and beans.
- Sustainable and smaller fish.
- Look for "no added salt" and/or BPA-free cans.

SNACK FOODS:

- Based on wholefoods.
- Energy content less than 600 kJ (140 Cal) per serve if weight is a concern.
- Avoid those with trans fats or partially hydrogenated vegetable oils.
- Look for options with the least saturated fat, sugar and sodium, and the most fibre per 100 g.

Further resources

More Food as Medicine

For more "Food as Medicine" information, links and resources, or to order additional copies of this book: www.foodasmedicine.cooking

How to find a qualified dietitian

In Australia, search for Accredited Practising Dietitian: www.daa.asn.au
In New Zealand, search for Registered Dietitian: www.dietitians.org.nz
In the United States, search for Registered Dietitian Nutritionist: www.eatright.org

Healthy cooking classes in Sydney

Join me at a Culinary Medicine Cookshop in Sydney, Australia. A combination of cooking class and nutrition workshop, these events are a unique way to learn about medicinal foods. In 2010, I was awarded the Dietitians Association of Australia President's Award for Innovation for these Cookshops. See the latest at: www.sueradd.com

Online nutrition research videos

For a snapshot of the latest findings in nutrition research, watch Dr Michael Greger's free videos at: www.nutritionfacts.org

Guide to chemicals in your environment

An independent US consumer guide to pesticides and other endocrine disruptors that lurk in your environment ranging from foods and non-stick cookware to personal care and cleaning products: www.ewg.org

Wild food app

Discover edible weeds and plants around you with "food as medicine" potential: www.wildfood.me

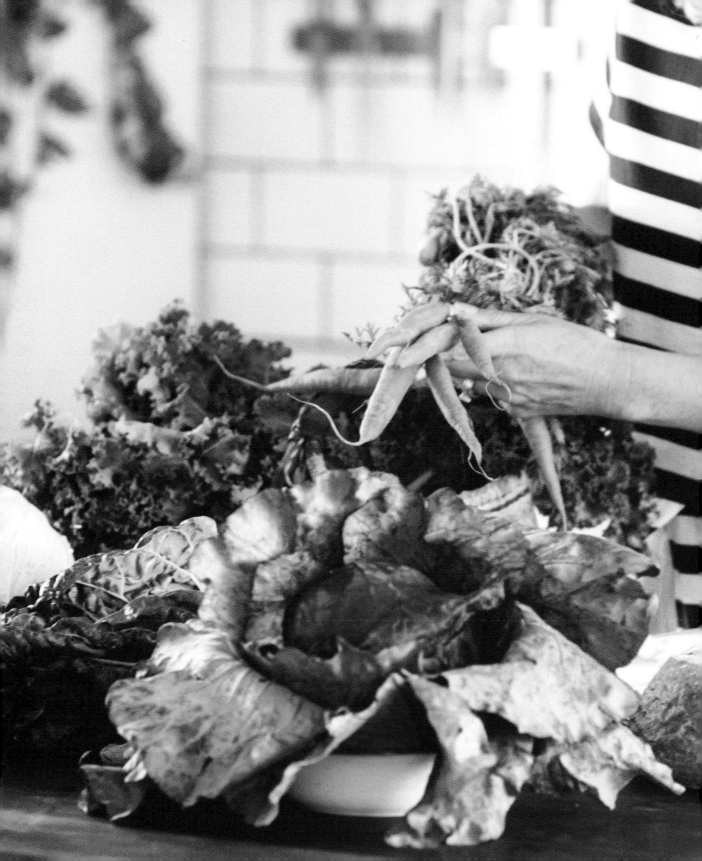

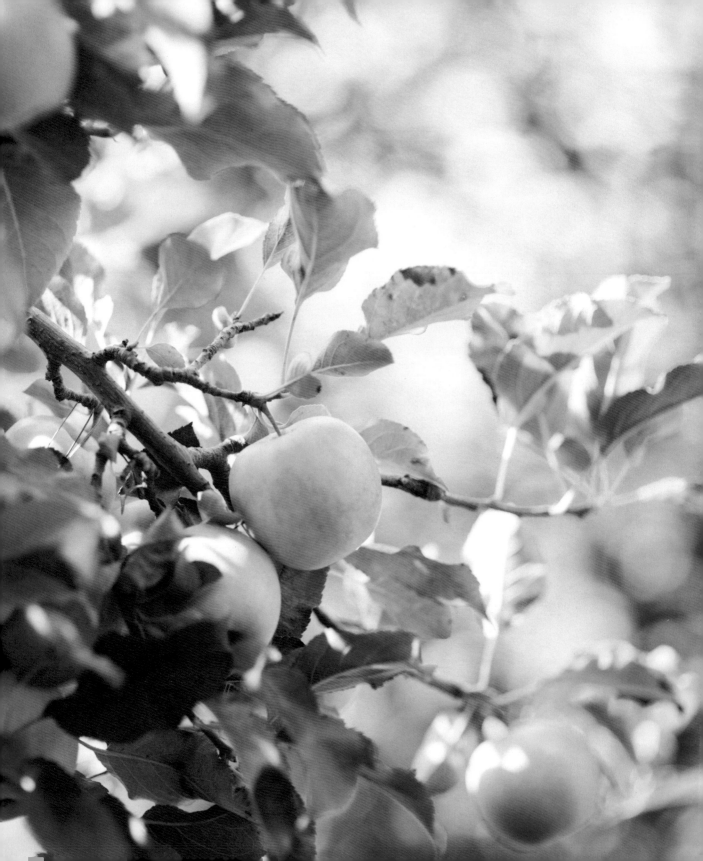

RECIPE AND KEY INGREDIENTS INDEX

(Recipe titles in bold)

CONVERSION CHARTS

Metric and imperial conversions
(These conversions are rounded for convenience)

Ingredient	Cups/Tablespoons/Teaspoons	Ounces	Grams/Milliliters
Cornstarch	1 tablespoon	0.3 ounce	8 grams
Cream cheese	1 tablespoon	0.5 ounce	14.5 grams
Flour, all-purpose	1 cup/1 tablespoon	4.5 ounces/0.3 ounce	125 grams/8 grams
Flour, whole wheat	1 cup	4 ounces	120 grams
Fruit, dried	1 cup	4 ounces	120 grams
Fruits or veggies, chopped	1 cup	5 to 7 ounces	145 to 200 grams
Fruits or veggies, pureed	1 cup	8.5 ounces	245 grams
Honey or maple syrup	1 tablespoon	0.75 ounce	20 grams
Liquids: milk, water, or juice	1 cup	8 fluid ounces	240 milliliters
Oats	1 cup	5.5 ounces	150 grams
Salt	1 teaspoon	0.2 ounce	6 grams
Spices: cinnamon, cloves, ginger, or nutmeg (ground)	1 teaspoon	0.2 ounce	5 milliliters
Sugar, brown, firmly packed	1 cup	7 ounces	200 grams
Sugar, white	1 cup/1 tablespoon	7 ounces/0.5 ounce	200 grams/12.5 grams
Vanilla extract	1 teaspoon	0.2 ounce	4 grams

Oven temperatures

Fahrenheit	Celsius	Gas Mark
225°	110°	¼
250°	120°	½
275°	140°	1
300°	150°	2
325°	160°	3
350°	180°	4
375°	190°	5
400°	200°	6
425°	220°	7
450°	230°	8

OVEN GUIDE: You may find cooking times vary depending on the oven you are using. For fan-forced ovens, as a general rule, set the oven temperature to 20°C (35°F) lower than indicated in the recipe.

Acknowledgments

I am so honoured to have colleagues and clients from a diverse range of professions—from educators and cooks to dietitians and writers—who have given generously of their time to review this cookbook and provide valuable feedback. They are listed in alphabetical order: Carol Boehm, Lindsay Christian, Sibilla Johnson, Nicole Kellow APD, Dr Grenville Kent, Dr Robyn Pearce, Tricia Pokorny, Courtney Thornton APD.

Thanks also to my family and friends, especially Dee Lazic, Angela Lazic, Linda Simpson, Sue Belosev, Nada Schmidt, Claudia Chakar, Nora Pertzel and Monic Saleh, who have contributed in meaningful ways, including recipe ideas, testing and media shoots.

Finally, I could not have done this without the enthusiastic support of my staff and clients at the Nutrition and Wellbeing Clinic who have willingly tested and eaten their way through all these recipes. I'm delighted to say they continue to use and enjoy them at home with their families.

Skyhorse Publishing books may be purchased in bulk at special discounts for sales promotion, corporate gifts, fund-raising, or educational purposes. Special editions can also be created to specifications. For details, contact the Special Sales Department, Skyhorse Publishing, 307 West 36th Street, 11th Floor, New York, NY 10018 or info@skyhorsepublishing.com.

Skyhorse® and Skyhorse Publishing® are registered trademarks of Skyhorse Publishing, Inc.®, a Delaware corporation.

Visit our website at www.skyhorsepublishing.com.

10 9 8 7 6 5 4 3 2 1

Library of Congress Cataloging-in-Publication Data is available on file.

Edited by Nathan Brown
Proofread by Lindy Schneider and Nathan Brown
Designed by Dominique Cherry
Design assistance by Daniele Howse
Cover Design by Daniel Brount
Food and Lifestyle Photography by Dominique Cherry
Food Styling by Claudia Martin
Food Preparation by Michael Demagistris

Print ISBN: 978-1-5107-5758-5
Ebook ISBN: 978-1-5107-5759-2

Printed in China